WRIGHT'S
VETERINARY ANAESTHESIA
AND ANALGESIA

This book was originally written to provide the student with an introduction to the subject and the practitioner with a clinical guide. Over successive editions this established framework has been retained, but with the considerable expansion of the subject the book has necessarily become a manual of reference to all with an interest in this field.

Much new material has been added for this edition, including an entirely new chapter on the artificial ventilation of the lungs. In particular the sections on basal narcosis, premedication, the anaesthetic agents and their administration, and relaxation of the skeletal muscles have been substantially revised and expanded to bring them into line with current developments. A number of new illustrations have been added, and old ones have been revised or replaced.

It is hoped that the new edition will provide a comprehensive and stimulating introduction to veterinary anaesthesia for students as well as remaining an up-to-date guide for veterinarians in the field.

Wright's
Veterinary Anaesthesia and Analgesia

Seventh Edition

L. W. HALL

M.A., B.Sc., Ph.D., M.R.C.V.S.

Fellow of University College, Cambridge, and
University Lecturer in the
Department of Veterinary Clinical Studies,
University of Cambridge

Baillière Tindall · London

© 1971 Baillière Tindall
7 & 8 Henrietta Street, London WC2 8QE

A division of Crowell Collier and Macmillan Publishers Ltd

I SBN 0 7020 0379–4

BY J. G. WRIGHT

First Edition, December 1941
Second Edition, January 1947
Reprinted, May 1948
Third Edition, October 1952
Fourth Edition, November 1957

Spanish Edition 1958

BY J. G. WRIGHT AND L. W. HALL

Fifth Edition, September 1961
Reprinted, February 1964

BY L. W. HALL

Sixth Edition, January 1966
Seventh Edition, September 1971

*Published in the United States of America
by the Williams & Wilkins Company, Baltimore*

*Made and printed in Great Britain by
William Clowes & Sons, Limited, London, Beccles and Colchester*

Contents

Preface

Throughout the revision of this book for the seventh edition, I have been conscious of the need to preserve the original framework of Professor Wright's book, which proved so useful both as a student textbook and as a manual of reference for veterinarians in general practice, while at the same time attempting to provide a comprehensive and stimulating introduction to the subject for intending specialists. I have, besides, endeavoured to incorporate in it those developments which have taken place over the past five years and also the suggestions made by various reviewers of the sixth edition.

The methods described and the views expressed are again based on my own experience of twenty years in the London and Cambridge schools, but, rightly and inevitably, the number of references to the works of others has increased. In preparing the material I have been constantly aware of the difficulty of avoiding oversimplification and inadequate preparation on the one hand, and complexity and lack of clarity on the other.

A good deal of new material has been added for this edition, including an entirely new chapter on the artificial ventilation of the lungs. In particular the sections on premedication and basal narcosis have been considerably expanded with the addition of some new drugs. There has also been substantial revision of the chapters on the anaesthetic agents and their administration, in order to bring them into line with current developments. The chapter 'Relaxation of the Skeletal Muscles during Anaesthesia' has been largely rewritten.

I have emphasized throughout the importance of simple monitoring equipment, suitable for use in the field; adoption of this practice will greatly increase the scientific aspect, and thus reliability, of veterinary anaesthesia, without in any way detracting from the art.

A number of new illustrations have been added throughout the book, and many of the old photographs and drawings have been revised or replaced.

I must thank Mr J. A. Taylor, F.R.C.V.S., for permission to reproduce his description of the innervation of the bovine limbs, and Mr J. A. Juby, of the British Oxygen Co. Ltd, for his never-failing help in the provision of illustrations, and also for supplying details on the standardization of cone and socket unions for Appendix 3. A number of new illustrations for the sixth edition were kindly supplied by Mr H. D. Williamson, M.S.R., and I am indebted to Mrs J. Day for the line drawings for the current edition. Figs 112 and 113 were prepared by Mr J. Patten, and Mrs J. Patten supplied the majority of the photographs. Dr Barbara Weaver very kindly provided a photograph of her large animal absorber unit (Fig. 103). I am indebted to Dr R. S. Comline, Miss G. M. Massey, Miss C. M. Trim and Mr R. G. Walter for reading parts of the manuscript and giving many helpful suggestions. Miss A. C. Donovan gave expert assistance in the reading of the proofs and the preparation of the index.

Cambridge   L. W. HALL
July 1971

1

General Considerations

Satisfactory anaesthesia for the performance of painful surgical interferences on animals is essential from two standpoints: the first, the humanitarian; and the second, that of technical efficiency. The problems which confront the veterinary anaesthetist differ in a number of ways from those of his medical confrère, for he is called upon to deal with a number of species which exhibit great variation in size, temperament and anatomical and physiological development. Not only does the response of each species to the various anaesthetic agents differ, but in addition there is marked individual variation within each particular species.

In man the anaesthetist may reasonably expect some cooperation on the part of the majority of his patients, whereas animals fear and resist the restraint necessary for the administration of anaesthetics, thereby increasing not only the technical difficulties associated with administration, but also the dangers which are inseparable from the use of anaesthetics. In man anaesthesia is often induced by inhalation of anaesthetic agents. When, however, a fully conscious animal is forced to inhale a strange, irritating vapour such as ether or chloroform it struggles, often violently, to escape, and to the classic stages of anaesthesia the veterinarian must add another—that of voluntary excitement and struggling. The risks associated with induction are greatly increased. Thus he exploits the use of cerebral sedatives and narcotics to the utmost, both to facilitate the completion of general anaesthesia, and as an adjunct to local analgesia in order to overcome that natural fear of restraint inherent in animals, and control any tendency to sudden movement during operation. Nevertheless, there must be no generalization in this respect, for in large and cumbersome animals, such as the horse, the locomotor incoordination and muscle weakness which may result from premedication in themselves cause risk to the animal. Many veterinary operators have to carry out their task without skilled assistance, and when employing the inhalation anaesthetics, after inducing anaesthesia themselves, have to depute the duty of continuing it to some lay attendant. For these reasons the continued development in recent years of safe, simple techniques of regional analgesia has been particularly welcome.

Terminology

There has been a tendency to standardize anaesthetic terminology in the medical literature and, if confusion is to be avoided, veterinarians must adopt this standardized terminology. The following definitions, while not perfect, do indicate the sense in which the various terms are now generally used.

Anaesthesia is the name given to the whole art and science relating to the production of insensibility.

General anaesthesia is a state of unconsciousness produced by a process of controlled, reversible intoxication of the central nervous system in which there is a lowered sensitivity to stimuli from the environment and a diminished motor response to such stimuli.

An anaesthetic agent is a substance which produces, in a controllable manner, both loss of consciousness and an absence of motor response to noxious stimuli.

An analgesic agent is a substance which temporarily abolishes awareness of pain.

A narcotic agent is any substance which can produce insensibility, or a stupor bordering upon it, from which simple stimuli such as noise can achieve at the most only temporary partial arousal. Thus, while all anaesthetic agents are narcotics, not many narcotics are anaesthetic agents. Confusion is common concerning the term narcotic as it has both this wide pharmacological meaning and a more restricted one in statutory legislation.

A hypnotic is a narcotic agent which is used to induce sleep (a state of unconsciousness which may be retarded as physiological and from which the subject can easily be awakened by a wide variety of stimuli).

A sedative is a narcotic agent which is used to calm a nervous, vicious or excited subject. Most sedatives cause drowsiness.

An ataractic is a substance which produces sedation without at the same time causing drowsiness. Such substances are popularly known as 'tranquillizers'.

A local analgesic is a substance which when applied about nerve terminals or nerve fibres temporarily prevents the conduction of impulses by the nerve tissue. Analgesia is produced by interference with the transmission of impulses concerned with the appreciation of pain.

Types of Anaesthesia

Broadly speaking, two distinct types of substances are used in anaesthesia. The first have a selective, transient paralytic action on sensory nerves and nerve endings. They are applied in aqueous or oily solution by topical application to mucous or abraded surfaces; by intradermal, subdermal or submucous infiltration; and by peripheral, paravertebral or spinal perineural injection. The anaesthesia, or analgesia as it is now described, thus produced is classified as local or regional. The alkaloid cocaine and its salts were the first of such agents to be employed, but more recently they have been largely replaced by synthetic substitutes, of which procaine hydrochloride and lignocaine hydrochloride are probably the ones most often used.

The second type of substance has a depressant, and ultimately paralytic, action on the central nervous system, producing progressive loss of consciousness and voluntary motor function. In the main these substances fall into two distinct groups: volatile or gaseous agents, typified by chloroform, ether and nitrous oxide, which are administered by inhalation; and nonvolatile agents, of which chloral hydrate and the derivatives of barbituric acid are the most important, which may be administered by a number of routes, including the stomach and rectum, and by subcutaneous, intravenous and intraperitoneal injection.

Thus anaesthesia may be classed into:

1. Local analgesia.
   (a) By surface application.
   (b) By intra- and subdermal infiltration.
   (c) Field anaesthesia: the blocking of an area by linear infiltration of its margins.
2. Regional analgesia.
   (a) By perineural injection.
   (b) Spinal block: (1) by epidural injection; (2) by intrathecal injection.
3. Sedation and narcosis.
   (a) In combination with local or regional analgesia.
   (b) As an adjunct to general anaesthesia.
4. General anaesthesia.
   (a) By inhalation.
   (b) By the oral, rectal, intravenous or intraperitoneal administration of a non-volatile anaesthetic.
   (c) By a combination of the two with or without premedication.

General Considerations in the Selection of the Anaesthetic Method

The first consideration will be the nature of the operation to be performed; its magnitude, site and duration. In general the use of local infiltration analgesia will suffice for simple interferences such as the incision of superficial abscesses, the excision of small neoplasms and the castration of immature animals. Nevertheless, what seems to be a simple interference may have special anaesthetic requirements. The equine capped elbow is an example, for with this lesion the degree of subdermal fibrosis is often such as to make local infiltration impossible to effect. Again, the site of operation, consequent on the complexity of the structures in its vicinity, may render operation under local analgesia dangerous because of possible movement by the conscious animal. The incision of a retropharyngeal abscess illustrates this point.

The likely duration of the operation will influence the selection of the anaesthetic especially when adopting general anaesthesia. For interferences of a few minutes' duration, such as the simpler dental operations, an ultra-short-acting non-volatile anaesthetic such as a thiobarbiturate may be selected. For longer interferences it may be decided to use a longer-acting barbiturate supplemented by local analgesia to give full anaesthesia for the contemplated duration of operation, or to induce anaesthesia with a thiobarbiturate and maintain it with an inhalation anaesthetic with or without tracheal intubation. In horses and cattle in which chloral hydrate has been used as the induction anaesthetic the relatively high toxicity of this drug must be borne in mind and thus for the continuation of anaesthesia it may be decided to switch to a volatile agent or one of the less toxic barbiturates. For major interferences under general anaesthesia, pre-anaesthetic medication will be considered, particularly when they are of long duration and it is required that the animal shall remain quiet for several hours after operation. Pre-anaesthetic sedation may significantly reduce the amount of general anaesthetic required; it may also increase the duration of anaesthesia. In addition, undesirable features of certain anaesthetics such as the provocation of salivation may be controlled by previous medication.

The species of animal involved is, of course, a pre-eminent consideration in the selection of the anaesthetic method. The operator will be influenced not only by size and temperament but also by any anatomical and physiological peculiarities of a particular species or breed. In general it may be taken that the larger an animal is, the greater are the difficulties and dangers associated with the induction and continuation of general anaesthesia. Methods which are safe and satisfactory for the dog and cat may be quite unsuitable for the horse or the ox. In a heavy and vigorous creature the mere upset of locomotor coordination may entail risks, as also may prolonged recumbency.

The Horse

In the horse, the necessity for adequate restraint, even for quite simple interferences, may necessitate casting to ensure the safety of the operator and of the patient. The process of casting the fully conscious horse is not only frightening to the animal but exposes it to danger of injury unless the assistance of an experienced casting team is available. It may be decided that the use of a muscle-paralysing drug as the means of casting the horse is no more distressing to the animal than is the use of casting tackle. It is probable that the former method entails less risk to the animal and it is certainly a great convenience to the operator, but the animal must always be the primary consideration in the selection of the method. The facility with which certain of the peripheral sensory nerves can be 'blocked' in this species of animal should always be borne in mind. Operations about the fore-feet, for example, can be satisfactorily performed with the animal standing under local block of the plantar nerves. An important consideration when selecting a general anaesthetic for the horse, particularly when it is proposed to use one of the non-volatile group administered in the standing position, is that induction shall be unassociated with narcotic excitement. Moreover, when using agents from which recovery is relatively slow it is important that this period also shall be free from excitement. A further requirement in the horse is that it shall be able to rise to its feet relatively soon after the completion of operation, at the outside within an hour or two, and that when it does so locomotor power and coordination shall have been regained to a degree whereby the animal is able to retain the standing position without floundering or falling. These requirements preclude the use of some of the non-volatile anaesthetics and also some of the sedatives in the horse.

Cattle and Sheep

In general, cattle and sheep are unsuitable subjects for inhalation anaesthesia unless endotracheal intubation is practised, and for field work, light general anaesthesia by intravenous injection gives satisfactory results. But it is in these species of animal that regional analgesia has attained its greatest development. For major abdominal interferences, paravertebral or lumbar epidural injections are most satisfactory; for obstetrical operations, caudal epidural analgesia is extensively employed, while for cornual and digital operations perineural block is suitable.

The Pig

The continuous squealing and struggling which restraint provokes in the pig make the operator disposed to adopt general anaesthesia in the adult animal for all but the most rapidly performed interferences. Fortunately the pig is a good subject for general anaesthesia using sedatives with inhalation or intravenous anaesthetics. In the *little pig* most of the interferences called for can be satisfactorily carried out under local infiltration.

The Dog

In the dog anaesthetic methods have now attained a degree of perfection whereby it is the inclination of the operator to induce general anaesthesia not only for practically all surgical interferences but in many instances for examination procedures also: exploration of the mouth, pharynx and oesophagus, abdominal palpation and radiography. It must be borne in mind that those breeds having a markedly brachicephalic type of skull with depression of the nasal bones—the bulldog, the Pekingese, etc.—are bad subjects for general anaesthesia in that relaxation of the jaw muscles may cause obstruction of the airway, and particular care will be required when using the slowly excreted intravenous agents. Endotracheal intubation is the only satisfactory way of maintaining a free airway in these breeds.

The Cat

The cat is often a difficult subject to anaesthetize quietly and safely, for restraint often provokes violent struggling and sometimes frenzy. Cats should always be handled quietly, using the minimum of restraint, and when this is done the most satisfactory method of inducing anaesthesia is by the slow intravenous injections of a barbiturate. For young cats, inhalation anaesthesia without the use of an intravenous induction agent is often used, and, in general, gives satisfactory results.

The variable reaction of the different species of animals, and of individuals, to the various anaesthetic agents must also be borne in mind. Sometimes the barbiturates, when used in sub-anaesthetic doses in the horse, provoke marked excitement, whilst a cat under the influence of large doses of morphine may become maniacal if stimulated.

Factors causing increased susceptibility to the toxic actions of anaesthetic agents include the following:

(*a*) Prolonged fasting, by depleting the glycogen reserves of the liver, greatly reduces the detoxicating power of that organ, and when using non-volatile agents in computed doses, allowance must be made for this increased susceptibility.

(*b*) Diseased conditions. Toxaemia causes degenerative changes in the parenchymatous organs, particularly the liver and myocardium, and thus great care must be taken when administering the non-volatile agents in computed doses to such subjects. In addition, when using non-volatile agents by intravenous injection, the injection should be made very slowly from the outset and careful assessment of the depth of narcosis or anaesthesia present made frequently. Quite often it is found that a toxaemic animal requires very much less than the normal dose. In those diseases associated with wasting there is often tachycardia and a soft, friable myocardium; animals suffering from such diseases are, in consequence, liable to develop cardiac failure when subjected to the stress of anaesthesia.

Examination of the Patient before Anaesthesia

Many operations are performed on normal, healthy animals. The subjects are generally young and represent good 'anaesthetic risks'. Nevertheless, enquiry should be made to ensure that they *are* normal—bright, vigorous and of hearty appetite. Should there be any doubt, operation is best delayed until there is assurance on this point. Many a reputation has been damaged by performing such operations as castration or spaying on young animals which are in the early stages of some acute infectious disease.

When an operation is to be performed for the relief of disease, considerable care must be exercised in assessing the risks which the particular animal carries in relation to the operation and anaesthetic. Once these are recognized the appropriate type of anaesthesia can be chosen and other measures enforced pre-operatively and post-operatively to diminish or, where possible, prevent them. The commonest conditions affecting the degree of risk are those involving the cardiovascular and respiratory systems, but the state of the liver and kidneys must also be taken into account.

History

The owner or attendant should be asked whether the animal has a cough. A soft, moist cough is associated with airway secretions which may give rise to respiratory obstruction and lung collapse when the cough reflex is suppressed by anaesthesia. Enquiry should also be made to determine whether the animal suffers from undue breathlessness, or respiratory distress, after exertion, since this sign may precede other signs of cardiac and respiratory failure by many months or even years.

Examination

The actual examination may be curtailed to one which is informative yet will not consume too much time nor unduly disturb the animal. While a more complete examination may sometimes be necessary, attention should always be paid to the pulse, the position of the apex beat, the presence of cardiac thrills, the heart sounds, the jugular venous pressure and any signs arising from the respiratory system. Examination of the urine for the presence of albumen and reducing substances is also valuable.

The rate of the pulse should be noted. Tachycardia is to be expected in all febrile and in many wasting diseases and under these circumstances is indicative of some degree of myocardial weakness. It can also be due to nervousness and where this is so it is often associated with rather cold ears and/or feet. Unless excessive, the presence of tachycardia need not unduly influence the choice of anaesthetic technique. Bradycardia may be physiological or it may indicate that complete atrio-ventricular block is present. When such a heart block is present there are usually some associated signs and, especially in large animals, careful inspection of the external jugular veins is a most

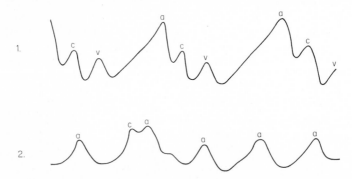

FIG. 1.—Pressure tracings.
(1) Tracing of the normal jugular pulse; (2) Tracing of the jugular pulse in a horse suffering from complete atrio-ventricular block.

helpful guide towards making the diagnosis. If the head is lowered to a position where jugular vein pulsation can be seen, it will be observed that while with physiological bradycardia the usual three waves appear in a regular sequence (Fig. 1), in cases of complete atrio-ventricular block two kinds of waves occur. The first is the larger and obvious pulsation caused by (1) the distension of the atrio-ventricular valves as they close producing a shock wave back in the jugular veins and (2) the pulse in the underlying carotid artery. The second kind of wave occurs at a regular but different rhythm and is due to contractions of the atria. In small animals, or in animals where jugular vein pulsation cannot be seen, an electrocardiogram may be the only way of determining whether bradycardia is physiological or is due to heart block.

In addition to observing the pulse waves, the jugular venous pressure should always be noted. When the animal is standing and the head is held up so that the neck is at an angle of about forty-five degrees to the horizontal, distension of the external jugular veins should, in normal animals, be just visible at the base of the neck. When the venous distension rises above this level, even in the absence of other signs, it indicates an obstruction to the anterior vena cava or a rise in the right atrial or right ventricular pressure. The commonest cause of a rise in pressure in these two chambers of the heart is probably right ventricular hypertrophy associated with chronic lung disease although congenital conditions such as atrial septal defects may also be indicated by this sign and it should be remembered that cattle suffering from constrictive pericarditis, or bacterial endocarditis, may have a marked increase in venous pressure.

The presence of a thrill over the heart is always a sign of cardiovascular disease and suggests an increased risk if the animal is to be subjected to anaesthesia.

Auscultation of the heart is, perhaps, only of limited interest in anaesthesia but the timing of any murmurs should be ascertained by palpation of the pulse while listening to the murmur. Diastolic murmurs are always indicative of heart disease and, while they may be of little importance in relation to cardiac function, it is unwise to come to this conclusion unless other signs, such as displacement of the apex beat, are absent. Systolic murmurs may or may not indicate the presence of heart disease, but if other signs are absent they are probably of no importance.

Accurate location of the apex beat is possibly the most important single observation in assessing the state of the cardiovascular and respiratory systems. It is displaced in most abnormal conditions affecting the lungs (e.g. pleural effusion, pneumothorax, lung collapse) and in the presence of enlargement of the left ventricle. In the absence of any pulmonary disorder a displaced apex beat is indicative of cardiac hypertrophy or dilatation.

Pulmonary disorders provide particular hazards for an animal undergoing operation or anaesthesia and any examination must be designed to disclose their presence or absence. The value of auscultation is, perhaps, limited but attention should be directed towards the length of the expiratory sounds and the discovery of any rhonchi or crepitations. If rhonchi and crepitations are heard excessive sputum is present, and the animal is either suffering from, or has recently suffered, a pulmonary infection. Prolongation of the expiratory sounds, especially when accompanied by high pitched rhonchi, indicates the existence of bronchospasm—a condition quite commonly encountered in elderly, 'broken-winded', brood mares. Unevenness of movement between the two sides of the chest is a reliable sign of pulmonary disease and one which is easily and quickly observed. The animal should be made to stand 'squarely' while the examiner stands first directly behind and then directly in front of it. In small animals unevenness of movement of the two sides of the chest is often better appreciated by palpation rather than by inspection.

The mouth should be examined for evidence of anaemia and the presence of loose teeth. Loose teeth may become dislodged during anaesthesia and inhaled into the tracheo-bronchial tree.

Urine testing is particularly important in dogs, since in those suffering from chronic nephritis the curtailment of water intake associated with anaesthesia and operation may give rise to a uraemic crisis. When urine examination suggests that chronic nephritis exists its significance must be explained to the owner of the animal. Urine testing may also uncover many undiagnosed cases of diabetes mellitus.

Provided that this brief examination of the animal is carried out thoroughly, and that the examiner has sufficient skill to realize the significance or insignificance of the findings, most of the conditions which have a bearing on the well-being of an animal during and after anaesthesia will be brought to light.

Significance of Conditions Found

During the course of even a brief examination the examiner will form some opinion of the animal's temperament. Animals which are unduly nervous or aggressive need special care in the immediate pre-operative period and many of them may be difficult to handle post-operatively. The appropriate choice of sedative medication can do much to facilitate the handling of such animals. An impression of the 'real' age of the animal as opposed to its chronological age will also have been gained. A dog aged 8 years, for example, may look 12 and is liable under stress to behave like a dog aged 12, whereas a dog aged 15 years which looks 5 years younger is again more likely to respond according to its appearance rather than its chronological age.

Heart Disease

As far as heart disease is concerned, a knowledge of the exact nature of the disease is less important in anaesthesia than is a knowledge of the effective function of the heart. A broad division into congenital and acquired heart disease is, however, of some value, In animals, acquired disease is more commonly encountered than is congenital disease, and is of more serious import since, unlike congenital disease, it tends to affect both the myocardium and the valves so that even in its earliest stages the heart muscle is weakened. Fitness for anaesthesia must be assessed from a knowledge of what the heart can do both at rest and at exercise set against such factors as the importance and urgency of operation and experience of how animals similarly affected have behaved in like circumstances. It is rarely possible to state emphatically that an animal will not tolerate anaesthesia because of heart disease. Of course, operations on large animals suffering from heart disease are seldom justifiable on economic grounds, but in small animal practice such considerations rarely apply. Provided that the anaesthetist is aware of the existence of a heart lesion and exercises care in the administration of the anaesthetic, these small animal patients will usually tolerate anaesthesia and operation quite well.

A feature of complete atrio-ventricular block is the occurrence of syncope due to ventricular asystole (Stoke-Adams attacks). In these attacks the animal loses consciousness, lies limp, still and pulseless, with fixed dilated pupils; breathing, however, continues. As a rule, ventricular contractions are resumed and recovery occurs quite spontaneously, but sometimes, ventricular fibrillation supervenes and the animal does not recover. These attacks may occur under general anaesthesia and not be noticed unless very careful attention is being paid to the pulse or an electrocardiogram is being recorded. Sudden asystole is also a feature of aortic stenosis and in this condition it may occur at any time, even when the animal is apparently at rest. It is uncertain whether such animals are more liable to sudden death when under anaesthesia than they are at any other time, but many have survived carefully administered general anaesthesia without incident. In these cases survival depends on the force of the ventricular contraction and agents such as thiopentone sodium, which are known to decrease this, must be used with caution.

Physiological bradycardia is associated with a marked ability to increase the cardiac output to meet extra demands, but the presence of heart block implies an inability to produce a more than fractional increase in output. Thus animals with physiological bradycardia are well able to withstand the stresses of anaesthesia, but animals with heart block are liable to develop circulatory failure when exposed to such strains as the vasodilatation induced by anaesthetic agents and hypovolaemia due to haemorrhage. Other important, common causes of fixed low cardiac output are constrictive pericarditis and mitral stenosis.

Hypoxaemia results from many pulmonary conditions. Horses afflicted with the condition commonly referred to as 'broken wind', and other animals suffering from conditions which give rise to bronchospasm may be difficult to keep well oxygenated during anaesthesia unless high concentrations of oxygen are administered. Pneumonia or lung collapse disturbs the ventilation–perfusion relationships within the lungs, and alveoli which are perfused with blood but not ventilated act as venous–arterial shunts. Significant desaturation of the arterial blood can result from this, even when cyanosis is not apparent.

Anaemia

All the various conditions of the heart and lungs which have been mentioned, and one other factor—the haemoglobin content of the blood—clearly affect the rate at which oxygen is made available to the tissues of the body.

Nunn and Freeman (1964) have drawn attention to the fact that this rate is equal to the product of the cardiac output and the content of oxygen in the arterial blood. Since the arterial oxygen content approximates to the product of the oxygen saturation and the quantity of oxygen which can be carried by the haemoglobin (about 1·34 ml/g of haemoglobin), the oxygen made available to the body can be expressed by a simple equation:

$$\text{Available oxygen} = \text{Cardiac output} \times \text{arterial saturation} \times \text{haemoglobin} \times 1\text{·}34$$
$$\text{(ml/min)} \qquad \text{(ml/min)} \qquad \text{(\%)} \qquad \text{(g/ml)}$$

This equation, of course, makes no allowance for the relatively small quantity of oxygen which is carried in physical solution in the blood, but it serves to illustrate the way in which the three variables combine to produce an effect which is often greater than is commonly supposed.

If any one of the three determining variables on the right-hand side of the equation is changed, the rate at which oxygen is made available to the tissues of the body is altered proportionately. Thus, if the cardiac output is halved, the available oxygen is also halved. If two determinants are lowered simultaneously while the third remains constant, the effect on the available oxygen is the *product* of the individual changes. For example, if the cardiac output and the haemoglobin concentration are both halved while the arterial oxygen saturation remains at the normal 95%, only one-quarter of the normal amount of oxygen is made available to the body tissues. If all three variables are reduced the effect is, of course, even more dramatic.

The full significance of these facts can, perhaps, be best appreciated if a hypothetical case is considered as an illustration. Taking figures quoted by Dukes (1955), if a 500 kg horse has a cardiac output of 30 litres/minute, a haemoglobin level of 15 g/100 ml of blood, and the arterial blood is 95% saturated, then the oxygen made available to the tissues of the animal is equal to

$$30,000 \times \frac{95}{100} \times \frac{15}{100} \times 1\text{·}34 \text{ ml/minute}$$

i.e. approximately 5700 ml/minute.

Thus, the oxygen made available to the horse would be adequate for its needs, since at rest its oxygen consumption is of the order of 1400 ml/minute, corresponding to an arterio-venous oxygen difference of 5 ml/100 ml of blood, and a mixed venous blood saturation of about 75%. (Because different organs extract widely differing amounts of oxygen from the blood, a mixed venous saturation of about 20% is about the minimum which can be tolerated by the body.)

If this hypothetical horse is now assumed to become anaemic so that its haemoglobin concentration falls by one-third to 10 g/100 ml of blood, and is anaesthetized with an agent which reduces the cardiac output by one-third to

20 litres/minute, and the arterial oxygen saturation decreases to 64%, then the oxygen made available to the tissues equals

$$20,000 \times \frac{64}{100} \times \frac{10}{100} \times 1\cdot34 \text{ ml/minute}$$

i.e. approximately 1700 ml/minute. Since the oxygen consumption is unchanged, making oxygen available at this rate would lead to the haemoglobin in the mixed venous blood being almost completely desaturated—a condition which is incompatible with life. It is important to note that none of the values substituted on the right-hand side of the equation would, in themselves, cause alarm. A reduction of one-third in the cardiac output is often encountered in anaesthesia, oxygen saturation of 64% may occur without cyanosis being apparent to the observer and haemoglobin levels of 10 g/100 ml are commonplace. Nevertheless, these three apparently mild departures from normal can in combination be lethal.

In most cases, especially when it is limited by disease, little can be done to increase the cardiac output, and this is the factor which determines the lowest permissible levels of the other two variables. The haemoglobin level, however, is capable of being raised and in a critical situation every effort must be made to do this. The concentration is often low pre-operatively and may be further reduced by transfusion of plasma or plasma volume expanders such as dextran. Pulmonary conditions which are likely to interfere with blood oxygenation should, if possible, be treated before anaesthesia to reduce the severity of their effect on this important factor. Where this cannot be done, the administration of high concentrations of oxygen during anaesthesia may be life-saving.

Renal Conditions

Chronic renal disease is common in dogs, and affected animals cannot produce concentrated urine. Dehydration from any cause deprives the kidneys of sufficient water for excretory purposes, so that urea and other waste products are retained, giving rise to uraemia. Curtailment of the water intake for a day when a general anaesthetic is administered may easily be responsible for uraemia in dogs suffering from chronic nephritis. Uraemia precipitates a vicious circle as it causes malaise and vomiting which not only themselves limit the water intake, but also produce further water depletion (Fig. 2). To guarantee that these animals receive an adequate fluid intake it may be necessary to administer fluid by intravenous infusion if the length of anaesthesia and/or the recovery period is prolonged. A uraemic circle can also be set up in animals suffering from chronic renal disease if the blood pressure falls as a result of haemorrhage and renal ischaemia ensues (Fig. 3). The replacement of blood as it is shed is very important in these animals.

Preparation of the Patient

Certain operations are performed in emergency when it is imperative that there shall be no delay, and but little preparation of the patient is possible.

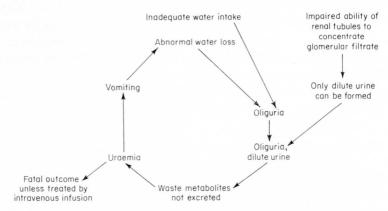

FIG. 2.—Diagram to illustrate how curtailment of the water intake may give rise to uraemia in dogs suffering from chronic nephritis.

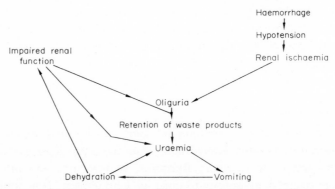

FIG. 3.—Diagram to illustrate the development of uraemia when an animal suffering from chronic nephritis is subjected to haemorrhage.

Among these operations are those for the repair of thoracic injuries, the control of severe, persistent haemorrhage, and certain obstetrical interferences where the delivery of a live foetus is of paramount importance. For all other operations time and care spent in pre-operative preparation are well worth while since proper preparation not only improves the patient's chances of survival, but also prevents the complications which might otherwise occur during and after operation. When operations are to be performed on normal, healthy animals, only the minimum of preparation is required before the administration of a general anaesthetic, but operations on dehydrated, anaemic, hypovolaemic or toxic patients should only be undertaken after careful preparation.

Food and Water

Food should be withheld from an animal on the day it is to undergo an elective operation under general anaesthesia. A distended stomach may interfere with the free movement of the diaphragm and hamper breathing. In cats, dogs and pigs, a full stomach predisposes to vomiting under anaesthesia and exposes the animal to the danger of inhaling vomitus. A full, or distended, stomach may rupture when a horse is forcibly cast or falls to the ground as anaesthesia is induced. In ruminants, a few hours of starvation will not result in any appreciable reduction in the volume of the fluid content of the rumen, but it seems to reduce the rate of fermentation within this organ, thus delaying the development of tympany when eructation is suppressed by general anaesthesia. Excessive fasting exposes the patient to risks almost as great as those associated with lack of preparation and should not be adopted. It has been customary to fast horses for as long as three days before the performance of such operations as ovariectomy and castration of abdominal cryptorchids with the object of overcoming the risk of confusion between faecal 'balls' in the small colon and the ovary or testicle. It is improbable that even after extensive fasting such as this the colon will be empty and the practice has little to commend it. In non-ruminants, free access to water should be allowed right up to the time when premedication is given, but in ruminants many surgeons consider that there is some advantage in withholding water for about six hours before abdominal operations.

Fluid and Electrolyte Balance

The water and electrolyte balance of an animal is a most important factor in determining the uncomplicated recovery or otherwise after operation. The repair of existing deficits of body fluid, or of one or more of its components, is complex because of the interrelations between the different electrolytes, and the difficulties imposed by the effects of severe sodium depletion on the circulation and renal function. Fortunately, in the majority of animal patients depletions are mild and of recent origin so that treatment by intravenous infusion with isotonic saline of 5% dextrose, depending on whether sodium depletion or water depletion is the more predominant, is all that is required. An anaesthetic should not be administered to an animal which has a decreased circulating blood volume, and every effort should be made to repair this deficit by the infusion of blood, plasma or plasma volume expander such as dextran, before anaesthesia is induced. In many instances, anaesthesia and operation may safely be postponed until the total fluid deficit is made good and an adequate renal output is achieved, but in cases of intestinal obstruction operation should be performed as soon as the blood volume has been restored. Attempts to restore the extracellular and intracellular deficits before an intestinal obstruction is relieved result in the further loss of fluid into the lumen of the obstructed bowel, making subsequent operation more difficult. When in doubt about the nature and volume of fluid to be administered, it is as well to remember that unless severe hypotension due to hypovolaemia is present, an animal's condition should not deteriorate from fluid imbalance, providing sufficient fluid is being given to cover current losses. These current losses include the inevitable loss of water through the skin and respiratory tract (approx. 20 ml/kg per 24 hours), the urinary and faecal loss, and any abnormal loss such as vomit.

Haemoglobin Level

As already mentioned on page 13 anaemia should be treated to raise the haemoglobin concentration to a normal level before any major operation is performed. When operation can be delayed for two or more weeks, the oral or parenteral administration of iron may raise the haemoglobin to a satisfactory concentration, but when such a delay is inadvisable the transfusion of red blood cells is indicated.

Treatment of Diabetes

It is sometimes necessary to anaesthetize a dog suffering from diabetes mellitus and if the condition is already under control no serious problems are likely to be encountered. However, if the normal dose of insulin is given, starvation before anaesthesia and inappetence afterwards may give rise to hypoglycaemia. For this reason it is advisable to reduce slightly the dose of insulin on the day of anaesthesia since hyperglycaemia is preferable to the opposite state. If an emergency operation has to be performed on an uncontrolled diabetic then the condition of the animal requires careful assessment and treatment. Ketonuria is an indication for treatment with glucose and soluble insulin, while overbreathing is a sign of severe metabolic acidosis. This must be treated by the infusion of sodium bicarbonate solution but the exact amount of bicarbonate needed in any particular case can only be calculated when the acid–base status is known from laboratory examination of an anaerobically drawn arterial blood sample. In veterinary practice, facilities for such examination of arterial blood samples are not generally available and metabolic acidosis has to be treated by infusing 2·5% sodium bicarbonate solution until the animal ceases to overbreathe. Because of the presence of an osmotic diuresis, many uncontrolled diabetics also require treatment for dehydration.

Clinical Measurement

Measurement of certain parameters of circulatory and respiratory function can provide data either to support a general clinical assessment of an animal's condition, or to suggest that this assessment should be modified. In very ill or badly injured animals these measurements, if made before, during and after operation, greatly increase the animal's chances of survival by enabling the whole procedure to be managed in a controlled, rational manner. In any animal, measurements made either at intervals or continuously throughout an operation can show the effects of anaesthetic agents and surgery on its physical state. It is regrettable that such monitoring has, in the past, seldom been employed in veterinary surgery because it was commonly believed that the expense and complexity of suitable measuring equipment prohibited its use outside very well equipped centres. It has now been realized that while measuring devices may be both complicated and costly, it is nevertheless possible to obtain much vital information from the use of a minimum of simple, inexpensive apparatus.

Many variables *can* be measured during anaesthesia, but anaesthetists differ in their views as to what *should* be measured. Some experienced anaesthetists take no measurements at all and claim (possibly with justice) that they can do better for their patients and provide a better service for surgeons if their attention is not distracted by having to use mechanical devices. Few anaesthetists regularly take measurements during minor surgical operations, but there is much to commend the practice of taking advantage of such operations to acquire skill in the technique of measuring. In circumstances in which measurements are mandatory (e.g. induced hypotension and hypothermia) it is clearly wise to avoid having to acquire skill with an anaesthetic technique and a measuring technique simultaneously. It is perhaps as well to take some measurements as a routine during even the simplest of procedures since it should be remembered that in anaesthesia just such procedures may become complicated and, therefore, interesting in a moment.

In order to make meaingful measurement in connection with anaesthesia it is necessary to know both what to measure and how to measure it. Measurement of the adequacy of respiratory function is, unfortunately, not easy. With the exception of the tidal and minute volumes in small animals, which can be measured with a Wright's respirometer (Wright, 1955), respiratory parameters do not lend themselves to measurement with simple devices in the absence of cooperation from the patient. The state of the circulation is much more easily assessed.

According to Lillehei (1964) the pulse volume reflects cardiac output; urine output parallels visceral perfusion; skin temperature indicates peripheral resistance. If, in addition, central venous pressure is monitored, the adequacy of the circulatory volume can be demonstrated. Pulse volume and skin temperature may be assessed by palpation; measurement of urinary output requires only the timed collection of urine voided or obtained by catheterization of the urinary bladder; measurement of the central venous pressure has recently been greatly simplified by the introduction of disposable, sterile packs prepared for transfusions. All these procedures can be carried out on the conscious animal prior to anaesthesia; their value during operation and in the immediate post-operative period cannot be overestimated, and all are well within the capability of veterinarians working outside large hospitals with the minimum of assistance. One other measurement, the determination of arterial blood pressure, cannot always be carried out on conscious animals, but is reasonably simple in unconscious or anaesthetized animals.

The Urinary Output

The urinary output depends on the renal blood flow which, in turn, depends on cardiac output and circulating blood volume, and thus it is a relatively sensitive indicator of the circulatory state.

Catheterization of the urinary bladder is a simple operation in most domestic animals, and the urine may be drained to a plastic bag for collection and subsequent measurement. Repeated catheterization not only disturbs sick or badly injured animals but also multiplies the risk of introducing infection into the bladder and traumatization of the urethra, so that either self-retaining catheters should be used or, once inserted, the catheter should be fixed in place with a suture or adhesive plaster. In restless animals where continuous drainage is difficult, the open end of the indwelling catheter may be clamped, the clamp being released every hour to drain the accumulated urine.

The Central Venous Pressure

Determination of the central venous pressure can be made quite rapidly. It is important as an indicator of the adequacy of the circulating blood volume and the ability of the heart to pump the venous return, but the circumstances of anaesthesia can also profoundly affect it. If it is allowed to rise unduly, the difficulty of certain operations may be greatly increased. It rises in the presence of respiratory obstruction or raised mean intrathoracic pressure, and a close correlation between the central venous pressure and the degree of bleeding at the site of operation is easily demonstrable.

Disposable venous manometer sets are available, but they are rather expensive for veterinary use. The complete apparatus can be made more cheaply from plastic three-way stopcocks, disposable giving sets and extension tubes (Fig. 4).

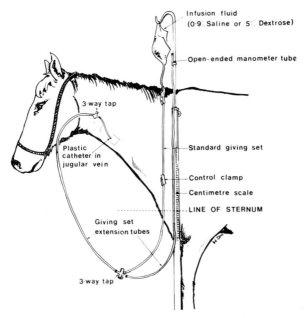

Infusion fluid
(0·9 Saline or 5% Dextrose)

Open-ended manometer tube

3-way tap

Plastic catheter in jugular vein

Standard giving set

Control clamp

Centimetre scale

LINE OF STERNUM

Giving set extension tubes

3-way tap

FIG. 4.—Apparatus for the measurement of the central venous pressure.

A polythene or nylon catheter (see Chapter 12) is introduced into the jugular vein and advanced until its tip lies in the anterior vena cava. The distance the catheter tip has to be introduced is, initially, estimated by measurement of distance, but once the catheter is connected to the manometer its position may be adjusted until the level of fluid in the manometer tube moves in time with the animal's respiratory movements. In dogs and cats the introduction of a catheter into the jugular vein is often greatly facilitated by laying the animal on its side and extending its head and neck over a pillow or sand-bag (Fig. 5). If the catheter is to be left in position for a long time it is kept patent with a drip infusion given through the three-way stopcock or the catheter is kept filled with heparin saline solution (10 i.u./ml) between measurements. Readings may be taken at any time. The drip is turned full on and the stopcock manipulated first to fill the manometer tube from the fluid reservoir and then to connect the manometer tube to the catheter. The fall of fluid in the manometer tube is observed and should be 'step-like' in response to respiratory pressure changes. The central venous pressure is read off when fluid fall ceases.

The actual reading obtained depends on the reference point taken to represent zero pressure. Probably the ideal reference point is the mean pressure in the right atrium, but for practical purposes the most appropriate appears to be the sternal manubrium, because this is easily located and seems

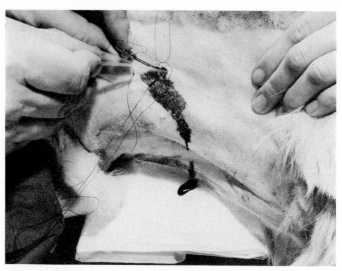

FIG. 5.—*Introduction of a catheter into the jugular vein of a dog through a MacGregor needle.* Note the small skin incision, the sutures laid ready to tie the catheter in place and the pillow under the dog's neck. The sterility of the catheter is maintained by keeping it inside its covering sleeve.

to be most constantly related to the position of the right atrium in all animals, irrespective of body position. In normal subjects standing quietly the pressure varies from animal to animal, but it is usually between 3 and 7·5 cm of water when using this reference point (Fig. 6). At the moment, the variations of normal resting central venous pressure seem to be as inexplicable as the normal variations of normal resting arterial pressure. In the dog and cat the value is relatively constant between 3 and 7·5 cm of water, no matter what the position of the animal's body; but in normal horses in lateral recumbency it is usually recorded as being between 25 and 35 cm of water, while in dorsal recumbency the reading may fall below the reference level.

Whilst a single central venous pressure reading may indicate that all is not well, it is the change in pressure during the intravenous administration of fluid which is most informative. When the administration of fluid improves an animal's condition (improved pulse volume, increase in skin temperature and urine production), therapy should be continued until the central venous pressure remains steady in the normal range. Excessive administration of fluid with overloading of the heart is extremely unlikely to occur if the central venous pressure is not allowed to exceed the upper limit of normality. If the apparent beneficial effects of fluid administration are short-lived and the central venous pressure falls quickly after an initial rise, it is likely that the blood is pooling in dilated peripheral vessels, i.e. the abnormality present is an increase in the vascular bed, and more fluid should be given. If an infusion or transfusion increases the central venous pressure without improving the animal's condition, then the cardiac pump mechanism is at fault. In this

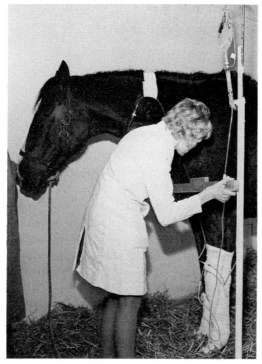

FIG. 6.—Measurement of the central venous pressure in a horse. Determination of the reference point by means of a spirit level.

situation an intravenous infusion of isoprenaline (1 mg in 500 ml of isotonic diluent) usually improves the cardiac output.

Since measurement of the central venous pressure reflects the filling pressure of the right side of the heart, it seems theoretically possible that left heart failure could precede that of the right side and precipitate pulmonary oedema without a rise in central venous pressure. Although this pattern has been recognized after cardiac surgery in dogs, there appears to be little evidence of its occurrence in other situations.

Arterial Blood Pressure

The measurement of arterial pressure can provide useful information and is mandatory when induced hypotension is employed to facilitate surgery. For accurate, continuous measurement, techniques involving cannulation of an artery are necessary, but for routine monitoring, indirect methods which do not depend upon needle puncture or cannulation of an artery are preferable.

(a) Indirect Measurement of Arterial Blood Pressure

Many attempts have been made to measure the arterial blood pressure in animals by indirect methods. These are modifications of the Riva–Rocci technique, involving occlusion of an artery by an inflatable encircling cuff and detection of returning blood flow distal to the site of occlusion as the occluding pressure is reduced. Many of these techniques have inherent inaccuracies and technical difficulties which render them unsatisfactory for clinical use in animals. For example, difficulty is encountered because inflatable cuffs slip down conical-shaped extremities as the pressure within the cuff is increased. Moreover, the detection of returning blood flow distal to the occluding cuff is not easy. Palpation of the pulse is often impossible, and its detection with sensitive pulse monitors is often difficult.

The auscultatory technique of sphygmomanometry is the most widely used method of indirect blood pressure measurement in man, and determines both the systolic and diastolic pressures. A stethoscope is placed over an artery distal to an occluding cuff. The pressure within the cuff is reduced slowly and is assumed to equal the systolic blood pressure when the first Korotkoff sound is heard. The cuff pressure is assumed to equal the diastolic pressure when the Korotkoff sounds either become muffled or disappear. This technique has been used in horses and is said to give results which correlate well with direct measurements from the same limb (Smith, 1969). The cuff (12×60 cm) is applied around the hind leg of the anaesthetized horse just above the hock and auscultation is performed over the anterior tibial artery. Measurements of the diastolic pressure is not as accurate as that of systolic pressure, and even systolic pressure readings have been found to be unreliable below 70 mm of mercury.

The change in pressure associated with a pulse, or the change in tissue volume, may be converted into an electrical signal with a suitable transducer. Pulse monitors involving carbon microphone transducers have been tested in dogs by Campbell, Lawson and Sanford (1964), who found the tail to be the best site for the cuff and pulse monitor. Artefacts due to movement of the tail often make it difficult to detect the first pulse wave as the pressure in the cuff is reduced, so that a clear-cut systolic point cannot be obtained.

Oscillometric methods have also been tried in animals (Romagnoli, 1953), but again the systolic and diastolic end points are not always obvious and, because the observer has to note changes in the amplitude of swing of the oscillometer needle, subjective bias enters into the results obtained.

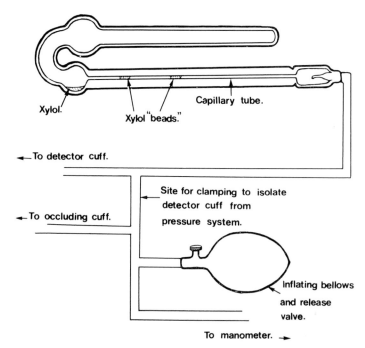

Xylol.

Xylol "beads."

Capillary tube.

To detector cuff.

To occluding cuff.

Site for clamping to isolate detector cuff from pressure system.

Inflating bellows and release valve.

To manometer.

FIG. 7.—'Newcastle' sphygmomanometer arrangement with xylol pulse detector. Note point of isolation of detector from pressure system.

The most satisfactory indirect method for determination of the systolic pressure in animals appears to be that using the xylol pulse indicator (Ashworth, Neligan and Rogers, 1959).* This apparatus has been used for measurement in dogs (Wilson and Clark, 1964), and Glen (1970) has both confirmed its accuracy in dogs and extended its use to other animals. Basically, the apparatus consists of an occluding cuff connected to a mercury manometer and a distal pulse-sensing cuff attached to the xylol pulse indicator (Fig. 7). The pulse indicator system (Fig. 8) can be isolated from the pressure system, and as the pressure in the occluding cuff is reduced, returning pulsations in the distal part of the body extremity are detected by movement of xylol

* 'Newcastle' sphygmomanometer. Chas. Thackray Ltd, Leeds.

'beads' in a capillary tube. The whole apparatus is simple, robust and self-contained. Artefacts due to movement of the extremities are easily recognized, so a clear-cut systolic pressure point is usually obvious.

In dogs, Glen confirmed that the detector cuff was best placed over the metacarpal region and the occluding cuff over the brachial artery, above the elbow, as described by Wilson and Clark. For accurate determination of the systolic pressure the occluding cuff must encircle the limb completely and a length of 25 cm has proved adequate for all sizes of dog. The width of the cuff also has an important bearing on the accuracy of the readings obtained.

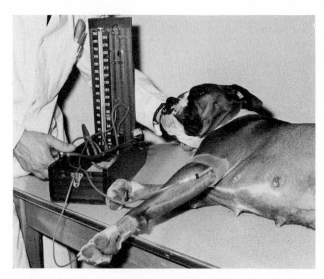

FIG. 8.—'Newcastle' sphygmomanometer arrangement in use on a conscious dog. Spencer Wells forceps used to isolate detector from pressure system.

A cuff 2·5 cm wide should be used for dogs weighing less than 12 kg and one 3·75 cm wide for heavier dogs. Cuffs 3·75 cm wide have been used on the tail in horses and cattle, and in sheep the 2·5 cm cuff applied around the tibial region just above the hock has proved satisfactory.

Both the occluding and detector cuffs are made of polyvinyl chloride and have a self-adhesive strap of the same material. The pressure within the system is raised to about 25 to 30 mm of mercury before the detector cuff is isolated from the rest of the system. As inflation of the occluding cuff continues, the xylol 'beads' move in the capillary tube to indicate an increase in volume of the body extremity as blood flows in after occlusion of the veins. Once arterial occlusion is complete the xylol column is stationary. As pressure is decreased in the occluding cuff, the xylol column either remains stationary or indicates a gradual decrease in volume of the extremity. When the pressure in the occluding cuff reaches systolic pressure, typical pulsations appear in the xylol column and the 'beads' move again to indicate a further increase in volume as blood flows in while venous occlusion is still complete. The proper site for a 'bead' of xylol at the end of cuff inflation is towards the closed end of the column (Fig. 8). If a 'bead' is not present in this region following inflation of the occluding cuff, one can readily be introduced from the reservoir by tilting the apparatus.

Estimation of the systolic pressure with this simple, inexpensive apparatus is easily taught to nursing staff and, in many cases, it can be performed on the conscious animal.

(b) Direct Measurement of the Arterial Blood Pressure

The direct continuous measurement of the arterial pressure is a monitoring technique little used outside the field of open heart surgery. The questionable safety and technical difficulty of arterial puncture or cannulation, together with the complexity and expense of measuring equipment, are the main reasons usually advanced for the limited use of this technique. However, if measurement of the mean, rather than systolic and diastolic, arterial pressure is accepted, simple and inexpensive equipment can provide direct, continuous

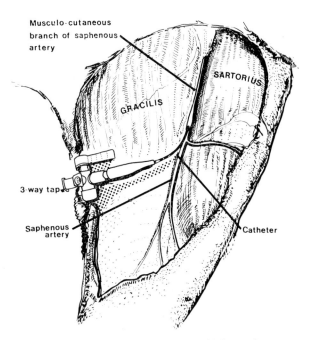

FIG. 9.—Dissection of the inner aspect of the thigh to show artery normally cannulated for direct arterial pressure monitoring in the dog.

monitoring for routine use in major surgery, in the care of animals in the immediate post-operative period, and for research purposes.

The technique is most commonly used in dogs, but it has also been employed in horses. Because the arterial cannula may be introduced under local infiltration analgesia, the technique can be applied in conscious animals. In dogs, the cannula is introduced into a superficial musculo-cutaneous branch of the femoral artery on the medial aspect of the thigh (Figs 9 and 10).

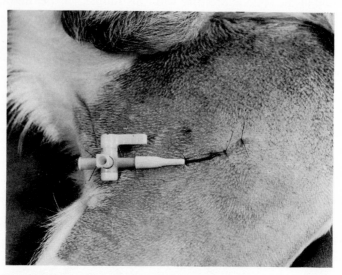

FIG. 10.—*Cannula for direct blood pressure measurement in a dog.* Cannulae in the superficial musculo-cutaneous arteries in the medial aspect of the thigh are well tolerated and accidental, unobserved withdrawal of the cannula from these arteries does not result in serious bleeding.

In horses, the submaxillary artery or a digital artery may be used. Following cleansing of the skin, a small nick is made with a scalpel blade just over the proposed site of arterial puncture. A disposable Guest cannula (see Chapter 12) mounted on a 2 ml syringe is then introduced into the lumen of the artery through the nick in the skin. As soon as the cannula is in the artery, the needle is withdrawn and the cannula pushed up the lumen of the vessel. A sterile, disposable, plastic stopcock is attached to the cannula and the stopcock and cannula flushed with a previously prepared heparin/saline solution to prevent clotting. The cannula is best fixed in position by suturing it to the skin with monofilament nylon (Fig. 10).

The monitoring apparatus is shown in Fig. 11. A number of variations are possible but the basic pattern is as shown. A standard type of anaeroid manometer has connected to it a 6 or 8 cm length of plastic drip tubing ending in a male Luer connection. This assembly may be kept, when not in use, in a covered container with formalin tablets. The remainder of the apparatus (two lengths of extension drip tubing and two disposable stopcocks) is available as presterilized and disposable items. After assembly the tubing is filled with heparin/saline solution until the meniscus lies 10 to 12 cm below the manometer. The solution can be introduced into both lengths of tubing by opening the appropriate ports on the stopcocks and injecting the solution from a 20 ml syringe through the stopcock. Both stopcocks have their side arms closed and the lower tubing is connected to the stopcock on the arterial cannula. This

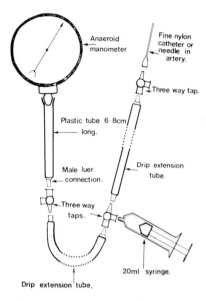

FIG. 11.—Apparatus for direct measurement of mean arterial blood pressure.

stopcock is opened and pressure readings should be obtained. There is an initial flow of blood into the lower tube as the air in the upper tube and manometer is compressed. This blood is flushed back into the animal by injection of heparin/saline solution through the middle stopcock. After this, flushing is only needed at infrequent intervals. The stopcock on the arterial cannula can be used for obtaining arterial blood samples and adds greatly to the convenience of setting up the apparatus and during transport of the animal from place to place.

The longer the air column between the meniscus of the heparin/saline solution and the manometer the greater the damping, but care should always be taken to ensure that the manometer does not become contaminated by heparin/saline solution because the air column is too short. An air column of about 8 cm seems to be optimum, and this can be adjusted by attaching a syringe full of air to the upper stopcock and introducing or removing air as required. The manometer must be attached to a suitable support so that the meniscus is at heart level.

This apparatus enables the pulse rate and mean arterial pressure to be kept under continuous observation. Used in conjunction with a central venous pressure manometer, an overall picture of cardiovascular dynamics is continuously available.

The main objection to the use of this technique is the technical difficulty of arterial cannulation and doubt as to its safety. The skill necessary to become proficient at arterial cannulation can be acquired with practice. There is little evidence of any serious complications arising after arterial cannulation. The most common complication is haematoma formation following with-drawal of the cannula, but this can be minimized by applying firm digital pressure to the puncture site for 5 minutes (by the clock) after removal of the cannula.

Electrocardiography

The use of the electrocardiograph during anaesthesia is often valuable and its value increases with the ability of the anaesthetist to interpret the informa-tion it yields. Many reliable instruments are available, with display by oscilloscope or direct writer, and their application encounters no special difficulties apart from the interference caused by surgical diathermy and other high frequency sources. In anaesthetized animals muscle potentials are not usually troublesome. Needle electrodes inserted into the muscles of the limbs, chest or withers are much more satisfactory than skin plate electrodes, provided that there is a really firm electrical contact between the needle and its connecting cable.

The artefacts commonly recorded during anaesthesia have been reviewed by Purchase (1963). Interference from the mains at 50 cycles/second is the most commonly observed abnormality, and results from earth loops, other electrical apparatus in close proximity (especially if the electric cables run parallel for any distance), close proximity of the mains cables to the recording leads of the electrocardiograph, poor contact between the electrodes and patient, and the use of endoscopic equipment. Earth loops occur if the animal is earthed to two separate points via the recording equipment. Earths are frequently at slightly different potentials, and a current may flow through the animal causing interference with the recording. Any current flowing at right angles to a loop so formed may induce electromagnetic interference. The high frequency discharge associated with coagulation or cutting with diathermy completely obscures the normal tracing. The amplifier of the instrument is not damaged but the pen or stylus of a direct writing machine can be wrecked. To safeguard the apparatus the pen should not be recording whilst diathermy is in use. The cutting movement of scissors used on the animal may produce spikes which are easily confused with the normal components of the electrocardiogram and the baseline may be distorted by movement of a large batch of instruments, such as haemostats, which are attached to the wound.

The significance of any abnormalities in the electrocardiogram is, of course, dependent on their cause and prognosis. Sinus tachycardia is frequently encountered during anaesthesia and is usually observed after the administration of atropine. An increase in heart rate may also result from surgical stimulation in an inadequately anaesthetized animal, or from sympatho-adrenal stimulation due to carbon dioxide retention. Sinus bradycardia is a normal consequence of some types of anaesthesia, but extreme bradycardia which cannot be overcome by the administration of atropine is usually only seen just before death.

Nodal rhythm is not of great significance and atrioventricular dissociation is only rarely seen during anaesthesia. Ventricular extrasystoles, on the other hand, are common. They may be isolated or occur alternately with sinus beats as in bigeminal rhythm. They may be unifocal or multifocal in origin. Ventricular extrasystoles are seen most commonly in animals anaesthetized with agents which sensitize the heart to the effects of adrenaline, which may be exogenous in origin (e.g. injected with local analgesic solutions), or endogenous due to reflex sympatho-adrenal stimulation. Sympatho-adrenal stimulation occurs during hypercapnia and hypoxia and thus is usually due to respiratory inadequacy.

Frequently the pulse and heart rates may differ considerably. If an extrasystole occurs during a period when the heart is empty, no peripheral pulse will be produced. Thus, the heart rate may be twice that of the pulse during bigeminy, and this condition might not be diagnosed by palpation of the pulse. Single extrasystoles are of no significance, and bigeminy is only important in that it may precede more serious events. Ventricular tachycardia is usually considered to be the immediate precursor of ventricular fibrillation and its occurrence must be regarded as a serious portent. Because these changes frequently result from sympathetic activity upon the sensitized myocardium, they often disappear if the depth of anaesthesia be reduced and adequate alveolar ventilation restored.

Alterations in amplitude of the electrocardiogram usually imply a change in the electrical axis of the heart and, as such, are of little significance. ST segment depression or elevation is considered by some to be normal in dogs, but changes of more than a few millimetres are indicative of myocardial hypoxia and, therefore, must not be ignored. T-wave changes appear to have no special importance and are seen during a variety of conditions.

Asystole and ventricular fibrillation indicate extreme myocardial changes rendering the heart incapable of acting as a pump. On occasion QRS deflections, which may appear to be normal, are recorded from animals long after the onset of circulatory arrest. These terminal signs of electrical activity are not associated with mechanical activity.

The Modern Approach to Anaesthesia

In 1952 Gray and Rees suggested that general anaesthesia involved three effects: (1) narcosis, (2) analgesia and (3) relaxation. They also pointed out that anaesthetic agents are general depressants, affecting the whole of the central nervous system (including the centres responsible for circulatory stability), the cardiovascular system and, to a lesser extent, the functions of the liver and kidneys. Thus, while these agents produce all three effects of anaesthesia, they do so quite indiscriminately—the need for more muscle relaxation implies deeper narcosis with consequent central nervous and cardiovascular depression. Since the introduction of muscle relaxants into anaesthesia in 1942, it has been possible to produce each of the three effects of anaesthesia independently of the other two by the use of agents which have almost a single action in the body. The patient thus anaesthetized can be maintained at a very light level of narcosis from which recovery of consciousness is rapid even after the longest surgical procedures, and has a comparative freedom from nausea or 'hang-over' after anaesthesia.

In Great Britain medical anaesthetists were quick to accept this approach to general anaesthesia, and a system based on the production of a light level of unconsciousness coupled with the use of muscle relaxants to provide both muscle relaxation and control of the patient's breathing was soon widely practised. The term 'balanced anaesthesia' was often applied to this system since it was considered to be a development, or improvement, of a system of anaesthesia described under this name by Lundy in 1927, and its use in veterinary practice was first reported by Hall and Weaver in 1954.

The use of the term 'analgesia' to describe one of the effects of general anaesthesia was, perhaps, unfortunate in that an anaesthetized patient is unconscious and must, therefore, be in an analgesic state. It is clearly more appropriate to use a phrase such as 'freedom from reflex response' to describe this component of general anaesthesia—meaning that noxious stimuli do not produce a reflex motor response in the patient. However, the concept of Gray and Rees can be extended to the whole subject of anaesthesia, and in this context the term 'analgesia' *is* appropriate since anaesthesia involves analgesia together with narcosis and relaxation. Clearly, when choosing the anaesthetic technique to be employed in any given case, it must be appreciated that not all these three components may be necessary. For many procedures it may be necessary to have the patient awake and standing (e.g. for rumenotomy in cattle), yet both analgesia and muscle relaxation must be provided. For other procedures, such as a minor operation on a horse's foot, analgesia alone may suffice, while for radiography the immobility due to unconsciousness is often all that is required.

Use and Abuse of Drugs in Anaesthesia

While the rationale behind the concept of modern anaesthetic practice is sound, there has been a regrettable tendency towards ever increasing complexity in the number of drugs given to animals to produce anaesthesia, and this has caused a number of senior workers to advocate a return to simplicity. Undoubtedly, if potentiation can occur in respect to desirable drug actions, it may also occur in relation to toxic effects. It is, therefore, likely that some of the difficulties encountered in anaesthesia today are produced by the anaesthetist in the sense that they are aggravated, if not caused, by the misuse of sedative, anaesthetic and analgesic drugs and their pharmacological antidotes. In the hands of the inexperienced or careless anaesthetist the apparently rational use of a combination of drugs, each employed for a specific purpose, can easily degenerate into polypharmacy in which the advantages of light, flexible anaesthesia become lost by the development of complications—the origin of which is promptly made more obscure by the administration of antidotes. This is not to say, however, that skilled anaesthetists should revert to deep general anaesthesia to produce satisfactory operating conditions, or avoid the use of muscle relaxants, for this would be a retrograde step, but the number of agents used in any one case should be kept to a minimum. The skilled anaesthetist, keeping to this minimum and using each agent for a specific purpose, can easily demonstrate that the advantages of modern anaesthesia can outweigh the alleged safety of the old, simple, depression techniques.

REFERENCES

ASHWORTH, A. M., NELIGAN, G. A. and ROGERS, J. E. (1959). *Lancet*, i, 801
CAMPBELL, J. R., LAWSON, D. D. and SANFORD, J. (1964). *J. small Anim. Pract.* 5, 255
DUKES, H. H. (1955). *The Physiology of Domestic Animals.* 7th Ed. London: Baillière, Tindall & Cox
GLEN, J. B. (1970). *Vet. Rec.* 87, 349
GRAY, T. C. and REES, C. J. (1952). *Brit. med. J.* 2, 891
HALL, L. W. and WEAVER, B. M. Q. (1954). *Vet. Rec.* 66, 289
LILLEHEI, R. C. (1964). *Surgery, St Louis,* 56, 182
LUNDY, J. S. (1942). *Clinical Anaesthesia.* Philadelphia: Saunders
NUNN, J. F. and FREEMAN, J. (1964). *Anaesthesia,* 19, 120
PURCHASE I. F. H. (1963). *Vet. Rec.* 75, 326
ROMAGNOLI, A. (1953). *Cornell Vet.* 43, 161
SMITH, M. (1969). *Nord. Vet.-Med.* 21, 312
WILSON, R. B. and CLARK T. J. (1964). *J. Amer. vet. med. Ass.* 144, 981
WRIGHT, B. M. (1955). *J. Physiol., Lond.* 127, 25

2

Local Analgesia

Many surgical procedures can be satisfactorily performed under local analgesia. Whether or not sedation is employed as an adjunct will depend on the species, temperament and health of the animal, and on the magnitude of the procedure. In adult cattle, many operations are performed on standing animals and since sedation may induce the animal to lie down, it is better avoided. In other animals sedation should be adopted for all but the simplest of procedures for by reducing fear and liability to sudden movement, efficient surgery is greatly facilitated. It must be remembered that some local analgesics (e.g. lignocaine) exert a sedative action when they are absorbed from sites of injection, and the dose of any sedative drug given must be reduced to allow for this effect.

There are several features of local analgesia which render it particularly useful in veterinary practice. Its use enables protracted operations to be performed on standing animals, and in large animals this avoids the dangers associated with forcible casting and prolonged recumbency. The surgeon can induce local analgesia and operate without the assistance of an anaesthetist. The techniques of local analgesia are not difficult to learn and do not involve the use of expensive or complicated equipment.

Mode of Action of Local Analgesics

The process involved in the excitation of a nerve cell, in the conduction of an impulse in a nerve fibre and in the blocking of this conduction by local analgesics are not yet completely understood.

The unit of nervous tissue consists of the nerve cell and its processes, the dendrites and the axon. The processes are dependent upon an intact connection with the nerve cell for survival and nutrition. Conventional theories of nerve function have long been based on the assumption that the surface membrane of nerve fibres and cells exists as a differentially permeable interface between tissue fluid and the liquid phase of the neuronal cytoplasm. However, modern cytological studies render it very unlikely that the external surfaces of nerve cells and fibres are bathed directly by tissue fluid, for it now appears that most neurones are entirely, or almost entirely, covered by supporting cells applied directly to their external surfaces. Thus, the diffusion barrier surrounding neurones must now be considered to involve these supporting cells and their membranes. The larger nerve fibres are surrounded by a coat of fatty material—the myelin sheath. The thickness of this sheath increases with the diameter of the axon it encloses, and it is composed of a number of lipoprotein lamellae which, in the case of peripheral nerve fibres, are laid down from the Schwann cells that enclose the axons. The myelin lamellae are not continuous along the entire length of the fibre, being interrupted at more or less regular intervals (the nodes of Ranvier) to leave short segments of the axons covered by the Schwann cells. Thus the axon is always separated from the surrounding tissue fluid by the thickness of the Schwann cell in which it is embedded, throughout the length of the unmyelinated fibres and at the nodes of Ranvier in myelinated fibres; and in the internodal segments of the latter, by the myelin lamellae also. Peripheral nerves are composed of fibres of many different diameters, the finest of which usually have no myelin within their Schwann cells, while the larger fibres are surrounded by increasing numbers of myelin lamellae. There is some correlation between fibre size and function, and the fibres in the spinal peripheral nerves may be classified into three broad groups in terms of diameter ranges, each of these groups mediating particular functions. Such an arbitrary division does, of course, give rise to some overlap. (Table 1.)

Table 1

RELATIONS BETWEEN NERVE FIBRE SIZE AND FUNCTION

The divisions are not absolute and there is a varying degree of overlap from one diameter group to the other.

Group	Fibre diameter range (μ)	Functions
I	15–25 (myelinated)	Somatic motor efferents Proprioceptive afferents
II	5–15 (myelinated)	Cutaneous afferents (except pain)
III <5	2–5 (myelinated) <2 (unmyelinated)	Pain afferents γ—motor efferents Pain afferents Post-ganglionic sympathetic efferents

In unmyelinated fibres the impulse travels along the axon as a localized propagating chemical change, surrounded by an electrical field more or less

2

spherically orientated around the axon as a core, but in myelinated fibres it cannot do so since the myelin acts as an insulator. Thus the ionic shifts which underlie the rising and falling phases of the action potential in myelinated fibres take place at the nodes, and in such fibres the electrical currents flow not between immediately adjacent zones of the axon, but from one node of Ranvier to the next. In myelinated fibres, therefore, the electrical fields have an elliptical geometry with one epicentre at a node of Ranvier and the other epicentre at the next node. Due to these differences, conduction in an un-myelinated fibre is continuous or linear, like a spark travelling along a fuse; but in a myelinated fibre it is discontinuous or saltatory, the impulse leaping from one node of Ranvier to the next.

The action of local analgesics is one of stabilization of the active membrane which surrounds the nerve fibre, but the actual mechanism by which this is brought about is unknown. They have no marked effect on the resting potential of neurones, nor do they decrease the oxygen consumption of resting nerve cells, but these two observations constitute the only established data relating to the action of these drugs in the body. The stabilization of the cell membrane can occur in the region of the cell body, the nerve ending and along the course of the cell processes. In the case of myelinated fibres, the inhibitory effect on the membrane occurs only at the nodes of Ranvier. All, including motor nerves, may be blocked and transmission at the neuro-muscular junction and at autonomic ganglia may be affected by a similar mechanism.

When a peripheral nerve is exposed to a local analgesic, conduction in its constituent fibres is blocked at a rate that is inversely proportional to their diameters. If a pool of local analgesic solution be infiltrated around a peripheral nerve, function fails first in the unmyelinated fibres in it, followed by loss of function in the smaller and then in the larger myelinated fibres. This sequence is due to the fact that Schwann cells containing myelin are relatively impervious to local analgesic solutions compared to those which contain little or no myelin. Therefore, once a drug has penetrated through the connective tissues of a nerve into the endoneural fluid, it can act upon the entire length of any unmyelinated fibres but only on the short segments of myelinated fibres at the nodes of Ranvier. As the number of nodes per unit length of an axon is greater in fine fibres than in thick ones, there will be more of such segments within the pool of solution in the finer fibres than in the thicker ones. For this reason also, local blockade of nerve fibres becomes more rapid and effective the greater the length of the fibres exposed to the action of the drug. An alternative to employing an increased concentration of drug to accelerate local analgesia is, therefore, to infiltrate along a greater length of the nerve with a more dilute solution.

Substances Employed

A remarkably large number of compounds with widely different molecular configurations are able to produce local analgesia, and this property has been attributed to agents of many varied classes. However, numerous compounds which from their general chemical structure might be expected to possess local analgesic properties are, in fact, inactive. Relationship between structure and function can only be found within narrow limits, and then only in a series of compounds which are almost homologous, e.g. the basic esters of benzoic acid and para-aminobenzoic acid. A very large number of substances have been isolated or synthesized and subjected to pharmacological tests for local analgesic activity, but the compounds which are used in clinical practice are very few in number.

Cocaine

Cocaine is an alkaloid obtained from the leaves of *Erythroxylon coca*, a South American plant. Reference to it has now become largely historical for it has become almost entirely replaced by synthetic substitutes. It was first introduced into surgery by Koller in 1884, and the late Sir Frederick Hobday popularized its use in veterinary surgery towards the end of the last century. The alkaloid itself is only very sparingly soluble in water, but readily soluble in fixed and volatile oils. The drug is chiefly used as an aqueous solution of its salt, the hydrochloride, applied to mucous surfaces. Cocaine hydrochloride solutions are decomposed by boiling and alkali causes precipitation. Solutions should be freshly prepared, using tablets sterilized by dry heat dissolved in sterile distilled water. Cocaine paralyses sensory nerve endings in a dilution of 1:3000, and its action is selective, for at this concentration it does not injure the tissues. Cocaine combines an analgesic action with a vasoconstrictor effect but unfortunately it is extremely toxic when injected. Small doses cause motor excitation, which may provoke exaggerated movement by the animal during operation. Toxic doses cause clonic convulsions followed by loss of consciousness and paralysis of the medullary centres. Hobday put the maximum quantities to be used by subcutaneous injection at the following:

| Horses | . | . | . | . | 780 mg | Small dogs | . | . | . | . | 45 mg |
| Large dogs | . | . | . | 120 mg | Cats | . | . | . | . | 15 mg |

For this reason cocaine is now only employed for surface analgesia of mucous membranes. A 4% solution is used for instillation into the eye, and from 10% to 20% for nasal and laryngeal work.

The toxic actions of cocaine have led to a search for synthetic substitutes which, while retaining its local analgesic properties or even improving on them, are in large measure free from these toxic effects.

Procaine

Procaine (syn. ethocaine hydrochloride) was introduced in 1905 under the trade name of Novocain, and largely replaced cocaine as a local analgesic. It is marketed, in some cases with slight variations in composition, under a large variety of trade names including Kerocain, Neotonocain, Novutox, Parsetic and Planocaine. As procaine hydrochloride (para-aminobenzoyl-diethylaminoethanol hydrochloride) it is included in the British Pharmacopoeia.

Administered by subcutaneous injection, procaine has an efficiency approximating that of cocaine, and it has the advantage of being considerably less toxic. When combined with adrenaline hydrochloride solution it is ten times less toxic than cocaine. Care should be taken, however, during administration that the drug is not accidentally introduced into a vein. A further advantage is that the drug, provided absorption is slow—and this is ensured by combining it with adrenaline—is rapidly and completely detoxicated by the liver, so that a second infiltration may be carried out in the course of an hour or so without a danger of toxicity by cumulation arising. Solutions can be sterilized by boiling, and are practically non-irritating. They are decomposed by alkali.

For general infiltration of the skin and gums in the dog and cat, 2% solutions combined with 1 in 100,000 adrenaline hydrochloride are employed and in this concentration the drug may be used almost *ad libitum* without danger. For epidural injection, 1 to 2·5% concentrations are used. For skin infiltration and perineural injection in horses and cattle concentrations of 4 to 5% are often employed, but it is unlikely that they are more effective than a 2·5% solution, and are certainly more toxic. Analgesia is present in about 5 minutes (in the case of epidural and perineural injection in about 10 minutes) and persists for an hour. Procaine has very little power of penetration, and for the anaesthetization of mucous surfaces is inferior to cocaine, its action on the cornea being one-sixteenth that of the plant alkaloid.

Among the solutions marketed under trade names with which veterinary surgeons may be familiar, and of which procaine hydrochloride is the active principle, are Chlorocain, Kerocain, Neocaine, Parsetic, Planocaine, and Novutox (this contains, in addition, quinatoxines and benzoic acid, and it is claimed that it remains sterile even after the rubber cap of the bottle has been punctured several times).

Tutocaine

Tutocaine is the hydrochloride of para-aminobenzoyldimethylamino-methylbutanol. It is considered by some workers to be more potent than procaine. Until recently it was extensively employed on the Continent, particularly in Germany, but it never found favour in Great Britain.

Amethocaine Hydrochloride

Amethocaine hydrochloride (Anethaine, Decicaine, Pantocaine, Ponto-caine, Rexocaine) is a member of the procaine series of compounds which is particularly useful for the desensitization of mucous membranes. A 1% solution is used for instillation into the eye, and a 2% solution is used for the pharynx, larynx and nasal mucous membranes.

Propoxycaine

This propoxy derivative of procaine, dimethylaminoethyl 3-propoxy-4-aminobenzoate hydrochloride (Ravocaine) is 8 to 9 times more active than procaine, but only twice as irritating. A solution containing 2% procaine with 0·4% propoxycaine and a vasoconstrictor has been described as being ideal for dental anaesthesia (Tainter, Wessinger and Lee, 1955), and this combination has been used in veterinary practice.

Cinchocaine

This was first introduced as Percaine by Uhlmann in 1929. It is known as Nupercaine, a name which prevents confusion with procaine, and in the United States as Dibucaine. The drug is quite different from either cocaine or procaine, and is a quinoline derivative—butyloxycinchoninic acid diethyl ethylene diamide. It is readily soluble in water and solutions may be boiled repeatedly for sterilization. It is very readily decomposed by alkali, and for this reason traces of hydrochloric acid are added to solutions which are to be stored. For the same reason Nupercaine must always be kept in alkali-free glass containers, and all syringes and needles used for injection of the solution must be sterilized by boiling in water which is free from bicarbonate. The drug is much more toxic than procaine, but this is counterbalanced by the smaller quantities used, for its minimal effective concentration is about one-fortieth that of procaine. In addition, the analgesia it produces lasts for very much longer. Nupercaine has been used for every type of local analgesia, but has been found to be most effective for surface and spinal analgesia.

Lignocaine Hydrochloride

Since its introduction into clinical practice in 1944 this compound has proved itself as a very effective local analgesic and has replaced procaine (and indeed most other compounds) in every field where local analgesia is used. It is also known as Lidocaine (U.S.P.), Duncaine, Xylocaine, Xylotox and

Versicaine. Chemically, lignocaine is diethylaminoacetyl-2,6-xylidine hydrochloride and as it is not an ester it is unaffected by pseudocholinesterase (procainesterase). It is extremely stable in solution and can be boiled with strong acids or alkalis for several hours without decomposing. This extraordinary stability places the compound in a class by itself, for solutions can be stored and resterilized almost indefinitely, without fear of toxic changes or loss of potency. Clinical experience has shown that lignocaine has a far shorter period of onset, a more intense action, and a longer duration of action than procaine. Spread through the tissues is much greater with lignocaine than with procaine, and injections made in the neighbourhood of a nerve trunk penetrate more effectively. This facility for tissue penetration has some important practical applications. It is unnecessary to add hyaluronidase to solutions of lignocaine for infiltration or nerve blocking purposes (as is often recommended with other agents) since the inherent spreading power of this agent is already adequate. Probably as another result of its tissue penetrating properties, lignocaine also has marked local analgesic activity when applied to the surface of mucous membranes or the cornea. Its activity on mucous membranes is similar to that of cocaine, while on the cornea a 4% solution of lignocaine is approximately equivalent to a 2% solution of cocaine.

Lignocaine is one of the few local analgesics which do not cause appreciable tissue damage or irritation. Concentrations as high as 8% cause no reaction whatever when applied to the cornea of a rabbit, and apparent tissue reaction after clinical use has not been reported. No proved case of allergy or hypersensitivity to the drug has yet been encountered.

It has been observed that moderate to large doses of lignocaine, such as may be administered in the course of major operations performed under infiltration analgesia, produce appreciable sedation and some general analgesia. At doses only slightly greater than those which produce sedation and general analgesia, however, the most notable central actions of lignocaine are respiratory depression and convulsions—the characteristic toxic effects seen after an overdose of almost all local analgesic drugs.

Lignocaine resembles procaine and procaine amide in having a regularizing action on cardiac arrhythmias. In large doses, lignocaine produces bradycardia and hypotension. A fall in blood pressure is one of the signs of clinical overdose. Lignocaine, in contrast to procaine, has no dilator effect on either arteries or veins.

The drug is rapidly absorbed from tissues and mucous surfaces. In dogs, after subcutaneous or intramuscular injection, the concentration of lignocaine in the blood reaches a maximum in about 30 minutes. The addition of adrenaline to the injected solution approximately doubles the time required for complete absorption. Ten per cent or less of an injected dose of lignocaine is excreted unchanged in the urine and the metabolism of lignocaine has, therefore, been the subject of much investigation, but its exact pathway has yet to be established. Liver is the only tissue which has been shown to metabolize lignocaine in significant quantities.

The toxic effects of lignocaine, in their usual order of appearance are:

1. Drowsiness.
2. Twitching and respiratory depression.
3. Convulsions and hypotension.

The appearance of toxic effects from lignocaine depends upon the concentration of the drug in the blood at any one time. It is clear, therefore, that the total amount of lignocaine injected is not the only significant factor; perhaps of equal importance is the rate of absorption from the site of injection. Both of these factors must always be borne in mind when lignocaine is used.

Dosage

The approximate maximum dose by infiltration is said to be:

Horses and cattle	6·0 g	equivalent to 300 ml of a 2% solution.
Dogs	0·6 g	equivalent to 30 ml of a 2% solution.

Mepivacaine Hydrochloride

This compound (Carbocaine) closely resembles lignocaine hydrochloride but is slightly less toxic. Dogs given intravenous injections of 29 mg/kg over a 20 minutes period convulse, and the convulsions are followed by sedation (Henn and Brattsand, 1966).

Bupivacaine Hydrochloride

Bupivacaine (Marcain) is 1-butyl-2', 6'pipecoloxylidide hydrochloride, a remarkably stable compound which is resistant to boiling with strong acid or alkali and shows no change on repeated autoclaving. It possesses, in greater or lesser degree, the general properties of a local analgesic drug.

The local analgesic effect of bupivacaine is similar in rate of onset and depth to that of lignocaine and mepivacaine, but is of much longer duration. The addition of adrenaline in low concentration has been shown to increase both the speed of onset and the duration of analgesia so that all solutions of bupivacaine available for clinical use contain adrenaline.

Bupivacaine is approximately four times as potent as lignocaine; hence a 0·5% solution is equivalent in nerve blocking activity to a 2% solution of lignocaine. It is generally agreed that bupivacaine provides a period of analgesia at least twice as long as that of lignocaine, and that it is exceptionally well tolerated by all tissues.

There are, as yet, few reports of the use of bupivacaine in veterinary anaesthesia, but it would seem to be indicated for use in situations where prolonged analgesia is required (e.g. for the relief of pain in equine acute laminitis).

Methods of Producing Local Analgesia

1. Surface Analgesia

Agents which cause freezing of the superficial layers of the skin are sometimes used for analgesia. Ice is the simplest, but generally volatile substances which cause freezing by their rapid volatilization from the surface of the skin are used. Ethyl chloride spray, ether spray and carbonic acid snow are examples. Their action is very superficial and transient, and their use is limited to the simplest forms of surgical interference, such as the incision of small superficial abscesses. Used too freely, they may cause considerable necrosis. In man, the thawing out after their use is known to be painful. Decicaine and lignocaine are sometimes incorporated in ointments and applied with friction to the skin. Some slight absorption occurs producing a local numbing which is useful for the relief of pruritis. Aqueous solutions of 2% lignocaine or 4% procaine may be applied topically for the relief of pain from superficial abraded or eczematous areas. The application is made by soaking a piece of absorbent wool or gauze in the solution and placing it on the affected area for about 5 minutes.

For analgesia of the mucous membrane of the glans penis and the vulva, solutions of cocaine or lignocaine may be applied in a similar manner. However, perhaps the most satisfactory agent to use on the glans penis and vulva is the preparation of lignocaine made for use in the urethra—a sterile carboxymethylcellulose gel containing 2% of the analgesic agent. (This gel possesses very good lubricating properties and is an excellent lubricant for urethral catheters.)

For procedures in the nasal chambers of the horse, or the transnasal passage of a stomach tube in dogs, spraying with a 4% solution of lignocaine or a 2% solution of cocaine provides satisfactory analgesia. In ophthalmic surgery 2% cocaine produces about the same degree of corneal analgesia as 4% lignocaine. This concentration of lignocaine is quite safe in the eye—it has no irritant effect and, unlike cocaine, lignocaine does not cause dilatation of the pupil or vasoconstriction. Perhaps the agent of choice for topical analgesia of the cornea, however, is a comparatively recently introduced compound, proxymetacaine hydrochloride (2-diethylaminoethyl-3-amino-4-propoxy-benzoate hydrochloride), known by the trade name of Ophthaine. The commercial preparation is a 0·5% solution which contains 2·45% glycerin as a stabilizer, and 0·2% chlorobutanol together with 1:10 000 benzalkonium chloride as preservatives. Using a single drop of this solution, the onset of corneal analgesia occurs in about 15 seconds and persists for about 15 minutes. This compound does not produce pupillary dilatation and is non-irritant, but its solution is rather unstable, having a shelf-life of only 12 months. Its use in animals has been described by Formston (1964).

Intrasynovial Analgesia

Surface analgesia is also employed for the relief of pain arising from pathological processes involving joints and tendon sheaths. A solution of local analgesic (lignocaine or procaine) is injected into the synovial cavity and then dispersed throughout the cavity by manipulation of the limb. If the synovial cavity is distended with fluid, it is first drained to ensure that the injected solution is not excessively diluted. Analgesia develops within 5 to 10 minutes after injection and persists for about 1 hour. The injection tenders the synovial membrane insensitive but it is not known whether the nerve endings in the underlying structures are affected.

The use of intra-articular injections of local analgesics in connection with the diagnosis of lameness was first introduced by Forssell at the Royal Veterinary College, Stockholm, in 1921, and his techniques, with only slight modifications, are still in use today. Clearly, almost every joint and tendon sheath in the body can be treated in this way (Westhues and Fritsch, 1960), but only the more important injections will be described in this book.

The pedal joint of the horse (coffin joint). A needle 7 to 10 cm long is inserted about 2 cm above the coronary band and 2 cm away from the midline, and directed onwards in a medial direction to contact the second phalangeal bone. It is run downwards over the surface of this bone until synovial fluid flows from it (Fig. 12). About 10 ml of solution are injected and the horse is then walked to distribute the injected fluid throughout the joint. By diffusion the synovial membrane around the navicular bone is also affected. The horse's foot should be held off the ground while the needle is being inserted in order to facilitate entry into the joint.

The proximal interphalangeal joint of the horse (pastern joint). By palpation the position of the medial and lateral collateral ligaments at their attachment to the first phalanx is located. The joint can be entered through the midpoint of an imaginary line drawn about 1 cm below these two points. The needle is inserted through the skin about 2 cm away from the midline and directed towards the midpoint of the imaginary line until synovial fluid is released (Fig. 12).

The metacarpo-phalangeal joint of the horse (fetlock joint). This joint is entered in the triangular space formed by the third metacarpal bone, the proximal sesamoid bone and the suspensory ligament (Fig. 12). This injection is made while the horse is standing on the limb.

The carpal joint of the horse. Only the proximal and middle joints need be injected since the distal joint communicates with the middle one between the third and fourth carpal bones (magnum and unciform). Both joint cavities can easily be palpated when the limb is flexed and the technique for injection is simple.

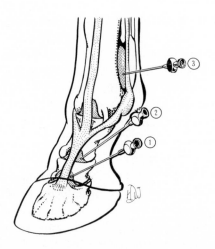

FIG. 12.—(1) Injection into the pedal (coffin) joint. (2) Injection into the pastern joint. (3) Injection into the fetlock joint.

The elbow joint of the horse. This joint is entered either in front of, or behind its lateral ligament. This ligament can easily be palpated as a tense, cord-like structure about 1 cm in diameter. The needle should be introduced in front of this ligament just under the easily palpated lateral condyle of the humerus and advanced obliquely and inwards along the bone until synovial fluid appears at the hub of the needle. The injection of 10 to 20 ml of local analgesic solution can then be made directly into the joint cavity. If the needle is introduced behind the lateral ligament, the solution is injected into the communicating bursa under the lateral flexor of the carpus (Fig. 13).

The shoulder joint of the horse. Entry into this joint is made between the anterior and posterior parts of the lateral tuberosity of the humerus (Fig. 13). The needle is directed backwards and inwards in a horizontal plane until synovial fluid appears at the hub of the needle. The tendon of the infraspinatus muscle can be palpated running just behind the site where the needle is introduced.

The tibio-tarsal joint of the horse. The best site for puncture of this joint

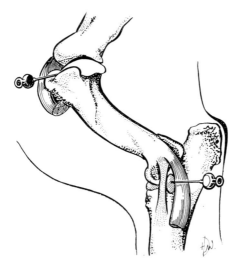

FIG. 13.—Injection into the elbow and shoulder joints. Illustration of the lateral aspects of the limb.

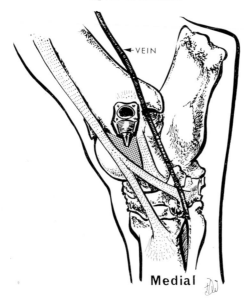

FIG. 14.—The approach to the tibio-tarsal joint of the horse.

capsule is located between the extensor tendons and the medial ligament of the joint, but care must be taken to avoid the vein (Fig. 14).

The stifle joint of the horse. This joint has three synovial sacs, one at the femoro-patellar articulation and two, one medial and one lateral, for the femoro-tibial articulation. The femoro-patellar joint capsule can be entered on either side of the middle ligament of the patella (Fig. 15). The medial joint sac is entered just behind the medial patellar ligament and just above the tibia (Fig. 15). The lateral sac is approached from between the lateral femoro-tibial ligament and the common tendon of the long digital extensor and the

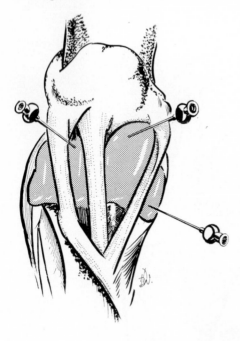

FIG. 15.—Injection of the stifle joint. The two upper needles illustrate the approaches to the femoro-patellar joint capsule, and the lower needle the approach to the medial sac of the femoro-tibial articulation.

FIG. 16.—The approach to the lateral sac of the femoro-tibial joint between the lateral femoro-tibial ligament and the common tendon of the long digital extensor and the peroneus tertius.

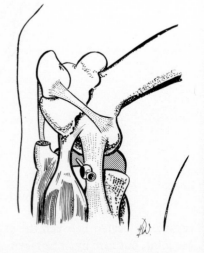

peroneus tertius. The needle should be inserted just above the margin of the lateral condyle of the tibia behind the groove for this tendon (Fig. 16).

Injection into the femoro-patellar joint capsule also affects the medial half of the femoro-tibial joint in those animals where these two joint capsules communicate.

The hip joint of the horse. A needle at least 15 cm long and 2 mm in diameter must be used and it is introduced through the notch between the anterior and posterior parts of the great trochanter of the femur (Fig. 17). The skin is incised under infiltration analgesia at the site of introduction of the needle and the needle is run along the neck of the femur until cartilage is touched, or synovial fluid issues from its hub.

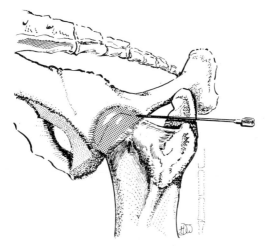

FIG. 17.—The approach to the hip joint in the horse.
The needle is passed between the anterior and posterior parts of the great trochanter.
(This is not an easy technique.)

Intra-articular injections in cattle and dogs. The techniques described for the horse are, with only minor modifications, applicable to cattle and dogs.

Injection into synovial sheaths. A needle can be introduced into synovial sheaths quite easily when they are distended with synovial fluid, but entry into a normal sheath is not easy. When searching for a synovial sheath the exploring needle should be connected to a syringe containing local analgesic solution and a slight pressure maintained on the syringe plunger. As soon as the needle enters the sheath the resistance to injection disappears and some of the solution enters the synovial cavity, lifting its wall away from the underlying tendon.

2. Infiltration Analgesia

By this method the nerve endings are affected at the actual site of operation. Most minor surgical procedures not involving the digits or teats can be performed under infiltration analgesia and the technique is also useful, in

conjunction with light basal narcosis, for major operations in animals which
are bad operative risks. Infiltration should, however, never be carried out
through, or into, infected or inflamed tissues.

Procaine hydrochloride has, for many years, been used for infiltration
analgesia, but the superior spreading power of lignocaine makes it a better
agent for this purpose. Suitable concentrations of lignocaine are 0·2 to 0·5%,
and stronger solutions than 0·5% should never be necessary. It is usual to add
adrenaline (1:400 000 to 1:200 000) to the solution, but this vasoconstrictor
should be omitted when there are circumstances present which may interfere
with healing, e.g. damaged tissue, possible contamination.

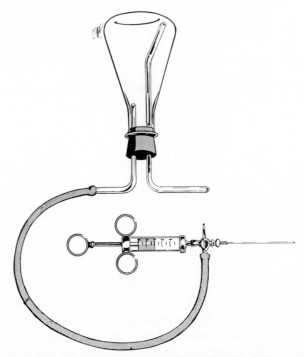

Fig. 18.—Apparatus for infiltration analgesia.

A hypodermic syringe and needle is all the apparatus strictly necessary for
the administration of local infiltration analgesia, but if the technique is to be
employed extensively some more specialized equipment is desirable. A dental
syringe, a 5 ml and a 10 ml hypodermic syringe and an apparatus which
enables the hypodermic syringes to be refilled rapidly (Fig. 18) enable the
infiltration to be performed quickly and efficiently. The dental syringe
introduced by R. B. Waite Company (Fig. 19) will be found to be useful for
simple skin infiltration. It comprises a metal case with a plunger into which
fits a glass 'cartridge' containing 2 ml of the local analgesic solution. The

ends of the cartridge are sealed by rubber bungs. The needle, which is of the fine dental type, is pointed at both ends and fitted with a metal collar about the middle. When assembling the syringe, the posterior pointed end of the needle penetrates the rubber bung and so enters the solution. The plunger of the syringe abuts on the bung at the other end of the cartridge which acts as a piston. Adaptors are supplied which hold the needle in position on the syringe and expose 1·0 or 2·0 cm of the shaft from the point.

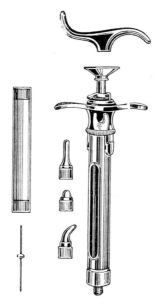

Fig. 19.—Waites' dental syringe, with adaptors, needle and cartridge of local analgesic solution.

The case, adaptor and needles are sterilized by boiling and the cartridges are sterilized by immersion in a disinfectant for the requisite period of time (e.g. at least 2 minutes in a 0·5% solution of chlorhexidine in 70% alcohol).

This syringe has many features which make it useful in veterinary practice. A new cartridge of sterile local analgesic solution is used for each case; if the syringe is allowed to fall, only a broken needle and cartridge results. The short, fine needle is ideal for skin infiltration since there appears to be little or no pain associated with its insertion through the skin, and considerable pressure can be applied to the plunger, which has a handle to fit the palm of the hand. There is no loss of solution due to an ill-fitting needle.

Technique of Local Infiltration

The limits of the area to be infiltrated are conveniently defined and marked for subsequent recognition by the use of intra-dermal weals. To produce an intra-dermal weal a short needle is held almost parallel to the skin surface with the bevel of its point uppermost away from the skin. The needle is thrust into the skin until the bevel is no longer visible and by exerting considerable pressure on the plunger of the syringe 0·5 to 1 ml of local analgesic solution is injected. The resulting weal is insensitive as soon as it is formed and if punctures are repeatedly made at the periphery of such weals, a continuous wheal can be produced along the proposed line of incision without the animal feeling more than the initial needle prick. Such intra-dermal infiltration is only easily performed in thin-skinned animals; in horses and cattle it is usual to simply mark the proposed line of infiltration by raising a weal at either end of the line.

Subcutaneous tissues are infiltrated by introducing a needle through the skin at the site of an intra-dermal weal. For infiltration of a straight line incision a needle about 10 cm long is introduced almost parallel to the skin surface and pushed through the subcutaneous tissue along the proposed line. Before injecting any local analgesic solution, aspiration is attempted to ascertain that the needle point has not entered a blood vessel. If blood is aspirated back into the syringe, the needle is slightly withdrawn and re-inserted in a slightly different direction. If no blood is aspirated, injection of the local analgesic is carried out as the needle is slowly withdrawn so that a stream of solution is deposited subcutaneously. About 1 ml of solution is required for every centimetre of incision. If the proposed incision is longer than the needle it may be infiltrated from its middle through one puncture site, the needle being introduced first in one direction and then in the opposite direction. Very long incisions will necessitate more than one puncture, but the needle may be reinserted through the extremity of an area which has already been infiltrated so that the animal only suffers the sensation of one needle puncture. Care should be taken to infiltrate an adequate area at the outset, so that there is no necessity for further infiltration as operation proceeds. It is always better to overdo local infiltration than to apply it inadequately and to use more of a dilute, rather than less of a concentrated, solution of local analgesic.

To infiltrate several layers of tissue, the procedure is to inject, from one puncture site, first the subcutaneous tissue and then, in succession by further advancing the needle, the deeper tissues.

Field Block

Field block consists of making walls of analgesia enclosing the operation field. It is accomplished by making fanwise injections in certain planes of the body so as to soak all the nerves which cross these planes on their way to the operation field, but no attempt is made to pick out the nerves individually. Usually the entire thickness of the soft tissues in which the nerves run is involved. Generally, walls of analgesia are created obliquely to the skin surface, involving only part of the tissues around the region, but meeting below so that the operation area is held in a sort of cup of infiltrated tissue (Fig. 20). If a vasoconstrictor is incorporated in the solution of local analgesic the principal advantages of field block are:

(a) Absence of distortion of the anatomical features in the line of incision.
(b) Ischaemia of the tissues within the blocked area.
(c) Muscular relaxation.
(d) Absence of interference with the healing of the wound which is often claimed to be the chief objection to direct local infiltration analgesia.

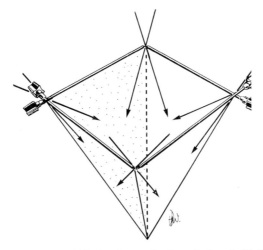

FIG. 20.—Technique of field block—the production of a 'cup' of infiltrated tissues.

The field block most commonly used in veterinary practice is probably that for rumenotomy and this block differs from the type of field block described above. Because of the course and distribution of the nerves supplying the operation site (see page 85) it can be accomplished by two linear infiltrations of the whole thickness of the body wall, one anterior to, and one above, the line of incision (Fig. 21). Up to 200 ml of local analgesic solution may be required for this block.

Ring block of an extremity is another special type of field block in which a transverse plane through the whole extremity is infiltrated with local analgesic solution and particular attention is given to the sites of large nerve trunks. The technique is more effective when the injection is made distal to a tourniquet. It is a type of block which is particularly useful for amputation of digits in cattle and it may also be used for operations on cow's teats. Vasoconstrictors should not be added to solutions used to produce ring block in teats, for prolonged vasoconstriction may result in ischaemic necrosis of the end of the teat.

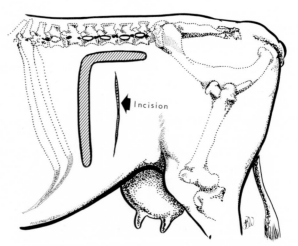

FIG. 21.—The L-block in cattle for operations through the flank.

3. Regional Analgesia

Regional analgesia is brought about by blocking conduction in the sensory nerve or nerves innervating the region where an operation is to be performed. The operative field itself is not touched while its sensitivity is being abolished and good analgesia results from the use of small quantities of local analgesic solution. The solution must, however, be brought into the closest possible contact with the nerve which is to be blocked, and special care must be taken to ensure that there is no sheet of fascia between the nerve and the site of deposition of the solution since solutions do not diffuse through fascial sheets. Success in regional analgesia comes only from practice, as does success in other techniques, but clearly it requires a thorough knowledge of the topographical anatomy of the nerves and the sites for injection. Moreover, no description, however long and detailed, or however well illustrated, can ever be more than a poor substitute for demonstration and tuition by an experienced practitioner.

It is quite beyond the scope of this book to give a complete account of all the nerve blocks that can be carried out, but in the following chapters various techniques will be described, arranged more or less on a regional basis. Selection presents difficulty in a book of limited scope and must be rather arbitrary, but two considerations have been borne in mind. First, the methods described are, with one or two exceptions, comparatively easy to carry out and may be attempted without apprehension. Secondly, they are all useful techniques which are suitable for inclusion in a general textbook of anaesthesia.

4. Intravenous Regional Analgesia

In 1908 Bier reported a technique of 'venous anaesthesia' and recorded 134 cases, but his technique seems to have been largely forgotten until it was revived by McK. Holmes (1964) who described its use in 18 men and 12 women. It has since been widely used in many parts of the world and, after modification, it has been employed in canine surgery with gratifying results.

The animal is restrained on its side and its systolic blood pressure measured (see page 22). The appropriate limb is held as high as possible above heart level for 2 to 3 minutes to partially exsanguinate it while a sphygmomanometer cuff is being applied. The cuff is placed around the forearm just above the carpus, or around the tibial region just above the hock, and is quickly inflated to just above the systolic blood pressure. An intravenous injection of 2 to 3 ml of 1% lignocaine is made through a very fine needle into any superficial vein which can be identified distal to the occluding cuff. The lignocaine should not include adrenaline which may impair its diffusion. Some animals show signs of slight discomfort as the injection is made, but the onset of analgesia up to the level of the cuff is rapid. Analgesia lasts as long as the pressure within the cuff is maintained above the animal's systolic pressure. Sensation returns to the foot within a few minutes after deflation of the cuff tourniquet.

In a series of 20 greyhounds, good results were achieved in 17 cases, while in 3, although the operation could be performed satisfactorily, the animal appeared to experience slight discomfort. The tourniquet was in place for 20 to 55 minutes and even during the longest of these operations there was no waning of analgesia. No harmful results were observed to follow the release of lignocaine into the general circulation, but it must be noted that none of the dogs were allowed to stand up for 2 to 3 minutes after removal of the tourniquet.

The major difficulty in the application of this technique in canine surgery is the identification of a suitable superficial vein distal to the occluding cuff. In greyhounds and other thin-skinned dogs this presents no problems, but in thick-skinned dogs it may be necessary to introduce an indwelling needle or catheter (see Chapter 12) before partial exsanguination of the limb.

The method appears to be both safe and simple for operations on the digits of tractable or sedated dogs, especially those unsuitable for general anaesthesia because of a full stomach or intercurrent disease, and the good analgesia and bloodless field produced are appreciated by the surgeon.

5. Local Analgesia of Fractures

A technique which does not fit readily into any system of classification, but which must be mentioned, is that of local analgesia for the relief of pain arising from fractured bones. The injection is made directly into the haematoma at the site of the fracture and deposition of the solution in the correct place is essential for success. The needle should be inserted as far into the haematoma and as near the bone ends as possible. The position of the needle should be verified by aspiration, when blood or blood clot should be drawn into the syringe. Lignocaine hydrochloride (1% solution without adrenaline) is the best agent to use. In small animal patients 2 to 5 ml, and in large animals 10 to 15 ml of solution are required. Analgesia follows 5 to 10 minutes after injection. Scrupulous asepsis must be observed when injecting into a fracture site as the consequences of infection are serious.

This technique is particularly suitable as a first aid measure and in the relief of pain arising from fractured ribs.

REFERENCES

BIER, A. (1908). *Arch. klin. Chir.* **86**, 1007
FORMSTON, C. (1964). *Vet. Rec.* **76**, 384
FORSSELL, G. (1923). *Berl. tierärztl. Wschr.* **171**, 183
HERN, F. and BRATTSAND, R. (1966). *Acta anaesth. Scand.* Suppl. **21**, 9
HOLMES, C. McK. (1963). *Lancet*, **i**, 245.
TAINTER, M. L. WESSINGER, G. D. and LEE, J. W. (1955). *J. Amer. dent. Ass.* **51**, 19
WESTHUES, M. and FRITSCH, R. (1960). *Die Narkose der Tiere*, Vol. 1, 'Lokalanasthesie'.
   Berlin: Paul Parey (Eng. ed. 1964, Edinburgh: Oliver and Boyd)

3

Regional Analgesia about the Head

The Horse

Regional analgesia about the horse's head was first recorded in America by Bemis (1917), who injected the infra-orbital and mandibular nerves for dental analgesia. The method has since been developed by Van den Eickhart, Shrader, Bolz and others.

Infra-orbital Block

Anatomical Considerations

The infra-orbital nerve is the continuation of the maxillary division of the fifth cranial nerve after it crosses the pterygopalatine fossa and enters the infra-orbital canal. The nerve emerges on the face as a flat band about 1 cm broad, through the infra-orbital foramen, where it is partly covered by the levator nasolabialis muscle. It is entirely sensory. During its course along the infra-orbital canal it supplies branches to the upper molar, canine, and incisor teeth on that side, with their alveoli and contiguous gum. The nerves supplying the first and second molars (PM. 1 and 2), the canine and incisors, arise within the canal about 2·5 cm from the infra-orbital foramen and pass forwards in the maxilla and premaxilla to the teeth. The nerves to cheek teeth three to six (PM. 3, M. 1, 2 and 3) pass directly from the parent nerve trunk in the upper parts of the canal (Fig. 22). After emerging from the foramen the nerve supplies sensory fibres to the upper lip and cheek, the nostrils and lower parts of the face.

It may be subjected to perineural injection at the following sites: (1) At its point of emergence from the infra-orbital foramen: the area desensitized will comprise the skin of the lip, nostril and face on that side up to the level of the foramen. (2) Within the canal, via the infra-orbital foramen, when in addition the first and second premolars, the canine and incisor teeth with their alveoli and gum, and the skin as high as the level of the inner canthus of the eye, will be influenced. (3) Within the pterygopalatine fossa at the point the nerve enters the maxillary foramen, in which case, in addition to the structures outlined in (1) and (2), the maxillary cheek teeth three to six will be desensitized.

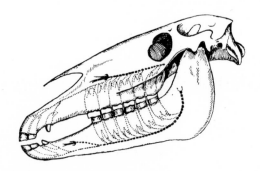

FIG. 22.—Scheme of distribution of dental nerves in the horse.

Technique

Sites 1 and 2: The infra-orbital foramen lies from 9 to 12 cm along an imaginary line running down the face from the inner canthus of the eye parallel with the interior aspect of the nasal bones. Or it may be located at a point 4 to 5 cm along a line passing obliquely forwards and downwards from the anterior end of the facial crest. The lip of the foramen can be detected readily as a bony ridge lying beneath the edge of the flat levator nasolabialis muscle. When it is desired to block the nerve within the canal it is necessary to pass the needle up the canal about 2·5 cm. To do this the needle must be inserted through the skin about 2 cm in front of the foramen after reflecting the edge of the muscle upwards. An insensitive skin weal is an advantage. For the perineural injection a needle 19 gauge, 5 cm long, is suitable. The quantity of local analgesic solution required will vary from 4 to 5 ml. For blocking the nerve at its point of emergence from the canal, the needle is introduced until its point can be felt beneath the bony lip of the foramen.

Site 3: This method was introduced by Bemis, and he describes it as follows: Select a point on the side of the face opposite the lateral canthus of the eye and just inferior to the facial crest, being careful to keep above the transverse facial vessels. Penetrate the skin with the needle (22 gauge, 10 cm long), keeping the point medially and slightly anteriorly, so that it will pass ventral to the border of the zygomatic process and drop into the pterygopalatine fossa just posterior to the maxillary tuberosity. Push in the needle until it strikes the perpendicular portion of the palatine bone in the region of the maxillary foramen at a depth of 6·5 to 7·5 cm, depending on the size of the animal. Following this technique, it is possible to avoid puncture of the vena reflexa, which lies just posterior to the point of injection; 4 to 5 ml of 2% procaine solution are injected, withdrawing the needle slightly as injection proceeds. Loss of sensation should be established after ten to twelve minutes, and should last a further twenty to thirty minutes.

Indications

Injection at Site 1 may be employed for interferences about the lips and nostrils, such as the suturing of wounds, the removal of polypi, etc. Extraction of the canine or incisor teeth is seldom indicated in the horse, and for extraction of molars general anaesthesia is preferred. Injection of the nerve within the pterygopalatine fossa is an uncertain and a possibly dangerous procedure. For trephining the facial sinuses, an indication advanced by German writers for infra-orbital block, local infiltration analgesia is quite efficient.

The Mandibular Nerve
Anatomical Considerations

The alveolar branch of the mandibular division of the fifth cranial nerve enters the mandibular foramen on the medial aspect of the vertical ramus of the mandible under cover of the medial pterygoid muscle. It traverses the mandibular canal, giving off dental and alveolar branches on that side, and emerges from the bone through the mental foramen. From this point it is styled the mental nerve. The nerves supplying the canine and incisor teeth arise from the parent trunk within the canal 3 to 5 cm behind the mental foramen, and pass to the teeth within the bone (Fig. 22).

(a) Mental Block

The mental nerve may be injected as it emerges from the mental foramen and analgesia of the lower lip on that side will ensue. Attempts may be made to pass the needle along a canal a distance of 3 to 5 cm, in which case the canine and incisor teeth will also be desensitized. The operation, however, is difficult to perform, and failure may occur.

Technique. The mental foramen is situated on the lateral aspect of the ramus in the middle of the interdental space. Through the skin locate and deflect upwards the pencil-like tendon of the depressor labii inferioris muscle until the bony lip of the foramen can be felt. The nerve may be detected as a thick strawlike structure emerging from it. From this point the technique is the same as that outlined for the infra-orbital nerve.

Indications. Suturing of wounds of the lower lip; wiring operations about the infra-orbital nerve.

(b) *Mandibular Block*

If the mandibular alveolar nerve is injected at its point of entry into the mandibular canal at the mandibular foramen, practically the whole of the lower jaw and all the teeth and alveoli on that side will become desensitized. The technique of the operation is difficult and uncertain, for the nerve enters the canal high up on the medial aspect of the vertical ramus.

Technique. Bemis describes the injection as follows, but comments that a better technique may be devised later. The mandibular foramen lies practically opposite the point of intersection of a line passing vertically downwards from the lateral canthus of the eye, and one extending backwards from the tables of the mandibular molar teeth. A point is selected on the posterior

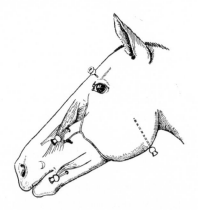

Fig. 23.—Perineural injection of the sensory nerves about the horse's head. Sites for insertion of the needle to block the supra-orbital, infra-orbital, mental and mandibular nerves.

border of the mandible about 3 cm below the temporomandibular articulation. Penetrate the skin with the needle and allow it to lie in the depression between the wing of the atlas and the base of the ear. Depress the point of the needle until it passes deep to the medial border of the ramus. Advance it to the depth and in the direction of the point of intersection of the previously mentioned lines, keeping the point as close as possible to the medial surface of the mandible, but, as the nerve lies medial to the accompanying artery and vein, the needle does not need to follow the bone closely. Following this method the needle should lie parallel with the nerve for a distance of 3 to 4 cm. Distribute 4 to 6 ml of analgesic solution along this length. German writers describe a modification. The approximate position of the foramen is located in the manner described by Bemis, but it is approached from the ventral border of the ramus, just in front of the angle. The point of the needle must penetrate a distance of 10 to 15 cm to reach the foramen (Fig. 23).

The chief indications are molar dental interferences in the lower jaw.

Supra-orbital Nerve Block

Anatomical Considerations

The supra-orbital (frontal) nerve is one of the terminal branches of the ophthalmic division of the fifth cranial nerve. It emerges from the orbit accompanied by the artery through the supra-orbital foramen in the supra-orbital process. It supplies sensory fibres to the upper eyelid and, in part, to the skin of the forehead. The nerve is injected within the supra-orbital foramen.

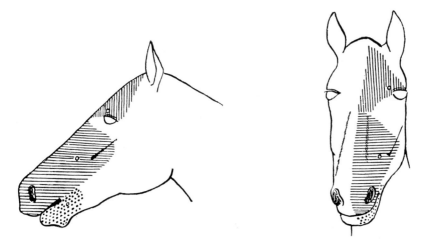

FIG. 24.—*Regional analgesia of the horse's head (after W. Bolz).*
Area of skin desensitization after blocking: (*a*) The infra-orbital nerve within the canal (transverse lines); (*b*) the supra-orbital nerve (vertical lines); (*c*) the mental nerve (spotted).

Technique

The upper and lower borders of the supra-orbital process, close to its junction with the main mass of the frontal bone, are palpated with the fingers. The foramen is recognized as a pit-like depression midway between the two borders. The skin is prepared and an insensitive weal produced. A needle, 19 gauge, 2·5 cm long, is passed into the foramen to a depth of 1·5 to 2 cm and 5 ml of analgesic solution injected (Figs 22, 23 and 24).

Indications

Operations about the upper eyelids; the suturing of wounds.

Retrobulbar Block

To block the nerves behind the eyeball a needle is introduced about 1·5 cm behind the middle of the supra-orbital process and pushed towards the last upper premolar tooth of the opposite side. After penetrating the tough periorbita, 20 to 30 ml of solution are injected. The nerves to the ocular muscles are blocked so that analgesia and paralysis of the eyeball is produced.

Indications

Enucleation of the eyeball.

The Ox

Cornual Nerve Block

This method, which was first developed by Emmerson in America, was introduced to British veterinarians by Browne of Dublin.

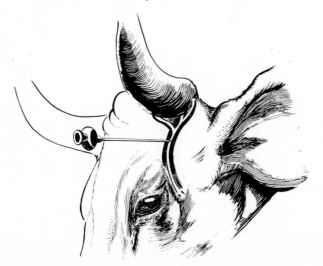

Fig. 25.—*Injection of the nerve to the horn core in the ox.*
In some animals the branch to the posterior part leaves the parent trunk anterior to the normal site for injection.

Anatomical Considerations

The horn corium and the skin around its base derive their sensory nerve supply from a branch of the superior maxillary division of the fifth cranial nerve. It emerges from the orbit, and ascends just behind the lateral ridge of the frontal bone. This latter structure can be readily palpated with the fingers. In the upper third of the ridge the nerve is relatively superficial, being covered by skin and a thin layer of the frontalis muscle only.

Technique

The site for injection is the upper third of the temporal ridge, about 2·5 cm below the base of the horn. The needle (19 gauge, 2·5 cm long) is inserted so that its point lies 0·7 to 1 cm deep, immediately behind the ridge, and 5 ml of local analgesic solution are injected. Browne stresses that the needle shall not be inserted too deeply, otherwise injection will be made beneath the aponeurosis of the temporal muscle and the method will fail. In large animals with well-developed horns, he advises that a second injection be made about 1 cm behind the first to block the posterior division of the nerve (Fig. 25). Loss of sensation develops in from ten to fifteen minutes and lasts about one hour. During recent years this form of nerve block has been widely used in this country for the dishorning of adult cattle. Under conditions of practice, however, the method is not invariably successful. Variability in the curvature of the lateral ridge of the frontal bone makes exact determination of the site of the nerve difficult, while in a struggling animal it may be difficult to ensure that the point of the needle is at the correct depth.

Lignocaine hydrochloride, on account of its great power of diffusion in the tissues, has come to be widely used for dishorning, generally as a 2% solution. While complete success has not been obtained, the degree of failure has been significantly less than with procaine.

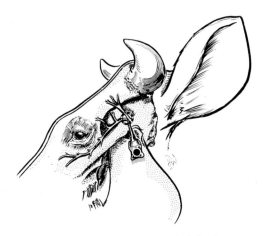

FIG. 26.—Auriculopalpebral block in the ox.

Auriculopalpebral Nerve Block

Anatomical Considerations

The nerve supplies motor fibres to the orbicularis oculi muscle. It runs from the base of the ear along the facial crest, past and below the eye, giving off its branches on the way.

Technique

The needle is inserted in front of the base of the ear at the end of the zygomatic arch and is introduced until its point lies at the dorsal border of the arch. About 10 to 15 ml of solution are injected beneath the fascia at this point (Fig. 26).

Indications

Prevention of eyelid closure during examination of, or interferences on, the eyeball. It does not produce analgesia of the eye or the lids. In conjunction with topical analgesia it is useful for the removal of foreign bodies from the cornea and conjunctival sac.

The Goat

Nerve Block for Dishorning

The sites for producing nerve blocks for the dishorning of goats have been described by Vitums (1954).

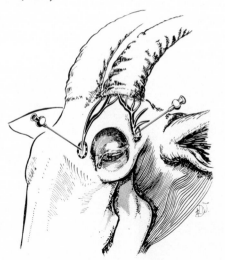

FIG. 27.—Nerve blocks for dishorning of goats.
The cornual branches of both the lacrimal and infratrochlear nerves must be blocked.

Anatomical Considerations

The nerve supply to the horns is provided by the cornual branches of the lacrimal and infratrochlear nerves. The cornual branch of the lacrimal nerve emerges from the orbit behind the root of the supra-orbital process. The nerve, covered by the thin frontalis muscle, divides into several branches, two of which course towards the caudolateral aspect of the base of the horn and supply mainly the lateral and caudal parts of the horn. The main trunk of the infra-trochlear nerve emerges from the orbit dorsomedially and divides into two branches, the dorsal or cornual branch, and the medial or frontal branch. The cornual branch soon divides, one division running towards the dorsal aspect of the base of the horn and ramifying in the dorsal and dorsomedial parts of the horn. The other division courses toward the medial aspect of the base of the horn and gives off branches to the medial and caudomedial parts of the horn. Both divisions are covered in part by the orbicularis and in part by the frontalis muscles.

Technique

The site for producing block of the cornual branch of the lacrimal nerve is behind the root of the supra-orbital process (Fig. 27). The needle should be inserted as close as possible to the caudal ridge of the root of the supra-orbital process to a depth of 1·0 to 1·5 cm.

The site for blocking the cornual branch of the infratrochlear nerve is at the dorsomedial margin of the orbit (Fig. 27). In some animals the nerve is palpable by applying slight pressure and moving the skin over this area. The needle should be inserted as close as possible to the margin of the orbit of a depth of about 0·5 cm.

About 2 to 3 ml of local analgesic solution should be injected at each site.

The Dog

Nerve Blocks for Dental Surgery

Prior to the development of the barbituric acid derivatives as general anaesthetics in the dog, perineural injection of the dental nerves received attention. Amongst those prominent in its study were Frank in America and Hinz in Germany. Today it is only likely to be used in cases in which general anaesthesia presents exceptional risks and only then when combined with sedatives such as morphine or chlorpromazine.

Anatomical Considerations

As in other species, the sensory nerves to the teeth are derived from the maxillary and mandibular branches of the fifth cranial nerve.

The maxillary nerve emerges from the cranium through the foramen rotundum, passes forwards in the pterygopalatine fossa, and is continued in the infra-orbital canal as the infra-orbital nerve. The nerves supplying the first and second molars leave the main trunk before it enters the canal. During its passage in the canal filaments are given off to the four premolars, together with their alveoli and contiguous gum. The nerve supply to the canine and incisor teeth is given off in the canal, and passes forwards in the maxillary and premaxillary bones.

The mandibular nerve passes downwards deep to the medial pterygoid muscle and enters the mandibular canal at the mandibular foramen on the medial aspect of the ramus. While in the canal it supplies fibres to the molar and premolar teeth, and gives off a branch which passes forwards within the ramus to supply the canine and incisors. These nerves are accessible to perineural injection at the following points:

1. *The infra-orbital nerve.* (*a*) In the pterygopalatine fossa at its point of entry into the infra-orbital canal. All the teeth in the upper jaw on that side will be desensitized. (*b*) In the lower part of the infra-orbital canal, injection being made through the infra-orbital foramen. Analgesia of the incisors, canine and first two premolars will develop.

2. *The mandibular nerve.* (*a*) On the medial aspect of the ramus at the mandibular foramen, when all teeth in the lower jaw on that side will be desensitized. (*b*) In the anterior part of the mandibular canal, injection being made through the mental foramen. Loss of sensation in the lower incisors, canine and first two premolars will supervene.

Technique

For complete blocking of the infra-orbital nerve Frank has developed a method of injection into the pterygopalatine fossa similar to that adopted by Bemis in the horse. A point is selected 4 cm below the lateral canthus of the eye (the head being held horizontal), in the space between the posterior border of the malar bone and the anterior border of the coronoid process of the mandible, and after preparation of the skin and the production of an insensitive weal, a needle, 22 gauge, 5 cm long, is inserted directly through the skin into the soft tissues occupying the space until its point has passed the edge of the malar bone. It is then redirected forwards, along an imaginary line that would reach the gingival margin of the upper incisor teeth, until its point reaches the maxillary foramen, at a distance of 2·5 to 4 cm from the point of insertion of the needle. 2 ml of a 2% procaine solution are injected, and the head inclined slightly downwards for several minutes (Fig. 28).

Injection into the lower part of the infra-orbital canal is made through the gum. The upper lip is retracted and the finger pressed against the gum immediately over the third premolar tooth at the line of reflection of the mucous membrane of the cheek. The lip of the intra-orbital foramen will be readily detected. After preparing the gum and making an insensitive weal, a 2·5 cm needle is inserted into the foramen and up the canal for a distance of 1 cm and 1 ml of solution injected (Fig. 28).

For complete blockage of the mandibular nerve, injection must be made at the mandibular foramen. If the finger is passed along the posterior part of the ventral border of the ramus a depression will be felt. The middle of this depression is the point for insertion of the needle. It is introduced at right angles to the ventral border of the jaw, and close against the medial aspect of the bone, for a distance of 1·5 to 2 cm, according to the size of the dog, and 2 ml of solution injected (Fig. 28).

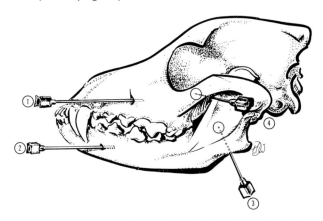

FIG. 28.—Perineural injections of the dental nerves in the dog.

Injection into the anterior part of the mandibular canal through the mental foramen is made through the gum. The foramen is situated immediately beneath the anterior root of the second premolar tooth. At this point there is a 'tied-up' reflection of the mucous membrane of the lip. The foramen cannot be felt with the finger, and a search must be made for it with the point of the needle. Having introduced the needle into the canal about 0·7 cm, 1 ml of solution is injected (Fig. 28).

When perineural injection is effectively performed, analgesia is complete at the end of ten minutes and persists for 20 to 30 minutes. Other than in exceptional circumstances, the dog should be narcotized before attempting the method.

Discussion

Infra-orbital injection at the infra-orbital foramen and mental injection are not difficult to effect, but the area desensitized is limited. Blocking of the maxillary nerve in the pterygopalatine fossa and of the mandibular nerve at the mandibular foramen presents considerable technical difficulties and there is no certainty that the analgesic solution will be introduced directly around the nerve. Moreover, the procedures are not free from risk. The author's conclusion is that in view of the facility with which general anaesthesia can now be induced, and the great advantages which accrue from having an animal unconscious when interfering with its mouth, uncertain procedures such as those just described have little place in surgery in the dog. Nevertheless, it must be recognized that there are still veterinarians who feel that these techniques are of value in frail elderly dogs, and it is for this reason that they are described.

Auriculopalpebral Nerve Block

Anatomical Considerations

The nerve runs behind the mandibular joint at the base of the ear and, after giving off the anterior auricular branch, proceeds as the temporal branch along the upper border of the zygomatic arch towards the orbit. Before reaching the orbit the nerve divides into two branches, which pass medially and laterally to supply the orbicularis oculi muscle.

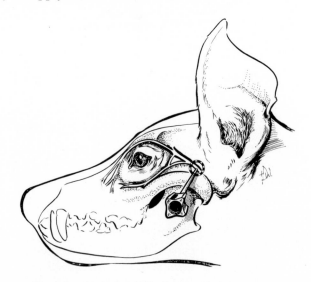

FIG. 29.—Auriculopalpebral nerve block in the dog.

Technique

The needle is introduced through the skin and fascia over the midpoint of the posterior third of the zygomatic arch (just where the arch can be felt sharply inwards) and 1 ml of solution is injected (Fig. 29).

Indications

The blocking of this branch of the facial nerve does not produce any analgesia. By paralysing the orbicularis muscle it facilitates examination of, and operations on, the eyeball. It is of particular value in preventing squeezing of the eyeball after intra-ocular operations.

REFERENCES

BEMIS, H. E. (1917). *Am. vet. J.* **51**, 188
———— GUARD, W. F. and COVAULT, C. H. (1924). *J. Am. vet. med. Ass.* **64**, 413
BOLTZ, W. (1930). *Berl. tierärztl. Wschr.* **46**, 539
BROWNE, T. G. (1938). *Vet. Rec.* **50**, 1336
FRANK, E. R. (1928). *J. Am. vet. med. Ass.* **73**, 233
VAN DEN EICKHART (1921). *Abstr. Am. vet. J.* **59**, 634
VITUMS, A. (1954). *J. Am. vet. med. Ass.* **125**, 294

4

Regional Analgesia of the Limbs

The Horse

Plantar Block

This is one of the most common forms of perineural injection employed in veterinary practice. According to the sites at which injection is made it is classified as high plantar, low plantar, and subcarpal plantar injection. The first is the most important.

Anatomical Considerations

The plantar (metacarpal or volar) nerves are those which confer sensibility to the digit. McFadyean describes the course of the *internal (medial) plantar nerve* of the fore-limb as follows: This is one of the terminal branches of the median nerve. Beginning at a variable point above the carpus, it passes within the carpal arch in close company with the large metacarpal artery, both resting on the side of the deep flexor tendon. Here the nerve crosses beneath the artery, to place itself behind it. Throughout the metacarpal region the same relationship is preserved, the nerve lying immediately behind the artery, in front of which is the internal metacarpal vein. Just above the fetlock the artery sinks in somewhat more deeply than the vein and nerve, and thereby allows these to approach each other. About the middle of the metacarpus it gives off a considerable branch, which winds obliquely downwards and outwards behind the flexor tendons, to join the external plantar nerve an inch or more above the *button* of the splint-bone. At the level of the sesamoid bones the trunk of the nerve divides into three digital branches, which are distinguished as anterior, middle and posterior. The posterior is much the largest. The middle is the smallest and most irregular, and all three branches are in close relationship with the digital vessels. The *anterior branch* descends in front of the vein, distributes cutaneous branches to the front of the digit, and terminates in the coronary cushion. The *middle branch*, which is small and irregular, descends between the artery and vein. It is generally formed by the union of several smaller branches which cross forwards over the artery before uniting, and it terminates in the sensitive laminae and the coronary cushion. The *posterior branch* lies close behind the artery, except at the fetlock, where the nerve is almost superposed to the artery. It accompanies the digital artery into the hoof, and passes with the preplantar branch of that vessel to be distributed to the os pedis and sensitive laminae.

The *external (lateral) plantar nerve* of the fore-limb is formed by the fusion of the termination of the ulnar nerve with one of the terminal branches of the median. These two branches unite at the upper border of the pisiform bone, beneath the middle flexor of the metacarpus (flexor carpi ulnaris). Behind the carpus the nerve inclines downwards and outwards, in the texture of the annular ligament that completes the tarsal sheath. In the metacarpal region it occupies, on the outside of the limb, a position on the flexor tendons analogous to that of the internal plantar nerve on the inside. Unlike the latter nerve, however, it is accompanied by only a single vessel—the external metacarpal vein, which lies in front of it. (Sisson points out that a small artery—lateral volar metacarpal artery—accompanies the nerve and vein from the carpus to the fetlock-joint on the external aspect of the limb.) At the level of the sesamoid bones it divides into three digital branches exactly similar to those of the internal nerve already described.

In the hind-limb plantar nerves result from the bifurcation of the posterior tibial (tibial) nerve when it gains the back of the tarsus. They accompany the perforans tendon in the tarsal sheath, and, diverging from one another, they descend in the metatarsal region, one at each side of the deep flexor tendon. Each is accompanied in the metatarsus by the metatarsal vein of that side, and by a slender artery from the vascular arch at the back of the tarsus. A little below the middle of the metatarsus the inner nerve detaches a considerable branch that winds obliquely downwards and outwards behind the flexor tendons to join the outer nerve above the level of the *button* of the splint-bone. At the fetlock each nerve, coming into relation with the digital vessels, resolves itself into three branches for the supply of the digit. (It will be recalled that in the hind-limb the main artery—the large metatarsal artery—passes downwards on the antero-external aspect of the limb in a groove formed on the outer side of the metatarsus by the junction of the large and outer small metatarsal bones. It passes to the back of the metatarsus by dipping under the free end of the splint-bone, and finally bifurcates above the fetlock, between the two divisions of the suspensory ligament, to form the digital arteries. In the pastern region the disposition of the nerve and vessels is the same as in the fore-limb.)

High Plantar Injection

Technique. The site for injection is from 5 to 7 cm above the fetlock joint. This ensures that the analgesic solution is in contact with the nerve about its point of division. It is located as follows: The groove, bounded anteriorly by the edge of the suspensory ligament and posteriorly by the deep flexor tendon, is detected with the finger. It is in this depression that the nerve and vessels lie, in the order from before backwards, vein, artery, nerve, the artery being more deeply situated than the other two structures. The nerve lies deep

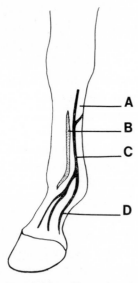

FIG. 30.—*Scheme illustrating the position and distribution of the plantar nerve in the horse.*

(A) Deep digital flexor tendon; (B) suspensory ligament; (C) the site of high plantar injection; (D) the site of low plantar injection.

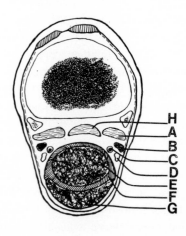

FIG. 31.—*Cross-section of horse's fore-limb in the lower third of the metacarpus.*

(A) Branch of suspensory ligament; (B) digital vein; (C) digital artery; (D) medial plantar nerve; (E) deep flexor tendon; (F) digital synovial sheath; (G) superficial flexor tendon; (H) intersesamoidean ligament.

to the subcutaneous fascia immediately in front of the anterior border of the deep flexor tendon. For thin-skinned horses a 21 gauge needle 1·2 cm long is used, and for heavy animals a slightly longer and stouter one (1·5 cm, 19 gauge). The point of the needle must be perfect. The skin over the site is clipped and cleansed, and a twitch applied to the animal. If it is considered advisable, the opposite fore-limb may be raised, although this is not usually necessary. The operator stoops down, facing the lateral aspect of the limb, and with a single thrust inserts the needle downwards and inwards, at an angle of 15 degrees with the vertical, to its full extent. In the great majority of cases the needle can be inserted without movement on the part of the animal.

With the animal standing on the limb, the skin and subcutaneous fascia are tense, and it is easy to penetrate the latter and thus ensure that the subsequent injection is in direct contact with the nerve. If the limb is held raised during insertion of the needle, the flaccidity of the skin may cause the point to enter the subcutaneous connective tissue and the method will fail. If blood escapes from the needle, it indicates that the vein (or possibly the artery) has been penetrated. The point of the needle was inserted to the correct depth, but its position was slightly wrong. It should be partially withdrawn, redirected a little to the posterior and reinserted. Whenever this accident occurs, it should be ensured that the needle has in fact been withdrawn from the vein by attempting to suck up a little blood into the syringe. The syringe is applied to the needle, and holding the joint between needle and syringe with the fingers of the left hand, the injection is slowly made with the right. The reason for holding the joint is that should the animal move suddenly, the risk of breaking the needle and/or the syringe is reduced. When dealing with coarse-limbed animals it may be decided, first, to provoke an insensitive skin weal, and then pass the needle through this at the appropriate angle until its point lies beneath the fascia. When it is intended to block both sides of the limb supplied by these nerves, the opposite side of the leg is similarly dealt with. When dealing with the medial nerve it is necessary to work 'around' the other fore-leg. With the horse standing squarely, the operator passes one hand around the front of the adjacent leg for inserting the needle, while the other is passed behind the limb for holding the syringe to the needle.

The injections completed, the twitch is removed and the animal allowed to stand quietly for 10 minutes. At the end of this time the limb is tested for sensation by pricking with a pin or needle. Any response to pricking around the coronet and heel indicates failure to block the nerve on that side. One indication of sensation is sufficient to prove this, and successive pricks only serve to agitate the animal. The most likely cause of failure is that the solution was injected into the subcutaneous connective tissue, and not beneath the fascia. Fortunately the skin at the site is now desensitized and a second and deeper injection can be made without restraint.

Dosage. The dose, using a 2% lignocaine hydrochloride solution, varies from 2·5 to 7·5 ml. The average hunter is given 5 ml over each nerve.

In the hind-limb the technique is similar, except that the procedure exposes the operator to a greater risk of injury, especially when dealing with a nervous animal. Thus not only must the animal be twitched, but a fore-limb raised in addition if the operation is to be carried out with the animal standing on the affected limb. It might with advantage be reiterated here that the degree of pain experienced will depend on the needle used, and thus it should be of the finest size compatible with strength, and its surface and point perfect. Should the operator feel indisposed to make the injection with the hind-leg free he may have it raised by an assistant, bearing in mind that he must insert the needle sufficiently deeply to penetrate the fascia. Bolz and Grebe (1932) point out that plantar block in the hind-limb does not give the same results as in the fore. The skin and deeper tissues on the anterior aspect of the hind fetlock and pastern are innervated by terminal branches of the deep peroneal (anterior tibial) nerve. They describe cases of lameness due to ringbone which have persisted after high plantar neurectomy. Fortunately the indications for the method are much less common than in the fore-limb.

An alternative site for injection in both the fore- and hind-limbs is where the nerve courses over the upper part of the fetlock. Although the nerve divides up into three branches at about this point the injection of 5 to 7 ml of analgesic solution still produces a complete plantar block. An advantage of this site is that when the limb is held up and the fetlock joint flexed, the nerves and their associated vessels can be palpated and thus their accurate location is easy.

Indications. 1. *Location of the site of lameness*: Plantar block is an invaluable aid to diagnosis of the site of lameness, particularly of the fore-limb, in those cases in which visual and manipulative examination fail to reveal it, or when doubt exists as to the significance of some obvious lesion. If a horse, previously lame, trots *sound* after bilateral high plantar block, it is irrefutable evidence that the cause of the lameness lies within the area desensitized. In the great majority of cases it is in the foot. Similarly unilateral block may give useful evidence as to whether or not an obvious lesion confined to one side of the foot, such as a tread, a corn or a quarter sandcrack, is the cause of lameness. Again, in cases of bilateral fore-foot lameness, analgesia of the more painful limb serves to demonstrate the existence of lameness in the other.

2. *To relieve pain and allow rest*: Plantar block is a valuable therapeutic measure in the treatment of acutely painful lesions about the foot, for by the relief of pain, of only for an hour or so, the animal experiences much-needed rest. The practice may be repeated daily for a few days in severe cases.

3. *Operative procedures*: Plantar neurectomy may be performed painlessly in either the cast or standing position. Operative procedures about the foot, coronet and heel, such as exposure of a corn or gathered nail-track, partial operations for quittor and sandcrack, are greatly facilitated by the procedure. In fact, most operations about the horse's foot are more conveniently performed with the animal standing.

Accidents and complications. Sudden movement by the animal, while inserting the needle or during injection, may cause the former to break at its junction with the adaptor. The accident is especially liable to occur if an attempt is made to carry out the operation without twitching the animal. A sufficient length of needle may remain exposed for it to be gripped with forceps and withdrawn. Removal will be facilitated by raising the limb, and thus easing the tension on the skin. Should the needle be completely buried, it is necessary to insert another needle into the subcutaneous connective tissue, provoke an insensitive weal, and make an incision 1 cm or so long, directly

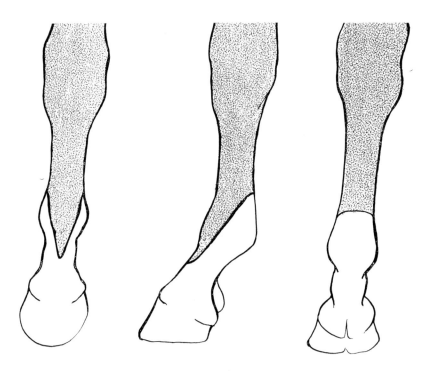

FIG. 32.—Area of skin desensitization (white) after bilateral high plantar block in the horse.

over the broken needle to expose it. The perineural injection is then made beneath the fascia.

The connective tissue of the horse's leg is especially susceptible to irritation, and it is usual for some inflammatory reaction to occur at the site twenty-four hours after perineural injection. Provided that asepsis has been observed, suppuration does not occur. An area around the site becomes diffusely swollen, hot and painful; in fact, an animal may become slightly lame particularly when high concentrations of local analgesic have been employed.

The reaction generally subsides in 48 hours or so without treatment. Should it be severe, it is best treated by kaolin poultice and bandage.

Care should be taken that a horse under the influence of plantar block is not exercised vigorously, for incoordinate movement may result in bone fracture. Cases involving the os pedis and the os suffraginis have been seen.

Low Plantar Injection

The posterior terminal division of the plantar nerve may be subjected to perineural injection in the pastern region. The site for injection is midway between the fetlock-joint and the coronet. The posterior border of the os suffragin is is located, and behind it the tense edge of the (at this point flattened) deep flexor tendon is palpated. The nerve lies immediately in front of the

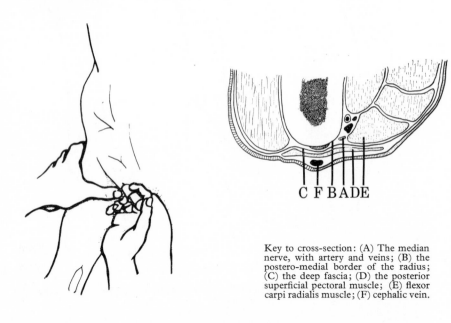

C F B A D E

Key to cross-section: (A) The median nerve, with artery and veins; (B) the postero-medial border of the radius; (C) the deep fascia; (D) the posterior superficial pectoral muscle; (E) flexor carpi radialis muscle; (F) cephalic vein.

FIG. 33.—The medial aspect of the horse's fore-limb, indicating the site for inspection of the needle for perineural injection of the median nerve.

tendon (Fig. 30). The technique of injection is similar to that described for high plantar, and from 2 to 4 ml of solution are injected. The area desensitized is limited to the posterior part of the foot and heel on that side. The indications for the procedure are not numerous, but it may be employed (bilaterally) to reduce the margin of error in the diagnosis of navicular disease. As sensation in the anterior and lateral parts of the foot and pastern remain, lameness due to osteo-arthritic changes about the pastern and pedal joints remains un-influenced.

Subcarpal Plantar Injection

Magee (1936) describes this form of perineural injection for the operation of *firing* the skin over the flexor tendons. 4 ml are injected over each plantar nerve just below the carpus, where the nerve is covered by the carpal sheath, and the fluid gently massaged downwards. 2 ml are also injected subcutaneously at the back of the tendons in line with the other two injections. If analgesia is not complete in fifteen minutes another injection is made over each plantar nerve half-way down the cannon. Fraser adopts a similar technique. Subcarpal block is difficult and uncertain, for the nerves are deeply placed and their exact position is difficult to locate. Moreover, the ulnar nerve supplies a considerable part of the supero-external aspect of the tendon region. It is probable that in the method described above the injections half-way down the cannon serve to block the region below these points, while the three injections higher up are, in fact, local infiltration.

Median Block

The best site at which to inject the median nerve is the one used for the operation of median neurectomy—that is, the point on the inner aspect of the limb about 5 cm below the elbow-joint, where the nerve lies immediately behind the posterior border of the radius and in front of the muscular belly of the internal flexor of the metacarpus, deep to the posterior superficial pectoral muscle and the deep fascia (see Fig. 33).

Location of the Site

With the animal standing squarely, the operator stoops adjacent to and slightly behind the opposite fore-limb. The posterior border of the radius where it meets the lower edge of the posterior superficial pectoral muscle is located. The point for insertion of the needle is immediately above the finger. A needle, 19 gauge, 2·5 to 3 cm long, is suitable. It is directed upwards and inwards at an angle of twenty degrees with the vertical, to ensure penetration of the pectoral muscle and the deep fascia. 7·5 to 10 ml of local analgesic solution are injected. To facilitate insertion of the needle to the proper depth it is best first to induce an insensitive skin weal.

The indications for blocking the median nerve alone are limited, for the surface area desensitized is little more than that obtained with internal high plantar block (see Figs 32 and 34). The chief indication for the procedure is the operation of median neurectomy, and when this is performed in the cast position the technique advised by Share-Jones (1932) is the most certain method of ensuring that the nerve is blocked. One or more skin weals are provoked and an incision of a length appropriate for the completion of the operation is made through the skin and pectoral muscle, exposing the deep fascia. A small incision in the latter is made, and through this the local analgesic solution is injected around the nerve. Ten minutes should elapse before operation is continued.

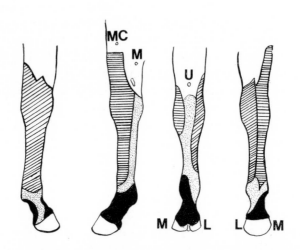

Lateral Medial Posterior Anterior

FIG. 34.—Desensitization of the fore-limb of the horse by perineural injection (after W. Bolz).

(a) Median nerve (black); (b) ulnar nerve (oblique lines); (c) musculocutaneous nerve (transverse lines); and (d) additional area desensitized when the three nerves are blocked simultaneously (spotted).

The Complete Desensitization of the Fore-limb below the Carpus

Bolz has shown that only by the simultaneous block of the median, ulnar and musculocutaneous (cutaneous branch) nerves can the entire manus be desensitized. He has plotted on the limb the area rendered insensitive by the injection of the nerves individually, and also simultaneously. These are well shown in the illustrations accompanying his article (see Fig. 34). In each case 10 ml of local analgesic solution (3 to 6%) are injected.

Sites for Perineural Injection of the Ulnar and Musculocutaneous Nerves

Ulnar. The centre of the posterior aspect of the limb, one hand's breadth above the pisiform bone, in the groove between the tendons of the middle and external flexors of the metacarpus, and beneath the deep fascia (Fig. 35).

Musculocutaneous. The internal aspect of the limb where the nerve lies on the surface of the radius half-way between the elbow and carpus, immediately in front of the cephalic vein.

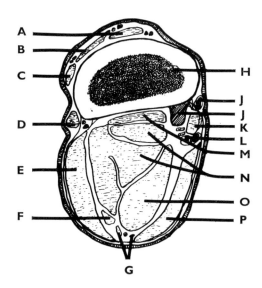

FIG. 35.—Cross-section of horse's fore-limb one hand's breadth above the pisiform bone (after dissections by C. W. Ottaway).

Posterior aspect of the limb, indicating site for injection of the ulnar nerve.

Key: (A) E. carp. rad.; (B) E. carp. obl.; (C) E. pedis; (D) Ext. lateralis; (E) Ulnaris lateralis; (F) F. perforans ulnar hd.; (G) Ulnar nerve and vessels; (H) Radius; (I) Cephalic vein; (J) Supracarpal lig.; (K) F. carpi rad.; (L) Median nerves and vessels; (M) F. perforans radial hd.; (N) F. perforans humeral hd.; (O) F. perforatus; (P) F. carpi uln.

Nerve Block of the Hind-limb

The technique of nerve block of the hind-limb has not been satisfactorily worked out. Bolz has referred to the variable results which follow plantar injection. Westhues and Fritsch (1960) have described techniques for blocking the tibial and peroneal nerves.

Tibial Nerve

Injection is made about 15 cm above the point of the hock, in the groove between the Achilles tendon and the long digital flexor. Palpation of the nerve at this site is facilitated by holding up the foot and slightly flexing the leg. Care must be taken to inject deep to the subcutaneous fascia or only the superficial branch of the nerve will be affected. About 20 ml of local analgesic solution should be injected at this site (Fig. 36).

Peroneal Nerve

The deep branch of this nerve is best blocked in the groove between the tendons of the long and lateral extensors above the lateral malleolus. The needle must be inserted to penetrate the deep fascia and about 10 ml of local analgesic solution injected (Fig. 36).

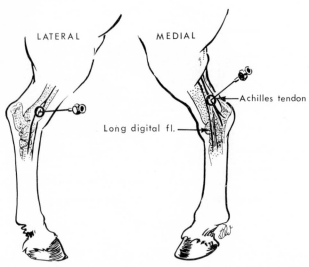

FIG. 36.—Sites for injection about (A) the peroneal nerve, on the lateral aspect, and (B) the tibial nerve, on the medial aspect of the horse's hind-limb.

Block of the tibial nerve above the hock, and of the deep peroneal nerve, desensitizes the posterior metatarsus, the medial and lateral aspects of the fetlock and the whole digit. To produce a complete block distal to the hock, these two nerves must be injected together with the saphenous nerve, the superficial peroneal nerve and the posterior cutaneous nerve (a branch of the tibial nerve).

The Ox

The nerve supply of the digits of the ox is much more complex than in the horse and regional analgesia is more difficult to produce. The skin below the carpus and tarsus is tense and the subcutaneous tissue is very fibrous, so that precise location of nerves is not easy. Many workers consider that simple ring block, in which a transverse plane through the whole extremity is infiltrated, is the most reliable way of producing regional analgesia of the digit. However, block of the individual nerves is more elegant.

An excellent description of the course of the nerves in the fore- and hind-limbs has been given by Taylor (1960):

Nerves of the Fore Foot

The dorsal metacarpal nerve is the continuation of the cutaneous branch of the radial. It runs over the dorso-medial aspect of the metacarpal bone in company with the dorsal metacarpal vein to gain the medial border of the tendon of the extensor *digiti tertii* (medial digital extensor) half-way down the metacarpus. It then crosses the tendon, runs on that of the common extensor and divides into the axial dorsal nerves of the third and fourth digits just above the fetlock. There are anastomoses between these and the axial volar digital nerves.

At about the middle of the metacarpus the dorsal metacarpal nerve gives off a medial branch. This runs in the groove between the bone and the suspensory ligament, over the inside of the fetlock and down as the abaxial dorsal nerve of the third digit.

The dorsal branch of the ulnar nerve completes the innervation of the dorsal aspect. It runs laterally in the groove between the metacarpal bone and the suspensory ligament and continues into the foot as the abaxial dorsal nerve of the fourth digit. It also supplies the lateral dew-claw, i.e. the fifth digit.

On the volar aspect the main parent of the digital nerves is the median. It supplies all of the volar part of the third digit, the axial part of the fourth digit, and contributes to the innervation of the abaxial part of the latter. It runs down the metacarpus somewhat deeply embedded in the local fascia alongside the medial border of the flexor tendons related to the superficial volar metacarpal artery. In the first part of its course it may be deep to the tendons. On reaching the distal third of the metacarpus the nerve divides in a variable manner, typically into medial and lateral branches. These eventually form 3 volar digital nerves and part of a fourth.

The medial branch continues the direction of its parent in the groove between suspensory ligament and flexor tendons. It runs over the sesamoid behind the medial digital vein to become the abaxial volar nerve of the third digit. Just above the fetlock the lateral branch is joined by the volar ramus of the ulnar nerve and then receives a branch from the medial nerve. On reaching the bifurcation of the flexor tendons it divides into the axial volar digital nerves of the third and fourth digits. Before it divides the nerve is related to the volar common digital artery and lies in fat below the strong fibrous plate associated with the dew-claws.

The volar branch of the ulnar nerve runs down laterally in the groove between the suspensory ligament and the flexor tendons. It joins, as already mentioned, the lateral ramus of the median and the abaxial volar nerve of the fourth digit is thus formed.

Nerves of the Hind Foot

On the dorsal aspect the superficial peroneal nerve runs downward on the extensor tendons giving off medial and lateral branches at the middle of the metatarsus though the lateral branch may be given off earlier.

It is accompanied laterally by the dorsal metatarsal vein and at the bifurcation of the long extensor it gives off the axial dorsal nerves of the third and fourth digits. It then turns into the interdigital space to join the deep peroneal nerve and the common trunk so formed divides into two branches that run back and deep to join the axial plantar digital nerves. The deep peroneal nerve runs down in the dorsal metatarsal groove where it is accompanied by the dorsal matetarsal artery. The lateral and medial branches cross obliquely to the respective sides of the metatarsus and enter the grooves between the bone and the edge of the suspensory ligament. They continue over the sesamoids, in front of the digital vein and become the abaxial dorsal nerves of the third and fourth digits. The two branches also supply the dew-claws and give off other nerves that run cutaneously down the digits.

On the plantar aspect the tibial nerve divides into the lateral and medial plantar metatarsal nerves which run down along the respective sides of the flexor tendons. The lateral nerve continues into the foot as the abaxial plantar nerve of the fourth digit. The medial plantar nerve gives off a branch that runs into the foot as abaxial plantar nerve of the third digit and then divides into the axial plantar nerves of the third and fourth digits.

Nerve Block in the Fore-limb

According to Taylor (1960) analgesia may be produced by injection at the sites indicated in Fig. 37. The dorsal metacarpal nerve is located by palpation at about the middle of the metacarpus, medial to the extensor tendon. The dorsal branch of the ulnar is blocked about 5 cm above the fetlock on the lateral aspect of the limb, in the groove between the suspensory ligament and the metacarpal bone. At this point the volar branch of the ulnar nerve may also be blocked, the two nerves being respectively situated in front of, and behind, the suspensory ligament. The axial volar aspect of the digits may be rendered analgesic by a single injection in the midline just above the fetlock. This injection will reach the lateral branch of the median nerve before it divides, or if it has already divided its two branches will still be close to each other. The two branches may also be simultaneously blocked on the midline just below the level of the dew-claws, i.e. after they have passed from below the fibrous plate of the dew-claws. The medial branch of the median nerve is

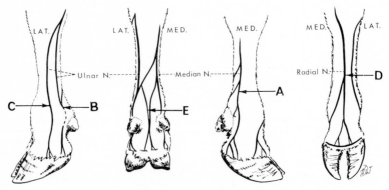

FIG. 37.—*Nerve block in the fore-limb of the ox.*
To block the whole of the digit, injections must be made at A, B, C, D and E. To block the medial digit, inject at A, D and E. To block the lateral digit, inject at points B, C, D and E.

blocked on the inside of the limb in the groove between the suspensory ligament and the flexor tendons about 5 cm above the fetlock. As practically the whole of the volar aspect, and a large part of the lateral aspect of the digits is supplied by the median nerve, the obvious point to make the injection is higher up the limb before the nerve divides. Unfortunately, at this point the nerve lies beneath the artery and vein and is not conveniently situated for injection.

To summarize: to block completely the whole of the digits, injections must be made at points A, B, C, D and E (Fig. 37). To block the medial digit, injections should be made at points A, D and E. To block the lateral digit, inject at points B, C, D and E.

Pincemin (1933) described a technique of six injections about the nerves below the level of the metacarpo-phalangeal articulations to produce analgesia of the claws alone. However, precise location of the sites for injection is not easy at this level.

Nerve Blocks in the Hind-limb

Collin (1963) reviewed the methods available for producing analgesia of the digits of the hind-limb and described a technique very similar to that of

Brown (1956). This technique involves blocking the tibial and external popliteal (common peroneal) nerves above the hock. Among the advantages offered by the technique are the following: only two injections are necessary; the injections are made into soft tissues, at a convenient level—this means that they are easily performed, thin needles may be used and they can be carried out in the standing animal with the very minimum of restraint; the position of the nerves is readily determined by reference to definite and palpable landmarks; there is only moderate interference with the nerve supply to muscles—the leg does not become paralysed and bears weight in an almost normal manner; most of the lower limb is rendered analgesic; the complications which may arise from the insertion of needles into diseased tissues of the digits are avoided.

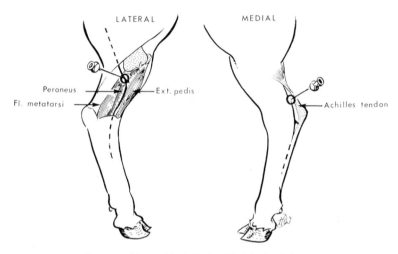

FIG. 38.—Nerve block in the hind-limb of the ox.
Injection of the common peroneal (external popliteal) nerve on the outer aspect of the limb, and of the tibial nerve on the inner aspect.

The peroneal nerve is blocked immediately behind the posterior edge of the lateral condyle of the tibia, over the fibula and before it dips down between the extensor pedis and flexor metatarsi muscles to divide into the deep and superficial peroneal nerves. The bony prominence can easily be palpated in most animals, and in some the nerve itself can be rolled against the bone as it passes superficially, obliquely downwards and forwards, at this point. A narrow gauge needle about 2·5 cm long is inserted through the skin, the subcutaneous tissue and the aponeurotic sheet of the biceps femoris until its point just touches the bony landmark and 20 ml of lignocaine hydrochloride solution are injected through it. Analgesia develops after 5 to 20 minutes. Paralysis of the nerve is shown by a loss of sensation in the exteroceptive area and a paralysis of the extensor muscles of the digit. The signs associated with this motor paralysis are that the animal can walk normally on a level surface but is inclined to stub the toe against obstructions so that the fetlock and phalangeal joints flex as was described by Keown (1956).

The tibial nerve is blocked about 10 to 12 cm above the summit of the os calcis on the medial aspect of the limb, just in front of the Achilles tendon. The Achilles tendon is grasped between the thumb and index finger of one hand while a needle, about 2·5 cm long, is inserted immediately below the thumb until its point can be felt just under the skin by the index finger. About 15 to 20 ml of local analgesic solution are injected at this site and the block takes 5 to 15 minutes to develop.

When both nerves are blocked (Fig. 38), there is complete loss of sensation from the fetlock downwards.

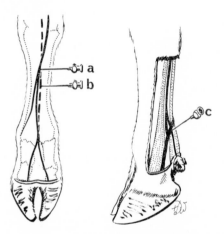

FIG. 39.—Nerve block of the distal part of the hind-limb in the ox. Technique of Raker.

(a) Injection of the superficial peroneal nerve; (b) Injection of the deep peroneal nerve; (c) Injection of the plantar metatarsal nerves.

Alternative Method

An alternative method for desensitization of the hind-limb below the fetlock joint has been described by Raker (1956). The superficial peroneal nerve is blocked in the upper third of the metatarsus where it lies subcutaneously over the midline of the dorsal aspect of the metatarsal bone. The deep peroneal nerve accompanies the dorsal metatarsal vessels in a groove on the anterior aspect of the metatarsal bone under the cover of the extensor tendons. Injection is made about half-way down the metatarsus beneath the extensor tendons. To facilitate this the needle is inserted from the lateral aspect of the bone and its point directed beneath the edge of the tendon. The plantar metatarsal nerves are blocked at the sites so familiar in the horse, i.e. in the depression on the medial and lateral sides of the limb between the suspensory ligament and the flexor tendons some 5 cm above the fetlock joint and deep to the superficial fascia. About 5 ml of local analgesic solution are injected over each nerve (Fig. 39).

Pincemin's technique is also applicable to the hind-limb but, as in the fore-limb, gives no analgesia above the claw itself.

The Dog

Brachial Plexus Block

A technique for the production of brachial plexus block has been described by Nutt (1962) and would appear to be a simple and safe method of attaining regional analgesia of the fore-limb.

With the dog standing on all four legs, the triangular area bounded by the anterior border of the supraspinatus muscle, the chest wall and the dorsal border of the brachiocephalicus muscle, is clipped and prepared for injection. The animal's head is held away from the side to be injected and the depression in the centre of the clipped area is palpated and the first rib is located. A 7·5 cm needle of 1·6 mm bore is inserted into the centre of the depression and guided backwards lateral to the chest wall and medial to the subscapularis muscle until its point is judged to be level with the spine of the scapula. After aspiration to confirm that the point of the needle does not lie within a blood vessel, 1 to 3 ml of lignocaine hydrochloride, according to the size of the dog, are injected through the needle. Onset of analgesia should be observed in most cases within 10 minutes of injection. There is a gradual loss of motor power, followed by complete relaxation and loss of sensation below and including the elbow-joint as the block develops. It is possible that paraesthesia occurs soon after injection, for some animals chew at the leg.

Certain complications may occur consequent upon this procedure. A major blood vessel may be punctured by the needle and a large haematoma develop as a result of this: the local analgesic solution may be injected intravascularly; the brachial plexus may be damaged, causing neuritis or permanent paralysis; the needle may enter the thorax and admit the entry of air into the pleural cavity; infection may be introduced into the axilla. However, if due care is exercised the technique may be regarded as a relatively safe procedure, of particular value where general anaesthesia is contra-indicated owing to the state of the patient when presented for surgery.

Nutt reports that fat dogs are difficult subjects on which to perform this block and says that some failures may be anticipated in these animals. However, it must be noted that he used very small volumes of a concentrated solution of lignocaine hydrochloride (3%). Tufvesson (1951) records the use of 10 to 15 ml of 2 to 3% procaine hydrochloride solution for this block. If this volume of solution can be injected into a dog's axilla, it would appear that Nutt might have obtained more certain results by the injection of 10 to 15 ml of 1% lignocaine hydrochloride solution containing 1:200 000 adrenaline to delay absorption and diminish the risk of toxic reactions.

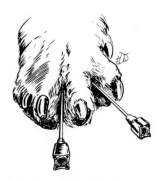

FIG. 40.—Injection of the digital nerves in the dog.

Infiltration of the Digital Nerves

The digital nerves are approached lateral and medial to the first phalanx of the digit to be rendered analgesic. A fine needle is introduced subcutaneously on each side of the digit (Fig. 40) and 2 ml of local analgesic solution are injected on each aspect.

REFERENCES

BOLZ W. and GREBE, W. (1932). *Tierärztl. Rdsch.* **38**, 101 and 119 (*Abs. Vet. Rec.* (1932), **12**, 588)
BROWN, C. W. (1956). Quoted by Arthur, G. H. (1960). *Vet. Rec.*, **82**, 1215
COLLIN, C. W. (1963). *Vet Rec.* **85**, 833
FRASER, A. C. (1940). *Vet. Rec.* **52**, 689
KEOWN, G. G. (1956). *Can. J. comp. Med. Sci.* **20**, 12
MCFADYEAN, J. (1922). *Anatomy of the Horse.* London: Baillière, Tindall & Cox
MAGEE, L. M. (1936). *Vet Rec.* **48**, 1131
NUTT, P. (1962). *Vet. Rec.* **74**, 874
PINCEMIN, Y. (1933). *Rec. med. vet.* **109**, 341
RAKER, C. W. (1956). *J. Am. vet. med. Ass.* **128**, 238
SHARE-JONES, J. T. (1932). *Vet. Rec.* **12**, 587
SISSON, S. (1930). *Anatomy of the Domestic Animals.* Philadelphia & London: W. B. Saunders
TAYLOR, J. A. (1960). *Vet. Rec.* **72**, 1212
TUFVESSON, G. (1951). *Nord. Vet. Med.* **3**, 183
WESTHUES, M. and FRITSCH, R. (1960). *Die Narkose der Tiere.* Vol. 1. Berlin: Paul Parey (Eng. ed. 1964. Edinburgh: Oliver & Boyd)

5

Regional Analgesia about the Trunk

The Ox

Paravertebral Block

By paravertebral block is understood the perineural injection of local analgesic solution about the spinal nerves as they emerge from the vertebral canal through the intervertebral foramina. The method has for some years been employed in human surgery both for operative interferences and as an aid to diagnosis.

Farquharson introduced the method into bovine surgery for the operations of laparotomy and rumenotomy and claimed for it the following advantages over field infiltration: the abdominal wall, including the peritoneum, is completely and uniformly desensitized. Muscular relaxation is produced and intra-abdominal pressure is decreased. The method is simple and safe, and quicker to effect, the post-surgical convalescent period is shorter and of no consequence. There is a saving of local analgesic solution.

Experience has indicated that Farquharson's claims were fully justified provided the technique of injection was exact and it has now become a commonly used method for laparotomies in cattle.

Anatomical and Physiological Considerations

The area of the flank bounded anteriorly by the last rib, posteriorly by the angle of the ilium and superiorly by the lumbar transverse processes, is innervated by the thirteenth dorsal and first and second lumbar nerves. In addition, the third lumbar nerve, although it does not supply the flank, gives off a cutaneous branch which passes obliquely backwards in front of the ilium. Operations involving the ventral aspect of the abdominal wall will require additional desensitization of the dorsal nerves anterior to the thirteenth. The last dorsal and first lumbar intervertebral foramina in the ox are occasionally double. The last dorsal foramen lies immediately posterior to the head of the last rib and on a level with the base of the transverse process of the first lumbar vertebra. The lumbar foramina are large and are situated between the bases of the transverse processes and approximately on the same level. The spinal nerves, after emerging from the foramina, immediately divide into a smaller dorsal and a larger ventral branch. The dorsal branch supplies chiefly the skin

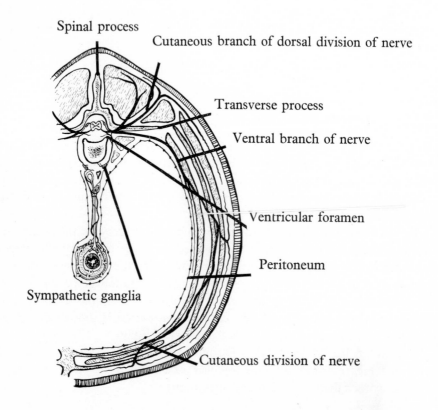

Fig. 41.—Innervation of the abdominal wall in cattle.

and muscles of the loins, but Formston points out that some of its cutaneous branches pass a considerable distance down the flank. The ventral branch passes obliquely downwards and backwards between the muscles and comprises the main nerve supply to the skin, muscles and peritoneum of the flank. The ventral branch is also connected with the sympathetic system by a ramus communicans. Paralysis of the nerves at their point of emergence from the intervertebral foramina will provoke desensitization of the whole depth of the flank wall and complete muscular relaxation. The effects of blocking the sympathetic fibres through the rami communicantes must be complex and require special study, but according to Farquharson the corresponding abdominal viscera are desensitized and intra-abdominal pressure is reduced.

It is obvious from such factors as the deep situation of the nerves and the lack of absolute precision by which 'landmarks' may be detected, that paravertebral block cannot be induced with absolute certainty. Formston considers the secret of success to be an appreciation not only of the depth at which the nerves are situated, but also that they lie beneath the intertransverse ligaments for it is improbable that analgesia will ensue if the solution is injected dorsal to those structures. Fortunately penetration to this depth is not attended by serious risks of injury to subjacent structures, for in the average

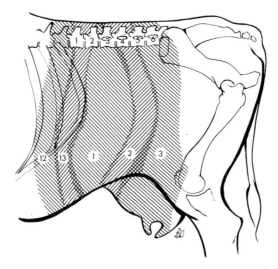

Fig. 42.—Regions of the flank involved after paravertebral block of the respective nerves.

subject the psoas and quadratus muscles are of considerable bulk. It is probable that blocking of the dorsal branch is automatic if the larger, ventral branch is effectively contacted, but if the dorsal branches only are injected, desensitization of the flank will be incomplete.

The number of nerves to be dealt with will depend on the site and extent of the incision to be made. The areas involved by blocking of the respective nerves are illustrated in Fig. 42. It will be seen that for rumenotomy, using the customary incision—parallel with and about 7 cm behind the last rib—analgesia of the thirteenth thoracic and the first lumbar nerves is adequate, whereas for Caesarean section by flank incision it will be necessary to inject the first, second and third lumbar nerves.

Technique

Farquharson locates the sites for injection as follows: By following the last rib with the index finger, the head of the rib can be felt about 5 cm lateral to the midline. This marks the site for the injection of the thirteenth thoracic nerve. To determine the sites for the lumbar nerves, a transverse line is drawn immediately behind the spinous process of the particular vertebra and the needle is inserted at a point on this line 5 cm from the midline. The nerves lie at a depth of about 5 cm.

Adopting Farquharson's method of siting, operators in the United Kingdom have had irregular results and both Formston and Brain have described

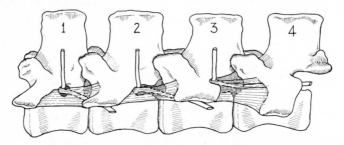

FIG. 43.—The first four lumbar vertebrae of the ox viewed from the left side and showing the positions of the ventral primary divisions of the spinal nerves in relation to the superior spinous processes.

alternative sites. In the Liverpool School the most regular results have attended the method recommended by Neal, which is as follows. For injection of the lumbar nerves the point of skin penetration is some 6 cm lateral to the centre point of the corresponding spinous process. Vertical insertion of the needle at this point causes it to penetrate the intertransverse ligament just behind the posterior edge of the transverse process and it is in this position that the ventral branch of the nerve lies. Should the needle strike the hinder edge of the transverse process it is redirected a little posteriorly (Fig. 43). Location of the position of the thirteenth thoracic nerve is more difficult because the anatomical features relating to the lumbar nerves do not apply. The point selected as being the most certain is 6 cm from the midline opposite the anterior extremity of the first lumbar spinous process. Inserted at this point the needle strikes the anterior edge of the first lumbar transverse process. It is then redirected a little forward and deeper just in front of the process, for it is at this point that the thirteenth thoracic nerve which crosses the costo-transverse space diagonally attains the edge of the first lumbar transverse process.

An insensitive skin weal is first produced, using a short and comparatively fine needle (20 gauge, 3 cm long) and injecting about 3 ml of solution. This serves to counteract spasm of the longissimus dorsi muscle during subsequent insertion of the long needle. After an appropriate pause, an 18 gauge needle, 8 cm long, is inserted directly downwards until its point strikes the transverse process or the intertransverse ligament. After penetration of the ligament 5 to 10 ml of solution are injected. During withdrawal of the needle a further 5 ml are infiltrated along its track. During the final withdrawal of the needle, the skin is pressed downwards to prevent separation of the connective tissue and the aspiration of air through the needle.

Dissections carried out at the Cambridge School (Fig. 44) indicated that a more certain location of the nerves might be obtained by always directing the needle towards the anterior border of the transverse process of the

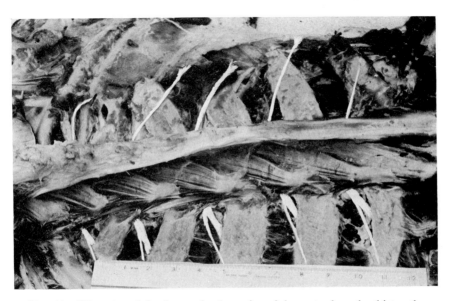

Fig. 44.—Dissection of the thoraco-lumbar spine of the ox to show the thirteenth thoracic and first four lumbar nerves (by courtesy of R. G. Walker).

vertebra behind the nerve to be blocked. For example, to block the first lumbar nerve it appeared that the needle should be directed to strike the anterior border of the process of the second lumbar vertebra about 5 cm from the midline. Moreover, it was noted that at such sites the anterior borders of the transverse processes were usually in the same cross-sectional plane of the body as the most prominent parts of their lateral borders. It seemed, therefore, that palpation of the most prominent part of the lateral border of the process would be of value in locating the site for the insertion of the needle. From these observations a technique was developed which has proved to be satisfactory even in the hands of inexperienced students.

In this technique, to block the thirteenth thoracic and the first, second and third lumbar nerves, skin weals are raised in line with the most obvious parts of the transverse processes of the second, third and fourth lumbar vertebrae, about 5 cm from the midline of the body. Location of the transverse process of the first lumbar vertebra is usually difficult so that in most cases the site for infiltration around the thirteenth thoracic nerve is found by simple measurement. The distance between the skin weals over the second and third lumbar transverse processes is measured and another skin weal is produced at a distance equal to this in front of the anterior weal to mark the site where the needle is to be introduced to strike the anterior border of the first lumbar transverse process. A stout needle (7 cm long, 3 mm bore) is inserted through each skin weal and the underlying longissimus dorsi muscle infiltrated with 2 to 3 ml of local analgesic solution injected through these needles as they are advanced to a depth of about 4 cm from the skin surface. The needles used for the injections around the nerves (10 cm long, 2 mm bore) have 'short-bevel' points so that penetration of the tough intertransverse ligaments can be appreciated as the needle is advanced. These needles are introduced through the holes made in the skin by the stout needles used for infiltration of the longissimus dorsi muscle, and advanced to strike the anterior border of the vertebral processes. Each needle is then redirected forwards over the edge of the process and advanced until it is felt to penetrate the intertransverse ligament. Injection of 15 ml of 2% lignocaine hydrochloride with 1:4,000,000 adrenaline is made immediately below the ligament and a further 5 ml of this solution are injected as the needle is withdrawn to just above the ligament. It is important to ensure that the needles shall be vertical when contact is first made with the anterior border of the processes for, as pointed out by Hickman (1953), if they are not, redirection forwards over the edge of the processes may cause their points to come to lie well away from the course of the nerves. Successful infiltration of the nerves is indicated first by the development of a belt of hyperaemia which causes an appreciable rise in the skin temperature. Full analgesia develops in about 10 minutes and persists for about 90 minutes. When a unilateral block is fully developed it produces a curvature of the spine, the convexity of which is towards the analgesic side.

A method of producing lumbar paravertebral block which utilizes a lateral approach to the nerves has been described by Magda (1949). The skin is clipped and disinfected at the ends of the first, second, third and fourth lumbar transverse processes and about 10 ml of local analgesic solution is injected beneath each transverse process towards the midline. The needle is withdrawn a short distance and redirected first forward and then backward, more analgesic solution being injected along each line of insertion. A total of about 20 ml of solution is used for each site and the last portion of each 20 ml is injected slightly above and posterior to the transverse process to block the dorsolateral branches of the nerves. Cakala (1961) considers this technique to be easier, safer and more satisfactory than that of Farquharson. Delahanty (1960) has also used a technique similar to that of Magda with very satisfactory results. Gianturco (1970) has described a method of blocking the thirteenth thoracic nerve, in which accurate location of the transverse process of the first lumbar vertebra is not required. He blocks the nerve just before it divides (Fig. 41), about 0·5 cm behind the posterior border of the last rib.

It is inevitable that failure or at least partial failure will sometimes attend attempts to inject local analgesic solution in the immediate vicinity of a series of nerve trunks situated at a depth of 5 to 7 cm from the surface of the body, however careful the technique of injection and no matter which method of approach is adopted. Among the factors which reduce the precision of the method are: the nerves traverse the intransverse spaces obliquely; in some animals the nerve roots are double, emerging from double foramina; it is difficult to ensure that the site of injection is the same as that assessed from the body surface; penetration of the muscular mass of the back tends to cause spasmodic contraction of the muscles with consequent modification of the needle track. However, there is no doubt that more regular results have followed the replacement of procaine by 2% solutions of lignocaine hydro-chloride, presumably due to the greater spreading power of lignocaine solutions.

Pudic (Internal Pudendal) Block

While epidural block is a reliable means of provoking exposure of the penis in the bull, it must be acknowledged that the method also has disadvantages, particularly in the heavier individuals. The chief of these is that the volume of the analgesic solution required to cause complete exposure may result in severe interference with the motor power in the hind-limbs, and in order to prevent injury to the limbs and pelvis it becomes necessary to keep the animal cast and restrained for several hours. But prolonged recumbency in a heavy bull, often associated with struggling, may result in injury elsewhere. Radial paralysis, fortunately only of a temporary nature, but alarming while it lasted, has occurred from this cause.

Larson has developed the method of bilateral pudic nerve block to bring about exposure of the bull's penis without causing locomotor impairment. He recorded an experience of 51 trials in 20 bulls, varying in weight from 550 to 1050 kg. The majority of instances were for the purpose of treating the penis and prepuce for *Trichomonas foetus* infection. In 34 cases (66%) exposure and desensitization of the penis were complete, in 15 partial exposure only was obtained but it was adequate for the purpose of carrying out treatment, while in two cases the method failed. No untoward sequelae in relation to the sites of injection or the penis itself are recorded and it is of interest to note that in two of the bulls the method was practised on ten occasions over a period of five months.

Exposure of the glans penis for examination is a frequent requirement of veterinary practice, particularly in cases of inability fully to protrude the organ, for the treatment of injuries and infections and for the removal of neoplasms. Since the publication of Larson's article the method has also been used in the cow in the treatment of prolapsed uterus and to prevent straining in inflamed conditions of the vagina.

Anatomical Considerations

The pudic nerve is made up of fibres arising from the ventral branches of the third and fourth sacral nerves. It passes downwards and backwards on the medial surface of the sacrosciatic ligament where it is in association with the middle haemorrhoidal nerve, to cross the lesser sacrosciatic foramen where it

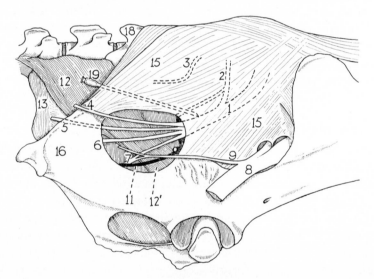

FIG. 45.—*Pudic nerve block in the bull* (after Larson, L. S., *J. Am. vet. med. Ass.*). Lateral view of dissection of pelvis; all muscles are removed to the level of the sacrosciatic ligament. The relation of the pudic nerve to the sacrosciatic ligament and fascia closing all but the extreme anterior part of the lesser sciatic foramen is shown. The needle is shown deep to the sacrosciatic ligament. (For key to numbers see Fig. 46.)

is accompanied by the internal pudic vessels and pass along the floor of the pelvis to the ischial arch supplying motor fibres to the urethra and the erector and retractor muscles of the penis and, with the middle haemorrhoidal nerve, sensory fibres to the skin on either side of the midline from beneath the anus downwards to the scrotum. Between the sacrosciatic ligament and the rectum in the region of surgical approach to the nerve lies the sheet-like coccygeal muscle. The pudic nerve lies between the ligament and the muscle, while the accompanying middle haemorrhoidal nerve lies deep to the muscle, that is between it and the rectal wall. The lesser sacrosciatic foramen is closed by a sheet of fascia which is an extension of the fascia of the coccygeal muscle. Habel has since pointed out that in addition to the pudic and middle haemorrhoidal nerves some fibres which enter into the dorsal nerve of the penis are obtained from a branch of the sciatic nerve which, leaving the parent nerve on the outer aspect of the sacrosciatic ligament, passes into the lesser sacrosciatic foramen and anastomoses with the ventral branch of the pudic nerve where that lies immediately above the internal pudic vessels close to the ventral border of the foramen.

Technique of Injection

The pudic nerve is first located per rectum. The hand is introduced as far

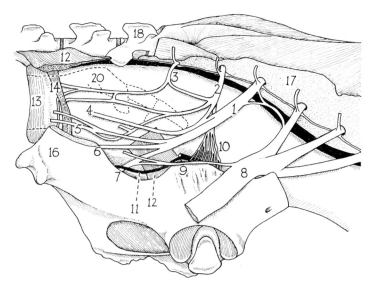

FIG. 46.—*Pudic nerve block in the bull* (after Larson, L. S., *J. Am. vet. med. Ass.*). Lateral view of dissection of pelvis with the sacrosciatic ligament removed showing the distribution of the sacral spinal nerves. The position of the hand palpating the pudic nerve is shown. The sacrum is partially chipped away to show the origin of the sacral spinal nerves.

Key to Figs 45 and 46: (1) Pudic nerve. (2) Middle haemorrhoidal nerve. (3) Caudal haemorrhoidal nerve. (4) (5) Proximal and distal cutaneous branches of pudic nerve. (6) Deep perineal nerve. (7) Nerve becomes dorsal nerve of penis. (8) Sciatic nerve. (9) Branch connecting sciatic nerve with branch of pudic nerve (7). (10) Pelvic nerve. (11) Internal pudic artery. (12) Coccygeus muscle. (Fascia of coccygeus muscle, extending anteriorly to fill in all but extreme anterior part of lesser sciatic foramen.) (13) External anal sphincter. (14) Retractor penis muscle. (15) Sacrosciatic ligament. (16) Tuber ischii. (17) Sacrum. (18) First coccygeal vertebra. (19) Needle in position. (20) Position of hand with fingers palpating pudic nerve.

as the wrist and the fingers directed outwards and downwards to detect the lesser sacrosciatic foramen. Its outline is not clearly identifiable, but its position is recognized by the softness and depressibility of the pelvic wall at this point. Moreover, the internal pudic artery which can readily be detected running along the lateroventral aspect of the pelvic cavity passes out of the pelvis at the anterior part of the foramen. Care should be taken not to introduce the hand too far, for on entering the rectum the foramen lies immediately ventrolateral to the fingers. The nerve can readily be felt, the size of a straw, lying on the sacrosciatic ligament immediately in front of and above the foramen. The pulsation of the artery which lies about a finger's breadth below the nerve will also be felt.

For the introduction of the needle, Larson, after a trial of several sites, selected the one via the ischiorectal fossa as the best. The ischiorectal fossa is the triangular depression bounded ventrally by the ischial tuberosity, laterally by the posterior border of the sacrosciatic ligament (sacrotuberous ligament) and medially by the rectum and tail 'head'. The site of insertion of the needle is at the point of deepest depression of the fossa immediately medial to the ligament and it is directed in a forwards and slightly downwards direction. During the whole procedure a hand is kept in the rectum. When the needle has penetrated to a depth of 5 to 7 cm, it will be felt through the rectal wall and its point is directed to the position of the nerve a little in front of the foramen. Here some 20 to 25 ml of local analgesic solution are injected. A further 10 to 15 ml are injected a little behind and above this point in order to block also the middle haemorrhoidal nerve which may carry some sympathetic fibres to the penis. Habel, in view of the fact that the results following Larson's technique are not always as good as might be expected, suggests from his anatomical experience that a third injection should be made after redirecting the needle a little ventrally just inside the lesser sacrosciatic foramen where the ventral branch of the pudic nerve can be palpated distal to the anastomosis previously referred to.

Larson very properly stresses the need for rigid surgical cleanliness throughout. In order to avoid the possible transfer of bacteria from the skin to the site of the nerve, he first introduces a short, stout needle through a dermal skin weal, to serve as a cannula for the needle which is used for injecting the nerve. He uses his left hand for the rectal palpation of both the right and left nerves and his right for making the injection. The onset of adequate exposure and desensitization for treatment is delayed for a period varying from 30 to 45 minutes after injection.

The method has been used in the Liverpool University School. Location of the pudic nerve was found to be relatively easy in adult bulls but some difficulty was experienced in yearlings. Location of the point of the needle through the rectal wall was not always easy, and it was thought there might be a danger, should the animal move suddenly during the procedure, of penetration of the rectum. The use of the left hand only in the rectum for locating the nerves on both sides and the use of the right hand for the injections was found to be awkward in the case of the left nerve and thus after thorough washing the hands were changed (Fig. 47). After a total injection of 40 ml of 2·25% procaine hydrochloride solution on each side, commencing exposure of the penis was observed after 30 minutes, while by 40 minutes the sigmoid

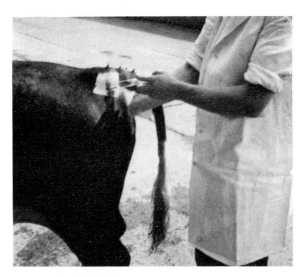

FIG. 47.—Injection of left pudic nerve in a yearling Hereford bull.

flexure was obliterated and interference with the organ provoked no response. The duration of effect was prolonged; in several cases the penis could still be exposed with ease after six hours while in a young bull there was still some relaxation of the retractor muscles after 24 hours.

In so far as Habel's criticism of Larson's method is concerned it is probable, having regard to the considerable volume of solution used in the method, that its dispersion is so widespread that the nerve anastomosis to which he refers is in many instances effectively blocked. In regard to an additional injection of the ventral branch of the nerve the risk of the injection being made into the vein or the artery should not be lost sight of, for the three structures are closely related at the site recommended. It should be mentioned in passing that there are records of central intoxication occurring after pudic injections in the human subject.

This technique of pudic block for provoking exposure of the penis in the bull is more exacting, more cumbersome and probably less certain than that of epidural injection. Nevertheless it overcomes that serious objection of anterior epidural analgesia, namely prolonged recumbency.

Lateral approach. A lateral approach to pudendal nerve block has been described by McFarlane (1963). In this technique one injection is made over the pudendal nerve just as it passes medial to the dorso-anterior quadrant of the lesser sciatic foramen, and a second injection is performed between the posterior haemorrhoidal and pudendal nerves. This latter injection necessitates penetration of the sacrosciatic ligament. The site of insertion of the needle is determined by using the anterior tuberosity of the tuber ischii as a fixed point and the length of the sacro-tuberous ligament as a radius. This distance is used to establish the site on a line drawn parallel to the midline, anterior to the fixed point. After clipping, cleaning and disinfecting, the site is marked by the subcutaneous injection of 2 ml of local analgesic solution. This injection makes subsequent manipulations less painful and renders the subject more amenable to handling. Either hand is then introduced into the rectum and the lesser sciatic foramen located. A 12 cm long, stout needle (1·8 mm bore) is inserted at the skin site and directed towards the middle finger held in the foramen until the point can be felt to lie alongside the nerve. About 10 ml of local analgesic solution are injected at this site. The needle is withdrawn 4 to 5 cm and redirected caudally and dorsally so that it penetrates the sacrosciatic ligament at a point about 2·5 cm above and behind the first site of injection. Five ml of solution are injected at this point, the needle is withdrawn and the sites massaged to spread the solution in the tissues. Similar injections are carried out on the other side of the animal. Using this approach McFarlane produced satisfactory exposure of the penis on 38 of 42 occasions, the 4 failures all occurring early on in the series due to faulty technique.

Local Analgesia for Castration of the Bull

For castration the site of the proposed incision in the scrotum may be rendered analgesic by the subcutaneous infiltration of local analgesic solution but this does not, of course, block the nerve fibres which run in the spermatic cord. These fibres may be blocked by the direct injection of 5 to 10 ml of local analgesic into each cord at the neck of the scrotum, or by injecting 5 to 25 ml (depending on the size of the animal) into the substance of each testicle. In this latter method the analgesic drug is said to pass out from the testicle along the lymph vessels and to block, after diffusion, the nerve fibres present in the cord (Rieger, 1954). The bulk of the drug is carried on in the lymph stream to enter the bloodstream and for this reason excessive dosage must be avoided or intoxication will occur.

For the closed or bloodless (Burdizzo) castration the skin of the neck of the scrotum must be infiltrated by subcutaneous injection and the spermatic cord itself is also infiltrated at the same site. About 10 to 20 ml of 2% lignocaine hydrochloride solution are used on each side.

The Sheep and Goat

Paravertebral Block

In sheep and goats lumbar paravertebral block is carried out using techniques similar to those employed in cattle. In most animals palpation of the transverse processes of the lumbar vertebrae presents no difficulty, and because the nerves lie nearer to the skin surface the injections can be made with greater precision than in cattle. For operations carried out through the flank the thirteenth thoracic and the first three lumbar nerves are blocked. For each of these nerves 5 ml of 1% lignocaine hydrochloride with 1:100,000 adrenaline are injected below the intertransverse ligament and a further 2 ml are injected above the ligament. An increase in the skin temperature due to hyperaemia can be detected very soon after injection and full analgesia is present about 5 minutes later. Analgesia persists for about 60 minutes.

Pudendal Block

A technique for producing pudendal nerve block in sheep has been described by McFarlane (1963). The site for the introduction of the needle is determined by using the anterior tuberosity of the tuber ischii as a fixed point and the length of the sacro-tuberous ligament as a radius. This distance is used to establish the site on a line parallel to the midline, in front of the fixed point. After clipping and skin disinfection a finger is introduced into the rectum and the slit-like lesser sciatic foramen is located on one side (usually about finger depth from the anus). The needle is inserted at the corresponding site and 7 ml of local analgesic solution (e.g. 2% lignocaine hydrochloride with 1:100,000 adrenaline) are injected at the foramen. After massage through the rectal wall to distribute the solution, the other side is injected keeping the same finger in the rectum. Complete analgesia and, in the ram, exposure of the penis follow within about 5 minutes of injection of the second side.

Local Analgesia for Castration

In Great Britain the Protection of Animals (Anaesthetics) Act, 1964 specifies that castration of male sheep over 3 months of age and of male goats over 2 months of age must be carried out under anaesthesia. Although general anaesthesia of short duration can be given for this operation, in practice it is likely that some form of local analgesia will be employed. Intratesticular injection would appear to be the most convenient procedure for use on the farm, although all of the methods described for the bull (page 94) are applicable.

Dosage for intratesticular injection depends on the size and age of the animal concerned and from 2 to 10 ml of local analgesic solution (2% procaine hydrochloride or 1% lignocaine hydrochloride) are injected on each side. The needle is plunged perpendicularly through the tensed scrotal skin into the testicle and the bulk of the dose is injected into the substance of the testicle. The line of the skin incision is infiltrated with the remainder of the dose after the point of the needle has been withdrawn to a subcutaneous position.

The Horse

Analgesia for Castration

Local analgesia for castration of the horse was introduced into Great Britain by Hudson in 1919. The operation was performed in the standing position, and 3 ml of a 5% solution of cocaine hydrochloride were injected into each testicle in the region of the epididymis. Since that time other techniques have been developed and various methods of local analgesia are now widely used throughout the world.

Wright (1952) gave an excellent description of the technique which he has employed since 1929. He operates on yearlings and two-year-olds in the standing position. The animal is placed with its right side against a wall or partition and a twitch is applied to its upper lip. After preparation of the skin of the scrotum, prepuce and inner aspect of the thighs, the operator stands with his left shoulder pressed lightly against the posterior part of the animal's left chest wall. The neck of the scrotum on the right side is gripped with the left hand and the testicle drawn well down until the skin of the scrotum is tense. An assistant, standing in readiness, carries a tray holding three syringes filled with 2% lignocaine hydrochloride or 5% procaine hydrochloride solution. Two of the syringes are fitted with short fine needles (1·2 cm long, 0·7 mm bore) and the third has a long slender needle (4·5 to 6·0 cm long and 0·9 mm bore) attached. Using the syringe as a handle, one of the short needles is thrust through the skin into the subcutaneous connective tissue about the middle of the ventral surface of the testicle, and one-third of the contents of the syringe is injected. It is important that the direction of the needle shall be almost parallel to the skin to ensure that its point lies in the subcutaneous connective tissue, for if it enters the dartos or the substance of the testicle itself, difficulty may be experienced in injecting the solution and, what is more important, the skin does not become analgesic. The animal usually moves as the needle is inserted and the operator must be prepared for this and apply continuous gentle pressure to the syringe to prevent the needle being withdrawn. (If it is necessary to make a series of stabs with the needle before injection is made the animal's resentment may, not unnaturally, become vigorous!) When injection is properly made the skin weal can be seen. The needle is withdrawn. While still holding the testicle, a minute is allowed to elapse for the injection to take effect. The needle is again inserted about 3 cm beyond the first site—that is, through the edge of the original weal—and a second injection made. In the case of big colts a third injection is made by reintroducing the needle through the first weal and directing it upwards and forwards.

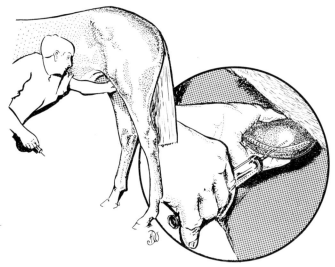

Fig. 48.—Injection into the substance of the testicles after linear infiltration of the scrotal tissues.

In this way an area of skin about 6 cm long and 2 cm wide is rendered analgesic. Care must be taken to ensure that reintroduction of the needle shall always be through skin which has already been desensitized, for colts will not tolerate unlimited needle-pricking of the sensitive scrotal skin. The reason that two 5 ml syringes rather than one 10 ml are used is that they are more easy to manipulate in this somewhat hampered position. The syringe with the long needle is taken up and the needle is thrust through the centre skin weal, through the substance of the testicle and epididymis, into the spermatic cord, and a further 5 ml of solution injected. This procedure is painless. The scrotum and testicle on the other side are then treated in a similar manner. Five minutes are allowed to pass before operation is commenced. Care must be taken to see that the incision is made through the infiltrated area, for by this time it may not be easy to detect. It is for this reason

4

that Wright stresses the importance of complete tension of the testicle in the scrotum and infiltration of the ventral surface of the scrotal sac. Under effective local analgesia the cremaster muscle is paralysed and the tendency for the testicle to be drawn upwards towards the external inguinal ring is overcome.

Using this method Wright has had very satisfactory results but he admits that in a few animals the cord has not been completely desensitized and some crouching and movement has been observed during crushing of the cord. He prefers to operate on mature subjects in the cast position and whenever possible uses chloral hydrate as an adjunct in these animals. The technique of injection of the scrotum and spermatic cord is the same as in the immature subject, and is more easily carried out because the animal is restrained.

German writers have described other methods of rendering the cord analgesic. One is the introduction of a needle through the neck of the scrotum into the vaginal sac. However, it is difficult to penetrate the sac with certainty since the needle tends to pass along the fascia. Another method is to make a small incision through the scrotum into the sac, and through this pass upwards towards the external inguinal ring a long, probe-pointed needle and inject the solution around the spermatic cord. This method, although effective, is only applicable when the animal is cast.

There is some evidence which suggests that intratesticular injection is an effective way of rendering the cord analgesic. Up to 20 ml of local analgesic solution are injected into the substance of the testicle, depending on the size of the animal.

The Pig

Analgesia for Castration

Local analgesia is quite suitable for the castration of male pigs up to about 5 months of age but general anaesthesia is probably more satisfactory for older animals. Intratesticular injection is probably the most practical method of local analgesia. A needle of suitable size is thrust perpendicularly through the tensed scrotal skin and advanced until its point lies in the middle of the testicle. Between 3 and 15 ml, depending on the size of the animal, of 2% lignocaine hydrochloride solution are injected into the testicle and a further 2 to 5 ml are injected subcutaneously beneath the scrotal skin as the needle is withdrawn. Both sides are treated in the same manner. Operation may commence about 5 minutes after completion of the injections.

The Dog

Paravertebral Block

Paravertebral block of the last 3 thoracic and first 4 lumbar nerves affords a useful, safe method of producing relaxation of the abdominal muscles. Used in conjunction with light general anaesthesia it produces excellent operating conditions for the surgeon working within the abdomen. The technique for blocking these nerves has been described by Micheletto (1954) and this technique has been slightly modified by several workers.

To block the eleventh thoracic nerve the twelfth rib is used as a landmark. This rib is traced upwards to the point where it disappears under the lateral border of the longissimus dorsi muscle. A skin weal is made over this point

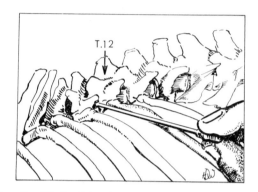

FIG. 49.—Block of the eleventh thoracic nerve in the dog.
The needle is advanced along the anterior border of the twelfth rib towards the body of the eleventh thoracic vertebra.

and through the weal a needle (about 7 cm long, 1 mm bore) is introduced to strike the anterior border of the rib. The needle is advanced carefully, keeping its point in contact with the anterior border of the rib, until its progress is arrested by the eleventh thoracic vertebra (Fig. 49). An injection of 2 ml of 1% lignocaine hydrochloride solution with 1:200,000 adrenaline is made at this point. The twelfth thoracic nerve is blocked in a similar manner, the thirteenth rib being used as the landmark.

To block the thirteenth thoracic nerve a skin weal is raised at the posterior border of the dorsal spine of the twelfth thoracic vertebra, and a needle is introduced through this and directed slightly caudally and laterally to strike the caudal articular process of the vertebra. The needle is then withdrawn slightly and advanced again over this process until it meets the transverse process of the first lumbar vertebra. After withdrawing the needle point about 1 cm, 2 ml of the local analgesic solution are injected. The lumbar nerves are treated in a similar manner, the landmarks sought being the caudal articular processes of the vertebrae immediately in front of the nerves to be blocked (Fig. 50).

For laparotomy, it is necessary to block seven nerves on each side of the

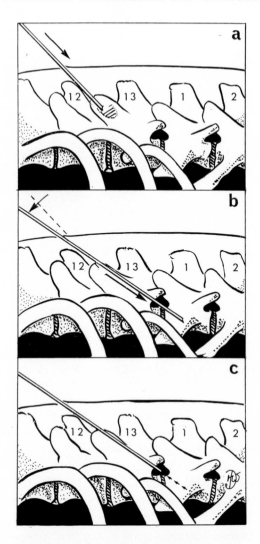

Fig. 50.—Block of the thirteenth thoracic nerve in the dog.
(a) Needle introduced to strike the caudal articular process of the twelfth thoracic vertebra; (b) Needle in contact with the transverse process of the first lumbar vertebra; (c) Needle withdrawn to site of injection.

body and, clearly, this is a time-consuming procedure. However, when combined with light general anaesthesia, it is a technique which is very useful under conditions of general practice, since it produces operating conditions equal to those obtained by the use of muscle relaxants; yet it does not necessitate the intermittent positive pressure ventilation of the lungs which must be employed when relaxants are used

REFERENCES

CAKALA, S. (1961). *Cornell Vet.* **51**, 64
DELAHANTY, S. (1960). Quoted by Cakala (1961) above
FARQUHARSON, J. (1940). *J. Am. vet. med. Ass.* **97**, 54
FORMSTON, C. (1945). Personal communication
GIANTURCO, R. (1970). Personal communication
HABEL, R. E. (1953). *J. Am. vet. Ass.* **128**, 16
HICKMAN, J. (1953). Personal communication
HUDSON, R. (1919). *Vet. Rec.* **32**, 1640, 274
LARSON, L. S. (1953). *J. Am. vet. med. Ass.* **123**, 18
MAGDA, J. J. (1949). *Sov. Vet.* **16**, 96
McFARLANE, L. S. (1963). *J. S. African Vet. Med. Assoc.* **34**, 73
MICHELETTO, B. (1954). *Annali Fac. Med. Vet.* **4**
NEAL, P. (1957). Personal communication
RIEGER, H. (1954). *Berl. Munch. Tierärztl. Wschr.* **67**, 107
WRIGHT, J. G. (1952). *Veterinary Anaesthesia.* 3rd Ed., p. 243. London: Baillière, Tindall & Cox

6

Spinal Analgesia

Spinal analgesia comprises the injection into some part of the spinal canal of a local analgesic solution, which by coming into contact with the spinal nerves temporarily paralyses them and gives rise to loss of sensation in those parts of the body from which the sensory portion of the nerves carries impulses, and motor paralysis of those parts supplied by the motor fibres. The method was first suggested by Corning in 1885, who found that the injection of cocaine solutions into the spinal canal of the dog was followed by paralysis of, and loss of sensation in, the animal's hind-limbs. This observation received very little attention until 1899, when Bier published his observations in the injection of cocaine solutions into the subarachnoid space in man.

Spinal analgesia is divided into two distinct types: (1) Subarachnoid injection in which the needle penetrates the dura mater and the arachnoid mater and the analgesic solution is introduced into the cerebrospinal fluid; (2) epi- (extra-) dural injection, in which the needle enters the spinal canal but does not penetrate the meninges, and the injected solution penetrates along the canal outside the dura mater.

It is the first of these methods which is still most commonly employed in human surgery. In veterinary practice subarachnoid injections were first performed in France by Cuille and Sendrail, who demonstrated the method in the horse, ox and dog, but consequent upon its difficulties and dangers, particularly in the larger species of animal, it has fallen into disuse and has been replaced by epidural injection.

Epidural injection was first demonstrated in the dog by Cathelin in 1901. Progress, however, was slow because of the toxicity of cocaine, but with the introduction of its less toxic synthetic substitutes, attention to the method was renewed. The practical application of epidural analgesia in veterinary surgery was developed in 1925, when Retzgen and others in Berlin employed it in the horse, and in the following year when Benesch of Vienna described its application in cattle using the first coccygeal interspace as the site of injection. The method was introduced into Great Britain by Brook in 1930, and this same worker has since contributed an extensive review of the subject (Brook, 1935).

Anatomical Considerations

The spinal cord is covered by three membranes, the dense dura mater, the arachnoid mater and the delicate pia mater, and lies within the spinal canal. The wall of the spinal canal is formed by the vertebral arches and bodies, the intervertebral discs and the intervertebral ligaments. The tube-like canal is somewhat flattened dorsoventrally and has two enlargements, one in the posterior cervical region, the other in the posterior lumbar region. The spinal cord and dura mater end at the lumbar enlargement and the canal itself tapers off behind this enlargement to end in the fourth or fifth coccygeal vertebra. In each vertebral segment the canal has lateral openings between the vertebral arches, the 'intervertebral foramina', through which pass blood vessels and the spinal nerves.

The Dura Mater

In the cranial cavity the dura mater is arranged in two layers, the 'perio-steal' and 'investing' layers, which are firmly adherent except where they split to enclose venous sinuses. The outer layer forms the periosteum of the inner surface of the cranial bones and in the spine acts as the periosteum lining the vertebral canal. The investing layer is continued from the cranium into the spinal canal but at the foramen magnum is firmly adherent to the margins of the foramen where it blends with the outer or periosteal layer. Between the two layers in the spinal canal is the extra- or epidural space, which anatomically would be better termed the 'interdural' space. Because of the adhesion between the investing layer and the periosteum at the fora-men magnum, solutions deposited correctly in the spinal epidural space cannot enter the cranial cavity or produce nerve block higher than the first cervical nerves.

The dorsal and ventral nerve roots issuing from the spinal cord penetrate the investing later of dura and carry tubular prolongations (dural cuffs, 'ink cuffs') which blend with the perineurium of the mixed spinal nerve.

The Arachnoid Mater

The spinal arachnoid mater is a continuation of the cerebral arachnoid. An incomplete and inconsistent septum divides the spinal subarachnoid space along the midline of the dorsal surface of the cord.

The Pia Mater

In the spinal canal the pia mater is closely applied to the cord and extends into the ventral median fissure. The blood vessels going to the spinal cord lie in the subarachnoid space before piercing the pia mater. They carry with them into the spinal cord a double sleeve of meninges.

The Epidural Space

The formation of the epidural space by the splitting of the two layers of the dura has already been described. The venous plexuses of the spinal canal lie in the epidural space and receive tributaries from the adjacent bony structures and the spinal cord. Although they form a network they can be subdivided into:

(i) a pair of ventral venous plexuses which lie on either side of the posterior longitudinal ligament of the vertebra, into which the basivertebral veins drain;

(ii) a single dorsal venous plexus which connects with the dorsal external veins.

Both (i) and (ii) connect with the intervertebral veins, and, although they are divisible into anatomical groups, all interconnect with one another and form a series of venous rings at the level of each vertebra. The accidental injection of local analgesic solutions into these veins may occur during the performance of an epidural block and be responsible for toxic manifestations.

In addition to the venous plexuses, branches from the vertebral, ascending cervical, deep cervical, intercostal, lumbar and iliolumbar arteries enter the intervertebral foramina and anastomose with one another, chiefly in the lateral parts of the epidural space.

The spaces between the nerves, arteries and veins in the epidural space are filled with fatty tissue the amount of which corresponds with the adiposity of the subject.

The Spinal Nerves

The phenomena which accompany paralysis of the spinal nerves are more complex than is the case with peripheral perineural injection, because of the varying types of fibre which enter into the formation of a spinal nerve. Sensory fibres are paralysed more readily and more rapidly than are motor fibres, while sympathetic fibres are still more susceptible.

Each spinal nerve results from the union of two roots—a dorsal, ganglionic or sensory root and a ventral motor root. In the horse, according to McFadyean, these roots perforate the dura mater separately and converge towards the intervertebral foramina, where they join, immediately external to the point where the dorsal root has the ganglion placed upon it. Sisson states that in the cervical, dorsal and anterior lumbar regions the bundles of both roots pass through separate openings in the dura mater in linear series before uniting into a root proper, but further back the bundles of each root unite within the dura mater. In the dog union is effected within the intervertebral foramina, except in the lumbar and coccygeal regions, where it takes place within the vertebral canal. The point regarding the site of fusion of the two roots is of practical significance—at any rate, in the small animals in which high epidural anaesthesia is often induced. It is the dorsal root which it is desired chiefly to influence, and thus when injecting volumes likely to permeate in front of the anterior lumbar region it is an advantage to place the animal on its back after injection in order to reduce the extent of the complicating factors which result from paralysis of the vasomotor fibres emerging with the ventral root.

Since epidural injection is generally made near the termination of the vertebral canal and the area in which analgesia and motor paralysis supervene will extend progressively forwards according to the quantity of solution injected, the distribution of the spinal nerves should be reviewed from behind forwards (see Table 2).

The Autonomic Nervous System

The phenomena which accompany spinal nerve block are not entirely due to paralysis of sensory and motor nerve fibres, since many of the spinal nerves which may be involved contain fibres of the autonomic nervous system. The autonomic nervous system is merely a convenient designation for a multitude of different types of efferent fibres which transmit impulses from centres in the brain to such structures as the blood vessels and the viscera. If these fibres are cut most of the structures supplied are capable of autonomic activity independent of any central control. The function of these nerve fibres varies according to the site at which they leave the spinal cord. The cranial and sacral outflow, the 'parasympathetic system', is, in general, concerned with vegetative functions such as digestion and excretion, whereas the thoracic and lumbar outflow, the 'sympathetic system', is more closely concerned with protective reflex activity.

The anaesthetist is more concerned with the sympathetic nervous system and there are two cell stations in this system. The first is in the lateral horn of the spinal cord and the second is in one of the sympathetic ganglia which lie outside the cord. The axon which passes from the lateral horn cell to its sympathetic ganglion is termed the 'pre-ganglionic fibre' and that which passes from the ganglion to the structure innervated is termed the 'post-

Table 2

DISTRIBUTION OF THE SENSORY AND MOTOR FIBRES OF THE SPINAL NERVES*

Spinal region	No. of nerve	Structures supplied	
		Sensory	Motor
Coccygeal	All	Greater part of tail	Coccygeal muscles
Sacral	5 and 4	Croup, base of tail; anus, vulva, perineum and adjacent parts	Anus, terminal part of rectum, vagina, penis, bladder, urethra
Sacral	3, 2 and 1	Dorsal branches—sensory to region of croup	
Lumbar	6, 5 and 4	Ventral branches—enter into the formation of the lumbosacral plexus	
Lumbo-sacral plexus	Post. gluteal nerve (1 and 2 S.)	Lateral and posterior parts of hip and thigh	Extensors of hip (in part)
	Great sciatic nerve 5 and 6 L., 1 S.)	Middle of tibial region to foot	Flexors of the stifle (in part); flexors and extensors of hock and digit
	Ant. gluteal nerve (5 and 6 L., 1 S.)	Lateral aspect of thigh	Flexors and abductors of hip
	Obturator nerve (4 and 5 L.)	Medial aspect of thigh	Adductors of hip
	Femoral nerve (4 and 5 L.)	Anterior and mesial aspects of limb as low as hock.	Flexors of hip (in part), extensors of stifle
Lumbar	3	Loins and croup, anterior aspect of stifle, scrotum, prepuce and inguinal region mammary gland	Sublumbar group (in part), post. parts of abdominal muscles
	2	Loins, flank, anterior and lateral aspect of thigh, scrotum, prepuce, mammary gland	Sublumbar group (in part), post. parts of abdominal muscles
	1	Loins, post. abdominal region, lateral aspect of thigh	Post. parts of abdominal muscles
Thoracic	Last two	Abdominal wall and flank	Abdominal muscles
	Mid-thoracic region to last pair	Anterior and ventral parts of abdominal wall	Intercostal muscles, anterior parts of abdominal muscles

* Free use has been made of standard veterinary anatomy and physiology textbooks in the preparation of this section.

ganglionic fibre'. The ganglia are situated on either side of the vertebral column. The fibres from the lateral horn cells at first join with those of the central ramus of the mixed spinal nerve to pass to the periphery. However, very soon after joining they leave the ventral ramus and pass to the ganglia in the white rami communicantes. The white rami are, therefore, connector fibres feeding the ganglia and they may synapse in the first ganglia they encounter, or they may run up or down the sympathetic chain to synapse in some distant ganglion. A few of the fibres do not synapse in these ganglia but pass on into the splanchnic nerves. From the ganglia in the sympathetic chain post-ganglionic fibres run in the grey rami communicantes back to the spinal nerve.

Distinct from the sympathetic nervous system but running with it are afferent fibres from the viscera. These visceral afferent fibres travel with the post-ganglionic fibres, but run in the opposite direction, passing through the ganglia, up the white rami and into the dorsal root of the spinal nerve. Their cell bodies are located in the dorsal root ganglia and an axon passes to a synapse in the lateral horn of the spinal cord. These fibres must not be confused with the post-ganglionic autonomic fibres (vasoconstrictor and vasodilator fibres) which also follow the dorsal root but whose cell bodies have not yet been precisely located.

The post-ganglionic fibres to a limb mainly pass with the spinal nerves to reach the cutaneous blood vessels, and the sweat and sebaceous glands in its distal four-fifths. The proximal one-fifth of the limb in the groin and axilla is supplied by fibres passing directly from the ganglia without joining the spinal nerves. Since the spinal nerve always carries sympathetic fibres, a peripheral nerve block always produces vasodilation in the distal part of the limb.

To the anaesthetist probably the most important components of the sympathetic system are the vasoconstrictor fibres. The largest vasometer nerves in the body are the splanchnic, which pass to the abdominal viscera. The area supplied by them is so great that their paralysis causes a fall in blood pressure. It is probable that this fall is most marked in herbivores, in which the abdominal viscera are large and their blood supply correspondingly great. It will thus be apparent that when the lumbar and thoracic nerves are blocked a marked fall in blood pressure will occur.

Spread of Solutions injected into the Epidural Space

The extent of neural blockade after injection of an analgesic solution into the epidural space is determined by a number of variables. Some of these variables are intrinsic to the animal, and some are extrinsic—variations of technique and drugs employed.

The intrinsic variables governing the spread of solutions in the epidural space are perhaps best understood if the space is considered to be a cylindrical reservoir, the volume of the reservoir being determined by factors such as the length and diameter of the cylinder and the size of the structures which it contains. Draining the reservoir are certain escape channels through which seepage and absorption of injected materials can take place. The rate of disappearance of solutions from the reservoir will depend on the patency and efficiency of the escape routes. The most important of these are the intervertebral foramina and the extradural venous plexuses, and any consideration of the spread of analgesic solutions must take account of any factors which affect these structures. Clearly, the extent of neural blockade will be governed, at least in part, by the speed at which nerves are blocked in relation to the rate with which the analgesic solution is removed from their vicinity. If this removal is fast compared with the speed of block, solutions may be removed so rapidly that there is no chance for them to spread and so produce widespread blockade. On the other hand, if absorption is slow there will be an opportunity for more prolonged contact between solution and nerves, so that the extent and intensity of spread is likely to be greater. The space in the epidural 'reservoir' is taken up by:

(1) Spinal cord and nerves, and cerebrospinal fluid, contained in their meninges.
(2) Fat and blood vessels—including the extradural venous plexuses which adjust alterations in venous pressure throughout the body, and which can undergo considerable distension in so doing (Batson, 1940).

The reservoir's exits through which injected solutions can escape are:

(1) The intervertebral foramina.
(2) The blood vessels and lymphatics which can absorb and remove drugs from the space. These vessels thus have a dual function, acting both as space-occupying structures and as escape routes at the same time.
(3) Possibly the dura mater, which may act as a partially permeable membrane, allowing some passages of solutions and drugs into the cerebrospinal fluid (Frumin, Schwartz, Burns, Brodie and Papper, 1953). The 'ink-cuff' area surrounding the spinal nerve trunks is particularly important in this respect (Brierley and Field, 1949).
(4) Solution and diffusion in the epidural fat.

Solutions which are injected into the epidural space spread up and down within it to an extent determined by these opposing factors. The larger the space-occupying structures, the less space remains to be filled and so the further a given volume will travel. Relatively little spread will take place, on the other hand, if the escape routes are patent and efficient, since solutions will pass out of the epidural space through these exits rather like water through holes in a bucket.

Age has an influence on the spreading of solutions in the epidural space. In young animals the capacity of the space is small, but it increases steadily to a maximum as the animal reaches maturity. In early adult life the size of the space and the patency of the escape routes are both maximal. The neurovascular bundles pass freely through widely patent intervertebral foramina and both venous and lymphatic drainage are maximal with all the adjustments of venous pressure which accompany active or violent behaviour. With advancing years aging process becomes apparent and conditions change. Blood flow becomes less brisk and opercula of fibrous tissue obstruct the intervertebral foramina, and, as the animal becomes more sedentary in habits, major adjustments of venous pressure become less frequent.

The length of the vertebral canal is, of course, an important factor governing the volume of the epidural space. Workers such as Harthoorn and Brass (1954) relate the dosage of local analgesic solution to the occiput–tail root measurement. Gravity also plays a part in the spread of solutions injected into the epidural space (Bromage 1962), although not all workers recognize its effects (Nishimura, Kitahara and Kusakabe, 1959).

Once an initial injection has created a solid area of analgesia, succeeding but much smaller injections given at the same site as the first injection produce an extension of the area of analgesia. This is difficult to understand since on consideration it would seem that the succeeding, smaller injections should be lost through the exits from the epidural space while still contained well within the area of spread of the first injection. However, the fact that these succeeding smaller injections do extend the area of block cannot be denied. A well recognized and commonly used method for exposing the penis in bulls makes use of this phenomenon. An initial injection is given and if, after a wait of 15 to 20 minutes, the penis is not extruded, further increments of 2 to 3 ml are injected into the epidural space at the site of the initial injection until the desired result is obtained. These succeeding injections seem to track along in the wake of the original 'path-finding' dose and pass onwards to extend the neural blockade.

It is well recognized that epidural block has a tendency to spread widely during pregnancy (Tufvesson, 1963), at least at term and when labour has begun. The reasons for this marked decrease in dose requirements at term still remain obscure. According to Bromage (1962) several factors are probably involved. One of the most important is the space-occupying and massaging effects of the distended venous plexuses in the epidural space, causing rhythmic pressure waves which tend to disperse solutions lying around them.

Increased vascularity of the meninges and changes in the cerebrospinal fluid have been invoked as an additional explanation for altered response to epidural injections in pregnancy (Marx, Zermaitis and Orkim, 1961). It is quite possible that changes of this nature may contribute to the enhanced spread, for if the coverings of the nerve roots are more permeable than usual, analgesic solutions will have a greater chance to penetrate the nerves within them.

Brook (1935) quotes the assertion of several practitioners that, in cattle, the concentration of the solution employed affects the extent of the block. Much more recently similar observations have been made in man (Bonica,

Backup, Anderson, Hadfield, Crepps and Monk, 1957; Bromage, 1962). This is difficult to understand. Why, for example, should 2 to 3 ml of 5% procaine injected into the caudal epidural space of a cow block as many segments as 10 to 12 ml of 2·25% procaine? As suggested by Bonica *et al.*, the explanation must be that there is a heightened tissue penetration when the more concentrated solution is employed.

Increased diffusion across the meninges into the cerebrospinal fluid was one of the first possibilities considered by Bromage (1962), but injections into the caudal epidural space in cows will not come into contact with the meninges until they reach the junction of the third and fourth sacral segments. Moreover, the observations of Foldes, Colavincenzo and Birch (1956) also suggest that diffusion across the meninges is unimportant. These workers took samples of cerebrospinal fluid at the onset of analgesia, and then at intervals until the block disappeared. They found that when the block had disappeared, the concentration of the drug in the cerebrospinal fluid was three times as high as when the block was first fully developed. From these results Foldes *et al.* concluded that the site of action of analgesics injected into the epidural space is primarily outside the dura-arachnoid and the spinal canal, involving the mixed nerves in the paravertebral spaces. However, there is strong circumstantial evidence against this conclusion. The volume of solution available for each paravertebral space after epidural injection is too small to account for the prolonged effective block which follows, and studies with radio-opaque materials suggest that the solution never reaches the paravertebral spaces in many instances (Bromage, 1954).

In 1962 Bromage proposed an explanation for one of the main pathways and sites of action of epidural analgesia which appears to reconcile all the clinical and experimental evidence which is available at present. This explanation was suggested by the work of Brierley and Field (Field, 1948; Brierley and Field, 1949; Brierley, 1950) on the passage of viruses into the central nervous system. They showed that the neighbourhood of the dural 'ink-cuffs' where the dorsal and ventral roots fuse is permeable to quite large particles, 0·5 μ in size, and that material can diffuse readily between the subarachnoid, subdural, and epidural spaces in this region. Moreover, they showed that extremely small quantities of radioactive substances, introduced without pressure into the subperineural spaces of the sciatic nerve, could enter the spinal cord, brain stem, and even the basal ganglia, in significant amounts after a short time. On the other hand, passage into the cerebrospinal fluid was slow, and maximum concentrations were not revealed until 50 to 60 minutes after injection (i.e. about the same time that elapsed before maximum concentration of chloroprocaine appeared in the cerebrospinal fluid in the experiments of Foldes *et al.*). The similarity of the time relations in these two series of experiments is very suggestive of an underlying mechanism common to both.

Moore, Hain, Ward and Bridenbaugh (1954) also carried out injection studies, using an oily solution of a local analgesic with methylene blue, on the peripheral nerves of monkeys. They too found very rapid spread from the peripheral nerves into the sub-pial spaces of the spinal cord.

Bromage suggested that this portal of entry into the neuraxis appears to be the key to the problems of unexpected variations in epidural spread. All earlier discussion and tentative explanations about the site of block in epidural analgesia had been dominated by the assumption that passage into the cerebrospinal fluid precedes neural fixation and blockade. Bromage contended that if this assumption is dropped in favour of the idea that passage into the cerebrospinal fluid follows or accompanies neural involvement after subdural and sub-pial spread, then all the available clinical and experimental findings fall into place. Analgesic solutions can reach the sub-perineural spaces by diffusion around the capillary and lymphatic channels of the vasa nervorum, at and beyond the dural 'ink-cuff' areas. Once inside the endoneural spaces, longitudinal capillary networks provide tissue interfaces along which the analgesic solutions can track up the spinal roots and into the sub-pial spaces of the cord itself. From there the concentration gradient allows a gradual diffusion out into the cerebrospinal fluid—but nerve block has already taken place.

It is clear that on this basis spread from the site of an epidural injection depends upon:

1. Spread within the epidural space itself. This is dependent on such factors as the volume of solution injected, the speed of injection, the patency of the intervertebral foramina, the posture of the animal, gravity and vascular absorption.

2. Spread in the subdural and sub-pial spaces. The amount of drug which reaches the sub-pial spaces will be proportional to the amount which is able to diffuse through the perineurium into the sub-perineural spaces. This, of course, is governed by the physical laws which affect diffusion, such as the area of contact, the concentration gradient and the duration of contact. Thus, ultimately, segmental spread is dependent on the mass of analgesic drug available for transneural diffusion in the epidural space. The appropriate mass of drug can be delivered in the form of a large volume of dilute solution (when it will travel widely in the epidural space but diffuse relatively poorly), or as a small volume of concentrated solution (when epidural spread will be small, but the concentration gradient for diffusion, steep).

The outcome of an epidural injection may, therefore, be regarded as dependent on the action of many different forces. If any of these are unusually weak, or strong, the result will not be as expected. Thus, epidural block can never be claimed to be a very precise technique, and the ability to achieve consistent results will depend on the ability to choose the appropriate dose of local analgesic drug for each occasion with intelligent anticipation.

The Duration of Epidural Blockade

The addition of a vasoconstrictor drug to the analgesic solution constricts the epidural blood vessels and reduces the blood flow through the epidural space. This, in turn, reduces the bloodstream absorption of the analgesic drug. Roberts (1952) found that using procaine hydrochloride alone for caudal epidural block in cattle, the average duration of the blockade was 1·9 hours, whereas when adrenaline was added to the analgesic solution the average duration was increased to 2·4 hours.

Posterior and Anterior Epidural Block

It is customary to classify epidural analgesia as anterior (high) and posterior (low), according to the distance forwards the analgesic solution spreads and thus the extent of the area in which sensory and motor paralysis subsequently develop. This will depend chiefly on the volume of solution injected, although, as has been pointed out above, the concentration and diffusibility of the drug and the rate of absorption from the space also play a part.

Posterior Block

If the motor control of the hind-limbs is uninfluenced the block is referred to as a 'posterior block'. Skin analgesia develops over the tail and croup as far as the mid-sacral region; the anus, vulva, perineum and the posterior aspect of the thighs lose sensation. Paralysis of motor fibres will cause the anal sphincter to relax and the posterior part of the rectum to balloon. Defaecation will be suspended and stretching of the vulva will provoke no response. The vagina will dilate and in animals at parturition 'straining' or 'bearing-down' ceases while uterine contractions are uninfluenced.

Anterior Block

'Anterior block' implies that some degree of interference with the control of the hind-limbs is present. The motor nerve fibres need not be blocked, for block of the afferent fibres alone will suffice to destroy temporarily the integrity of the reflex arcs involved in the maintenance of muscle tone. If the lumbar and thoracic segments are blocked, the sympathetic outflow will be affected and hypotension will result. Block of cardiac accelerator nerves prevents the operation of the normal compensatory mechanism (increase in the heart rate) and the hypotension associated with anterior epidural analgesia is then unaccompanied by tachycardia. Clinical experience would appear to indicate that in healthy animals the hypotension which may be produced by anterior blocks results in no harm, and indeed is often helpful since it tends to reduce haemorrhage at the operation site. Nevertheless, during any anterior block careful attention should be paid to the state of the circulation, for death can occur from a quite small loss of blood at the operation site since the animal cannot compensate for reductions in the volume of circulating blood.

REFERENCES

BATSON, O. V. (1940). Am. Surg. 112, 138
BENESCH, F. (1926). Wien. tierärztl. Wschr. 13, 130
BIER, A. (1899). Dtsch. Zschr. Chir. 51, 391, 882
BONICA, J. J., BACKUP, P. H., ANDERSON, C. E., HADFIELD, D., CREPPS, W. F. and MONK, B. F. (1957). Anesthesiology, 18, 723
BRIERLEY, J. B. (1950). J. Anat. (Lond.) 82, 203
——— and FIELD, E. J. (1949). J. Neurol. Neurosurg. Psychiat. 12, 89
BROMAGE, P. R. (1954). Spinal Epidural Analgesia. Edinburgh: Livingstone
——— (1962). Br. J. Anaesth. 34, 161, (c) 418
BROOK, G. B. (1930). Vet. Rec. 10, 30
——— (1935). Vet. Rec. 15, 549 et seq.
CATHELIN, M. F. (1901). C. r. Soc. Biol. Paris, 53, 452
CORNING, J. L. (1885). New York med. J. 42, 483
CUILLE, J. and SENDRAIL (1901). Rev. vet. 98
FIELD, E. J. (1948). J. Anat. (Lond.) 82, 153
FOLDES, F. F., COLAVINCENZO, J. W. and BIRCH, J. H. (1956). Curr. Res. Anesth. Analg. 35, 33
FRUMIN, M. J., SCHWARTZ, M. BURNS, J. J., BRODIE, B. B. and PAPPER, E. M. (1953). J. Pharmac. 109, 102
HARTHOORN, A. M. and BRASS, W. (1954). Vet. Rec. 66, 117
McFADYEAN, J. (1922). The Anatomy of the Horse. London: Baillière, Tindall & Cox
MARX, G. F., ZERMAITIS, M. T. and ORKIN, R. R. (1961). Anesthesiology, 22, 348
MOORE, D. C., HAIN, R. H., WARD, A. and BRIDENBAUGH, L. D. (1954). J. Am. med. Ass. 156, 1050
NISHIMURA, N., KITAHARA, T. and KUSAKABE, T. (1959). Anesthesiology, 20, 785
RETZGEN, B. (1925). Quoted by Westhues, M. and Fritsch, R. (1960). Die Narkose der Tiere. Vol. 1. Berlin: Paul Parey (Eng. edn. 1964, Edinburgh: Oliver & Boyd)
ROBERTS, S. J. (1952). J. Am. vet. med. Ass. 82, 336
SISSON, S. (1938). The Anatomy of the Domestic Animals. 3rd ed., p. 832. London: Saunders
TUFVESSON, G. (1963). Local Anaesthesia in Veterinary Medicine. p. 44. Stockholm: Astra Ltd.

7

Caudal Epidural Analgesia

The Ox

In the ox the spinal cord ends in the region of the last lumbar vertebra but the meningeal sac is continued as far as the junction of the third and fourth sacral segments. The diameter of the neural canal as it passes through the sacrum is approximately 1·8 cm in the posterior part and 2 cm in the anterior. In the lumbar region the dimensions of the canal are much greater, its width at the last segment being 4 cm. This helps to explain why paralysis of the spinal nerves as far forward as the first sacral is effected with comparatively small quantities of local analgesic solution (20 ml), whereas paralysis of the anterior lumbar nerves necessitates the injection of much larger quantities (100 ml or more).

Caudal epidural injection is made through the space between the arches of the first and second coccygeal vertebrae—i.e. beyond the termination of the spinal cord and its meninges. This site is selected in preference to the sacrococcygeal space because it is larger and thus more easily penetrated, and, in fat animals particularly, is more easily detected. Location of the site for the introduction of the needle is not difficult and the operator may be guided by one or more of the following ways:

1. The tail is gripped about 6 in from its base and raised 'pump-handle fashion'. The first obvious articulation behind the sacrum is the first intercoccygeal.

2. Standing on one side of the animal and observing the line of the croup, the prominence of the sacrum is seen. Casting the eye back towards the tail, the next prominence to be observed is the spine of the first coccygeal bone. The site is the depression immediately behind it.

3. The posterior prominence of the tuberosity of the ischium is palpated and a point selected 4 to 4½ in in front of it. A line drawn directly over the

back from this point passes, in a medium-sized animal, through the depression between the first and second coccygeal spines.

The dimensions of the opening in the dorsal wall of the neural canal are approximately: 2 cm transversely and 2·5 cm antero-posteriorly. The depth of the canal is about 0·5 cm. The canal is occupied by six caudal nerves, together with a vein on each side. The aperture between the two vertebral arches is closed by the interarcual ligament and the space between the vertebral spines is occupied by connective tissue. Surmounting the spines is a

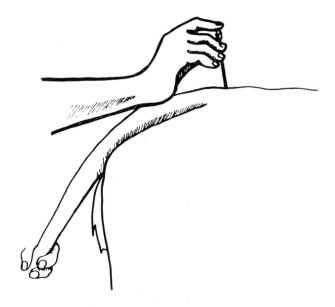

FIG. 51.—Caudal epidural injection in the ox.
The site for insertion of the needle.

variable amount of subcutaneous fat covered by the skin. The distance from the surface of the skin to the floor of the canal varies from 2 to 4 cm. The floor comprises, about the centre of the space, the intervertebral cartilaginous disc, and in front of and behind this, the upper surface of the vertebral centrum.

Apparatus Required

A hypodermic syringe having a metal nozzle. 'All glass' syringes are unsuitable because of the fragility of the nozzle. The 20 ml size is most appropriate, for in the majority of cases the bulk of the injection will be between 10 and 20 ml. When larger quantities are required it is refilled. A

short and comparatively fine needle (19 gauge, 2 cm long) serves for penetrating the rubber cork of the bottle containing the local analgesic or for
passing through the neck of the ampoule, and also for making the subcutaneous weal prior to insertion of the epidural needle. For the epidural injection
a longer and slightly stouter needle is required (18 gauge, 6 cm long). Its
point should be cut at an angle of 45°, for if the ordinary needle with the fine,
tapering point is used, the latter soon becomes 'turned' due to its striking the

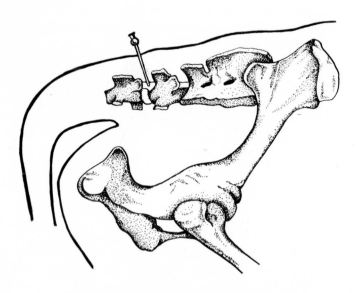

Fig. 52.—Caudal epidural injection in cattle.
Insertion of the needle into the first intercoccygeal space.

floor of the canal. A special bovine epidural needle has been introduced by
Brook, 8 cm long by 1·27 mm external diameter, marked in centimetres and
fitted with a stilette.

Technique of Injection

An insensitive skin weal is made with the object of preventing movement
during insertion of the epidural needle and thus ensuring that the latter is
introduced in the correct position and direction. For insertion of the epidural
needle the tail is allowed to hang naturally. The point of the needle is applied
to the centre of the depression between the first and second coccygeal spines,
taking care that it is exactly in the midline. If the dermis is tough and considerable pressure is necessary to pierce it, the thumb and forefinger of the
left hand are used to grip the needle immediately beneath its adaptor in

order to steady it while pressure is applied to the adaptor with the fingers of the right hand. The needle is thrust downwards and forwards at an angle of 15° with the vertical, until its point impinges on the floor of the canal. Often contact with a caudal nerve causes the animal to move suddenly, and the operator should be prepared for this.

Provided that the needle has been inserted in the proper position and direction, there is no doubt that it has entered the epidural space. Sometimes, however, the point of the needle has traversed the space and penetrated the intervertebral disc. This is detected, on attaching the syringe and attempting to inject the solution, by the great resistance offered to the plunger. Should this error occur, the needle should be slightly withdrawn and the syringe reapplied. When the point of the needle lies in the neural canal there is, for all practical purposes, no resistance, and the injection can be made quite easily. Sometimes blood escapes from the needle due to rupture of a vein. In this event the analgesic solution can still be injected without harm, or, if it is thought preferable, the needle can be withdrawn, cleansed of blood clot and reinserted. The rate of injection should be comparatively slow, and a volume of 15 ml occupies 10 to 15 seconds. When large quantities—30 ml or more—are to be injected, it is preferable that the solution shall previously be warmed to body temperature.

Solutions Used

Procaine hydrochloride, or slight modifications of it, was until recently almost invariably employed for the induction of epidural analgesia, but lignocaine hydrochloride is now widely used.

Posterior Block

By this is meant that motor control of the hind-limbs is uninfluenced. Using a 2% procaine hydrochloride solution, the maximum volumes which may be administered with reasonable certainty that the animal will be able to maintain the standing position are:

Heifers	. 10 ml
Medium-sized cows	. 10 „
Large cows	. 15 „

Exceptional cases are encountered in which considerably greater amounts can be given. When 0·75 to 1% solutions are employed, the range of dosage may be increased to 12 to 20 ml; while if high concentrations of 3 to 5% are used, the range should be reduced to 5 to 10 ml.

When 2% solutions of lignocaine hydrochloride are used the total dose lies between 5 and 10 ml, depending on the size of the animal.

Provided that the concentration used has been sufficient to paralyse completely the sensory fibres, skin analgesia of the following area will develop: the tail and croup as far as the mid-sacral region; the anus, vulva and perineum; the posterior aspect of the thighs. Paralysis of the motor fibres will cause the anal sphincter to relax and the posterior part of the rectum to balloon. Defaecation will be suspended. Stretching of the vulva will provoke no response and the vagina will dilate. In parturition cases 'straining' ceases, but uterine contractions will be uninfluenced.

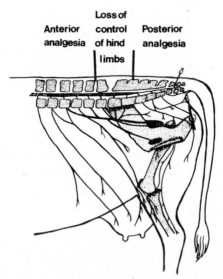

FIG. 53.—Epidural analgesia in the cow.
Scheme illustrating the distribution of the spinal nerves involved in posterior and anterior analgesia.

Indications

(*a*) *Obstetrics.* To overcome straining for the manipulative correction of malpresentations and the performance of the more simple embryotomical operations; operative treatment of parturient injuries; reduction of the prolapsed uterus.

(*b*) *General.* Surgical operations on the tail (5 to 10 ml sufficient). Suture of tears of the perineum and vulva, horn gores etc., Götze's operation for reconstruction of the perineum. Examination of the vagina and external uterine cervical os in fractious animals. Retraction of the uterine cervix. Albrechtson's uterine irrigation treatment. Ovariectomy.

Onset and Duration of Analgesia

The onset of muscular paralysis of the tail occurs in from 1 to 1½ minutes, and affords reliable evidence that the injection has been correctly made. When procaine is used analgesia attains its maximum extent in the course of 15 to 20 minutes, and persists for about an hour, after which there is progressive recovery. The animal is normal again by the end of the second hour.

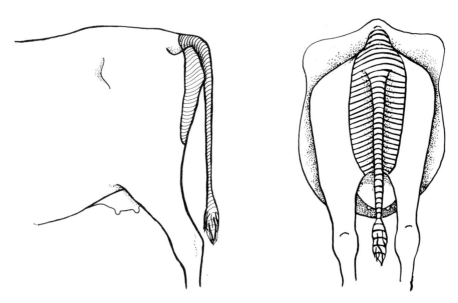

FIG. 54.—Area of skin desensitization after the epidural injection of 10 ml of 2% procaine solution in a four-year-old shorthorn cow of average size. The animal remained standing.

Paralysis of the Bull's Penis

The introduction of epidural analgesia was immediately followed by its use as a means of causing relaxation and exposure of the penis in the bull. At first, relatively large volumes of solution were used to ensure complete relaxation of the organ and Brook recommended a dosage of 25 ml of 2·25% procaine solution for small bulls and up to 70 ml for large ones. But these doses caused marked motor disturbance of the hind-limbs and it was necessary that the animal should be cast and restrained for several hours to ensure it did not sustain injury. It is probable that these quantities were used because it was not realized that there was a greater delay in the onset of relaxation of the penis than in sensory and motor paralysis of the tail. Howe advised that an initial minimal dose should be given and the needle left in position and if extrusion did not occur after the elapse of an appropriate interval additional small doses should be given until extrusion occurred, for in this way exposure of the penis could be obtained with the animal still standing. Edgson and Scarnell employed this method for the treatment of the penis of bulls infected with *Vibrio foetus*. They desired a degree of analgesia whereby the penis could be extracted from the sheath but the bull retained sufficient motor control of the hind-limbs to remain standing. For this purpose an average young Ayrshire bull weighing about 500 kg was given 10 ml of a 5% procaine solution without adrenaline and as a rule it was necessary to wait 15 to 20 minutes before the penis could be extracted. If, after this time, the penis was not sufficiently relaxed a further injection of 2 to 3 ml was given. In the Liverpool School a 3% lignocaine solution with 1:50,000 adrenaline has been used for surgical operations on the penis. It was possible to provoke complete relaxation and desensitization with the animal still able to maintain the standing position although there was some locomotor incoordination. It would seem that the dose capable of causing complete relaxation of the penis is very close to that which will cause a degree of incoordination which necessitates casting and restraint. As yet we have no accurate method of determining dosage in relation to weight and other measurements and it is probable there will be cases in which too much or too little has been given, but using the solution previously mentioned the dose for bulls up to 600 kg is tentatively put at 1 ml/50 kg. Penile relaxation attained its maximum some 25 minutes after injection; return of tone commenced in 2 hours and was complete in $4\frac{1}{2}$ hours.

For this particular purpose epidural analgesia has, nowadays, been replaced to a large extent by pudic nerve block, sympathetic blockade or by the use of tranquillizers such as the phenothiazine derivatives.

Anterior Block

The degree of motor interference in the hind-limbs will vary from a partial paralysis affecting primarily the flexors of the stifle-joint, and the flexors and extensors of the hocks and digital joints, to complete paralysis. In partial cases, attempts to move may be associated with spasmodic flexing and extending of the hocks, and arrangements should be made either to support the animal in the standing position or restrain it by hobbles in the recumbent. Plenty of straw bedding should be available to prevent the animal bruising itself when it goes down. In complete cases the animal should be kept on its breast with the hind-limbs placed beneath it for a period of 10 to 15 minutes to ensure the onset of bilateral analgesia. When unilateral analgesia only is required, the animal should be restrained on its side, with the appropriate side downwards, until the full development of analgesia, after which it is turned over. Loss of sensation spreads progressively forwards according to the dose, over the croup, between the hind-limbs to the inguinal regions, prepuce and scrotum, the hind-limbs, mammary glands, and finally flanks and abdominal wall to the region of the umbilicus. The duration of paralysis is longer. The animal will be unable to rise for two hours or so, and incoordination may persist for 3 to 4 hours or even longer. When full anterior epidural analgesia is attained, as is the case when the method is used for the operation of digital amputation, it is imperative that the limbs shall be kept in hobbles, with the animal in breast recumbancy, until it is certain that full motor function of the hind-limbs has returned, for otherwise attempts to rise may result in severe injury. The tail serves as a good guide. When power has returned to it, it may be taken that the animal can rise and stand.

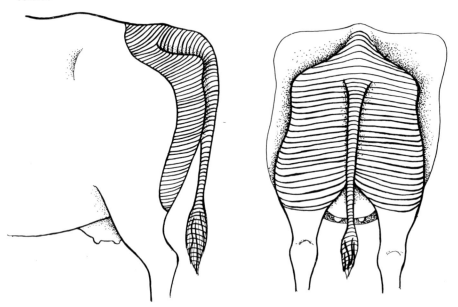

FIG. 55.—Area of skin desensitization after the epidural injection of 17 ml of 2% procaine solution in an adult (fat) Ayrshire cow. Coordination of the hind-limbs was interfered with to a degree whereby the animal was unable to maintain the standing position, although it kicked vigorously when down.

Indications

(*a*) *Obstetrics.* Difficult manipulative reposition, extensive embryotomy and amputation of the prolapsed uterus. Caesarean section.

(*b*) *General.* Examination of and operation on the penis. Cutting operations about the prepuce and inguinal regions. Castration. Operative interferences on the udder. Operations on the hind-limb such as amputation of the digit.

Dosage

For difficult obstetrical interferences and amputation of the uterus Benesch advises 60 to 100 ml of 1% Tutocaine solution, and for Caesarean section 120 to 130 ml. Frank and Roberts claim that 40 ml of 2% procaine are adequate for Caesarean sections in heifers, and 50 ml for older animals. They make the incision a little to the right of the midline immediately in front of the udder. For amputation of the udder Frank advises 40 ml of 3% procaine solution. It is improbable that this volume serves completely to desensitize the anterior quarters of the gland, for their innervation is derived from the anterior lumbar region, and it is suggested that the dosage recommended for complete desensitization of the hind-legs is more appropriate. To ensure complete analgesia of the hind-limbs for the operation of amputation of the digit Klarenbeek and Hartog employ 150 to 200 ml of a 1%, or 100 to 140 ml of a 1·5% solution. Experience in the Liverpool School has been that the effective quantity of a 2·25% procaine hydrochloride solution is from 100 to 150 ml according to the size of the cow. No ill-effects have been seen.

For severe operations requiring anterior block, chloral hydrate by the mouth in doses of 30 to 60 g or Xylazine (see page 161), 0·1 mg/kg by intramuscular injection, should be given.

ANTERIOR BLOCK: DOSAGE TABLE
(Millilitres of 2% procaine solution)

	Difficult reposition, extensive embryotomy, castration	Amputation of digit, amputation of udder, Caesarean section
Small sized adults	40	100
Medium sized adults . . .	75	120
Large sized adults . . .	100	150

Accidents and Complications

Benesch, whose opinion must receive the greatest respect, for it was he who was chiefly responsible for the introduction of epidural analgesia into bovine practice, states that its application, when properly performed, is entirely free from danger. Klarenbeek and Hartog, referring to the use of anterior block in cattle, state that several hundred operations have been performed under it with very satisfactory results, and no damage could be seen. Wright has observed no ill-effects attend its use, other than a temporary lameness in a cow which fell awkwardly. Cuille and Chelle have noted that sometimes the tail is carried in a twisted manner, but with normal mobility, for 5 to 6 days following injection, after which it becomes normal again, and they ascribe it to injury of the coccygeal nerves during injection. Brook has recorded a case in which permanent paralysis of the tail followed epidural injection for the delivery of a dead and oedematous foetus. The animal was unable to elevate the tail even during defaecation and urination, with the result that excoriation of the tail and perineum developed. There was some lateral mobility. A hard, diffuse and painful enlargement developed in the region of the first coccygeal spine. Gold has encountered a similar case in which permanent paralysis of the tail supervened, and in addition a sinus developed and persisted at the site of injection.

It is probable that infection of the neural canal with the subsequent inflammatory changes is the cause of these cases. Fortunately the accident is rare, but every effort must be made to avoid it, for it detracts greatly from the animal's value. The greatest care must be taken that the analgesic solution is not a source of infection. It may be assumed with confidence that when prepared by a manufacturing house of repute, the solution is sterile when received, but the danger is that it will become contaminated during use. When a bottle of analgesic solution is employed, the rubber cork should be thoroughly cleansed and the needle used to penetrate it must be sterile. For this reason a separate needle for this purpose should be carried. It is preferable when using comparatively small volumes (10 to 20 ml) to employ ampoules. There is a grave risk that asepsis will break when dealing with a dead and putrid foetus, particularly if a vaginal examination has been made prior to the induction of analgesia, or if a second injection is required after operation has commenced. In these cases the hands should be thoroughly scrubbed in hot antiseptic solution before handling the epidural instrument and care taken to avoid fingering those parts of the needle which are to penetrate the tissues.

When inducing full anterior analgesia, the possible development of hypotension must be borne in mind. Although Wright has seen no signs of hypotension when using volumes of 100 to 150 ml for amputation of digits, Swangarde has recorded the condition in bulls after doses of 150 to 200 ml of 2% solution. Symptoms are those of collapse, with a racing heart and small pulse, and rapid and shallow respirations.

Hypotension may be combated by the intravenous or intramuscular injection of vasopressors. For many years methylamphetamine was used as a vasopressor during epidural analgesia but, because it became a popular drug of addiction due to its ability to produce an elevation of mood and general euphoria in man, it is now not generally available. It has been replaced by other compounds such as metaraminol bitartrate and methoxamine hydrochloride which are equally effective, if not better, vasopressors.

Metaraminol bitartrate (Aramine) is a sympathomimetic amine which has a dual action in that it increases both the force of myocardial contraction and peripheral resistance. It has no central excitatory effect; side-effects such as tremor and tachycardia are not seen. Unlike adrenaline, metaraminol has no effect on blood sugar. It is best given to cattle by intravenous injection in doses up to 20 mg, after which the maximum effect takes 1 to 3 minutes to develop and lasts for about 25 to 30 minutes.

Methoxamine hydrochloride (Vasoxine, Vasylox) is another sympatho-mimetic amine but its main action is one of peripheral vasconstriction. It does not effect the force of myocardial contraction and is devoid of stimulatory action on the central nervous system. When given to adult cattle by intra-venous injection in doses of 30 to 60 mg it acts almost immediately and its action lasts about 1 hour. Alternatively, it may be given in doses of up to 60 mg by intramuscular injection.

The Horse

In the horse epidural block has not attained the prominence that it has in the bovine animal. This is readily understandable, because the interferences for which this form of analgesia has proved so useful in cattle are less often necessary in horses. In addition, not only are many horses unsuited tempera-mentally for puncture with needles in the vicinity of the hind legs but the epidural cavity is less easy to locate in the caudal region so that the technique is more difficult than in cattle. At the same time it must be noted that workers with considerable experience of the method in horses are enthusiastic as to its value.

Location of the Site

The spinal cord and its meninges end in the mid-sacral region and the arrangement of the spinal nerves in the neural canal behind this point is similar to the cow. Epidural injection is made in the first intercoccygeal space. The depression between the first and second coccygeal spines can generally be felt with the finger when the tail is raised, even in the heavy breeds, about 2·5 cm in front of the commencement of the tail hairs, although in fat animals it may be impossible to detect any of the sacral or coccygeal spines. Upward flexion at the sacrococcygeal articulation is seldom discernible; in fact, in many animals this joint is fused. Cuille and Chelle (1931) locate the site as follows: a line drawn over the back joining the two hip-joints crosses the midline at the level of the sacrococcygeal joint. Immediately behind this may be felt the superior spine of the first coccygeal bone, and the space immediately posterior to it is the site for the introduction of the needle. Browne (1938) points out that the space is opposite the caudal fold which is formed at each side of the root of the tail when the latter is raised. The interarcual space is smaller than in the ox and may be more difficult to locate with the needle, particularly in well-developed and fat animals in which the root of the tail is well covered by muscle and fat. Should the direction in which the needle is inserted be inappropriate in relation to the site of skin puncture, its point may strike the upper aspect of one of the vertebral arches, while, should its direction deviate slightly to one side of the midline, it may strike a transverse process. The question of restraint during injection must be considered. In the case of quiet animals the raising of a fore-limb may be sufficient, but in others it will be necessary to augment this by a twitch. The site is prepared and an insensitive skin weal provoked. The depth of the neural canal from the surface is greater than in the ox (4 to 8 cm) and a longer needle is necessary (8 to 10 cm). The operator stands on the left side of the animal adjacent to the hind-limb. The point of the needle is inserted in the centre of the depression between the first and second coccygeal spines and pressed downwards at right angles to the general contour of the croup until the floor of the neural canal

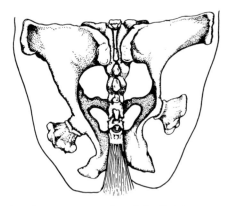

Fig. 56.—Illustrating the sacrococcygeal and the first intercoccygeal spaces in the horse.

is struck. Sometimes it is possible to detect a 'popping' sensation as the inter-arcual ligament is penetrated. The surest evidence, however, that the canal has been entered is the almost complete absence of resistance to injection of the solution. Should any resistance be encountered, the needle should be partially withdrawn and redirected. Browne advises a different method. The point of the needle is inserted at the posterior part of the intercoccygeal depression and directed downwards and forwards at an angle of 30° with the horizontal, taking care to maintain the direction of the needle exactly in the midline. The point glides along the floor of the neural canal, so that the needle can be inserted freely to its full length (the steep downward and backward direction of the canal at this point allows of this). He points out that if the direction of the needle is nearer the vertical, its point abuts against the floor of the canal and it is difficult to ascertain whether or not the canal has been entered.

Posterior Block

With the horse standing, posterior block only should be induced, for if motor control of the hind legs is interfered with the animal may become agitated with alarming consequences, and a sudden fall may cause injury. When it is necessary to induce anterior block, the animal must first be cast and restrained, and it is advisable to administer a narcotic such as chloral hydrate in addition.

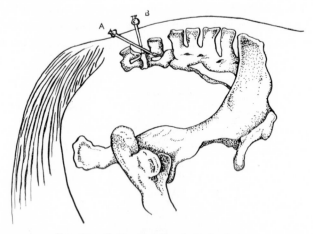

Fig. 57.—Epidural analgesia in the horse.
The site for insertion of the needle and the direction of penetration (A) by Benesch's method and (B) by Browne's method.

Indications

(a) *General.* Amputation of the tail (an operation which, in Great Britain, may only be performed for surgical reasons). Operations about the anus, perineum and vulva. Suture of wounds. Operation for prolapsed rectum. Caslick's operation for vaginal windsucking.

(b) *Obstetrical.* To overcome straining during the manipulative correction of the simpler forms of malpresentation of the foetus, and for partial embryotomy.

Dosage

2 to 2·5% procaine hydrochloride solutions:

	Amputation of tail	Operations on vulva, perineum	Obstetrics, manipulation
Foals	3 to 5 ml	Small animals 10 ml	15 ml
Older animals	10 to 15 ml	Medium 15 ml	20 ml
		Heavy Up to 25 ml	Up to 30 ml

According to Tufvesson (1963) up to 10 to 12 ml of 2% lignocaine hydrochloride solution can be injected in large horses before there is a risk of hindlimb incoordination.

Anterior Block

The chief indications for anterior block in the horse are obstetrical—difficult manipulative repositions and extensive embryotomy—although Frank mentions its adoption for the operations of scrotal hernia and cryptorchidism. To avoid any risk of injury during the period of recovery, restraint should be maintained for at least 3 hours to ensure that when the animal makes the effort to do so it will be able to regain and maintain the standing position. Casting should be carried out on a deep straw bed. On no account should efforts be made to make the animal rise before it attempts to do so itself.

Dosage

For severe obstetrical interferences doses of 50 to 120 ml of 1% solution should be adopted, and for cutting operations 30 to 80 ml of 2%, according to the size of the animal.

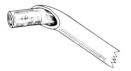

FIG. 58.—Catheter emerging from tip of Tuohy needle.

Tufvesson (1963) states that for analgesia of the hind quarters to the level of the costal arch at least 100 to 150 ml of 2% lignocaine hydrochloride solution are required.

Should signs of hypotension develop, the methods of correction to be employed are the same as those already described on page 123.

The Sheep

For intravaginal obstetrical procedures caudal epidural analgesia may be induced by the injection of 3 to 4 ml of local analgesic solution into the epidural canal through the sacrococcygeal space. This is a valuable technique and if careful aseptic precautions are observed no complications are encountered. Once again lignocaine hydrochloride is the drug of choice but 2 or 3% procaine hydrochloride may be used.

For the symptomatic relief of painful conditions of the vagina and rectum which provoke severe and continuous straining the technique of continuous caudal epidural block can be extremely useful. A fine nylon catheter is introduced through a Tuohy needle (Figs 58 and 68) at the sacrococcygeal space and advanced for 6 to 8 cm up the epidural canal. The needle is then withdrawn leaving the catheter in situ. Local analgesic solution (3 to 4 ml) is injected through the catheter whenever the animal shows signs of sensation returning to the pelvic organs. If all injections are made with aseptic precautions and the free end of the catheter is maintained in a sterile condition—bound up in a sterile gauze swab, for example—between injections, analgesia can be safely maintained for many hours by this technique.

Bradley (1966) reported that the injection of 0·75 to 1 ml of 5% procaine hydrochloride with adrenaline at the sacrococcygeal space produced excellent analgesia for the docking of lambs' tails.

The Dog

In the dog caudal epidural injections may be given between the sacrum and the first coccygeal vertebra or between the first and second coccygeal vertebrae. The same principles are followed as in the larger animals. The procedure is technically easy and the dose administered should not exceed 1 ml of 2% lignocaine hydrochloride solution. This block is useful for docking the tail in adult dogs and for other surgical operations upon the tail.

REFERENCES

BENESCH, F. (1938). *Proc. XIIIth Int. vet. Congr. Zurich*
——— (1951). *Veterinary Obstetrics*. London: Baillière, Tindall & Cox
BRADLEY, W. A. (1966). *Vet. Rec.* **79**, 787
BROOK, B. G. (1935). *Vet. Rec.* **15**, 601, 605, 606
BROWNE, T. G. (1938). *Vet. Rec.* **50**, 1617
CUILLE, J. and CHELLE, P. (1931). *Rev. gen. Med. vet.* **40**, 393
EDGSON, F. A. and SCARNELL, J. (1955). *Vet. Rec.* **67**, 469
FRANK, E. R. (1928). *J. Am. vet. med. Ass.* **72**, 336
——— (1931). *Vet. Rec.* **11**, 867
——— and ROBERTS, S. J. (1940). *N. Am. Vet.* **21**, 9 and 469
GOLD, T. N. (1940). Private communication to J. G. Wright
HOWE, G. Quoted by Brook, G. B. (1935)
KLARENBEEK and HARTOG (1938). *Proc. XIIIth Int. vet. Congr. Zurich.* Quoted by Wright, J. G. (1952). *Veterinary Anaesthesia*, 3rd Ed., London: Baillière, Tindall & Cox
TUFVESSON, G. (1963). *Local Anaesthesia in Veterinary Medicine*. Stockholm: Astra Ltd.

8

Lumbar Epidural Analgesia

Injection of local analgesic solutions into the epidural space in the caudal region affords a very safe method of inducing epidural analgesia, but it is not always easy to produce satisfactory anterior blocks when this site of injection is used. Consequently, when an anterior block is essential, some workers make the injection at the lumbosacral foramen. However, needles introduced through the lumbosacral foramen may enter the subarachnoid space and once this has been entered it is no longer safe to proceed with the induction of an epidural block until the puncture in the dura has become sealed. The patency of the hole in the dura persists for several hours and if an immediate spinal block is considered to be essential, a deliberate, controlled subarachnoid block must be performed. It is because subarachnoid block can be adequately managed only in relatively small animals, in which full use can be made of gravity to control the extent of neural blockade, that injection at the lumbo-sacral foramen is normally only employed in sheep, small pigs and dogs.

Injection into the epidural space in the anterior lumbar region has been employed to produce analgesia of a number of body segments in cattle. By careful control of the dose of local analgesic injected it is possible to produce a belt of analgesia around the animal's trunk without interfering with the control of the hind limbs. This type of spinal block may be referred to as 'lumbar segmental epidural analgesia'. Although not an easy technique to perform it is one which warrants inclusion in any discussion of lumbar epidural analgesia.

Lumbar Segmental Epidural Analgesia in the Ox

The desensitization of the flank in cattle by the extradural injection of local analgesic solution into the vertebral canal in the anterior lumbar region was first described in 1948 by Buchholz working in the Giessen School.

Later the Russian writers Magda, Shalduga and Voskovoinikov (1952)

5

described their technique and Arthur (1956) in the London School introduced the method to English veterinarians. By a single injection, analgesia of the whole of the flanks may be attained with the animal still able to maintain the standing position and operations such as Caesarean section and rumenotomy performed. Buchholz injected 10 to 15 ml of a 2% Tutocaine solution, Magda and his colleagues 10 ml of a 4% procaine hydrochloride solution, while Arthur has employed 3% lignocaine hydrochloride and 5% procaine hydrochloride, varying the volume injected according to the size of the animal; a

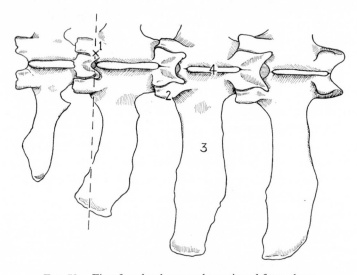

FIG. 59.—First four lumbar vertebrae viewed from above.
(1) Point of insertion of spinal needle through skin. (2) Articular processes. (3) Transverse process. (4) Spinous process.

yearling heifer receives 6 ml and an adult cow 10 ml. St. Clair and Hardenbrook in the United States who were investigating the method at about the same time as Arthur have since recorded very similar findings. 10 to 12 ml of a 4% procaine solution were sufficient to desensitize the sublumbar area in the average-sized animal. With 15 ml the hind-limb was usually weakened and with 20 ml the animal was unable to stand. Usually 10 ml of 2% lignocaine gave satisfactory results.

Technique

Arthur's technique is as follows: with the animal standing, the site for insertion of the needle is just to the right of the lumbar spinous processes on a line 1·5 cm behind the anterior edge of the second lumbar transverse process (Fig. 59). An initial skin weal is produced using a fine needle and a longitudinal skin incision some 2 to 3 cm long is made to facilitate penetration by the spinal needle. The spinal needle (14 gauge, 12 cm long) is directed downwards and inwards at an angle of 10 to 13° with the vertical for a distance of 7·5 cm (Fig. 60) at which point the needle has entered the neural canal. By adopting the preliminary skin incision the spinal needle can be moved with relative ease and the operator is able to appreciate the differences in resistance offered by the muscle and the interarcual ligament respectively. Even when small quantities of local anaesthetic are injected along the track of the needle, penetration of the interarcual ligament is apparently painful and thus the animal should be effectively restrained by the head. It should be noted that the intervertebral space through which the needle must pass to enter the epidural space is actually an interosseous canal formed by the bases of the

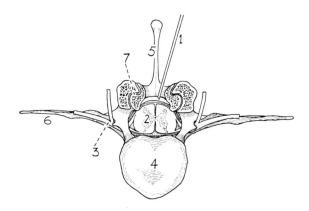

FIG. 60.—Transverse section through the joints between the articular processes of the first and second lumbar vertebrae. The body of the first lumbar segment is viewed from its posterior aspect.

(1) Needle in position. (2) Spinal cord surrounded by meninges. (3) Left 1st lumbar nerve. (4) Body of 1st lumbar vertebra. (5) Spinous process. (6) Transverse process. (7) Sectioned interlocking articular processes.

spinous processes in front and behind and by the intervertebral articular processes laterally. In an adult Jersey cow this canal measures 1 cm deep, 0·8 cm long and 0·5 cm wide (these dimensions will be considerably greater in the average Friesian or Ayrshire cow), and unless the needle is properly inclined its point will abut on the lateral wall of this canal rather than enter the neural canal (Fig. 60). Immediately the needle is felt to penetrate the interarcual ligament, the stilette is withdrawn and if air is heard to enter the needle it is certain evidence that the epidural space has been entered. Alternatively, in the absence of inspiration of air, and if no fluid flows from the needle, a trial injection is made. If the needle is in the epidural space scarcely any pressure on the plunger is needed. If, on withdrawing the stilette cerebrospinal fluid flows from the needle, the latter should be quickly but gently withdrawn until the flow ceases and then injection made. (Arthur records three cases of accidental puncture of the subarachnoid space but no ill-effect resulted.)

Effects

Lumbar segmental epidural injection results in a broad belt of analgesia encircling the abdomen and involving the whole depth of the wall including the parietal peritoneum. Analgesia develops some ten minutes after injection and persists for about three hours.

Further observations recorded by Arthur include a case of a small Guernsey

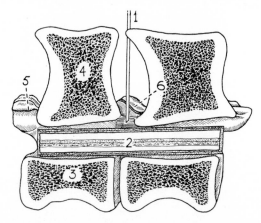

FIG. 61.—Vertical median section of first and second lumbar vertebrae. (1) Spinal needle penetrating ligament between vertebrae. (2) Spinal cord and meninges. (3) First lumbar body. (4) Spinous process. (5) Anterior articular process. (6) Interlocking articular processes.

cow in which the injection of 10 ml caused a partial paralysis of the left anterior crural and obturator nerves in addition, which resulted in 'dropping' of the stifle with abduction of the limb and a tendency to fall on to the left side. In several cases only unilateral analgesia developed, usually of the left side but occasionally of the right. This unilateral action may be due to an insufficient volume of local anaesthetic solution as was indicated by a cow in which 7 ml provoked unilateral analgesia only but an additional 3 ml, without altering the position of the needle, caused a complete belt of analgesia. A feature of unilateral block is a pronounced bending of the spine with the convexity of the curve on the desensitized side. Two interesting side-effects on the sympathetic nervous system were noted. The first was the passage of urine within a few minutes on the onset of analgesia, due presumably to paralysis of the sympathetic fibres controlling the trigonum, and the second an increase in skin temperature behind the site of injection to some 4°F. No clinical

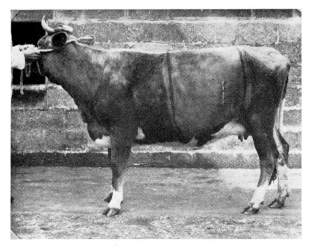

FIG. 62.—Lumbar segmental epidural analgesia (Arthur, G. H., *Veterinary Record*). Position of needle and area of flank desensitization after the injection of 10 ml of 3% lignocaine.

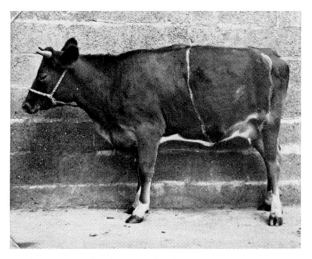

FIG. 63.—Lumbar segmental epidural analgesia (Arthur, G. H., *Veterinary Record*). A small Guernsey in which 10 ml of 3% lignocaine caused left anterior crural and obturator paralysis in addition to flank analgesia.

evidence of hypotension due to paralysis of the splanchnic nerves was observed. Arthur's conclusion is that preliminary trials of the method have confirmed its value for operations about the flank and udder performed with the animals standing.

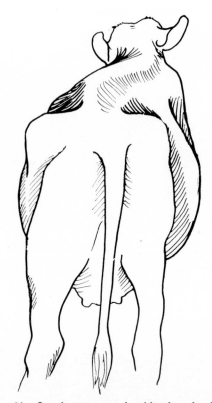

FIG. 64.—Lumbar segmental epidural analgesia.
Unilateral analgesia of left side with spinal curvature towards the unaffected side.

Lumbar Epidural (and Subarachnoid) Analgesia in Sheep

Both epidural and subarachnoid spinal nerve blocks provide excellent conditions for intra-abdominal, pelvic or hind-limb surgery. In sheep restraint of the head and fore-limbs is simple and if the animal is made comfortable upon the operating table it will not interfere with the surgeon's work by struggling. Provided that careful technique and the most scrupulous asepsis are employed there is very little risk to the animal. The vast majority of the complications which have been described as occurring after spinal nerve blocks can be traced to faulty or clumsy technique or to the introduction of infection into the epidural or subarachnoid space.

Lumbar Epidural Analgesia

Although the needle may be introduced between any two lumbar vertebrae there is less risk of puncturing the meninges if it is introduced through the lumbosacral space. The site for lumbosacral injection is located as follows: the anterior border of the illium on each side is located by palpation. A line joining these crosses the spinous process of the last lumbar vertebra. The needle is introduced immediately behind this.

Procedure

A large area around the site of injection is clipped and the skin thoroughly cleaned and disinfected. The sheep is then restrained in lateral recumbency with the lumbosacral spine in full flexion (Fig. 65). The restraint must be good, for the animal usually attempts to move as the needle penetrates the ligamentum flavum and movement at this juncture may result in accidental puncture of the dura mater.

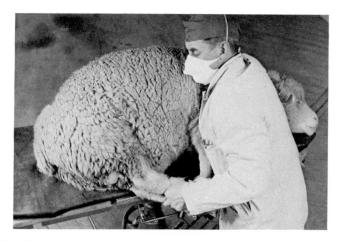

Fig. 65.—Method of restraint for lumbar epidural injection in sheep. The attendant's left hand holds the hind legs, while his right arm restrains the shoulder region of the animal.

With full aseptic precautions, the site for the introduction of the epidural needle is infiltrated with 2 or 3 ml of local analgesic solution using a very fine needle. A large-bore needle is introduced through the insensitive zone made by this injection and then withdrawn to leave a clearly defined skin puncture. The epidural needle (6 cm long, 16 b.w.g. with a fitted stilette) is inserted through the skin puncture and directed towards the lumbosacral space (Fig. 66). When the needle point is judged to have entered the tough ligamentum flavum the stilette is removed and a 20 ml syringe containing about 5 ml of air is attached to the needle. The needle is advanced cautiously with one hand while the thumb of the other hand maintains a continuous pressure on

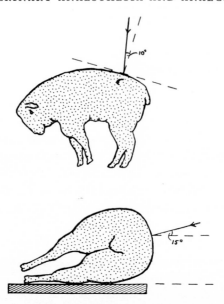

FIG. 66.—Direction of insertion of needle for lumbar epidural injection in sheep.

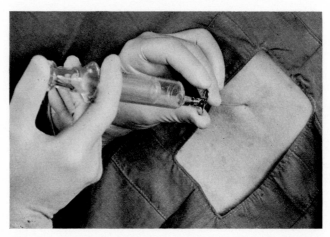

FIG. 67.—Loss of resistance test for location of the epidural space.

the plunger of the syringe (Fig. 67). The sudden loss of resistance to injection of the air when the needle emerges from the ligamentum flavum is immediately apparent by movement of the syringe piston. This loss of resistance indicates that the epidural space has been entered and the injection of air tends to force the dura away from the advancing needle point. Next, an attempt is made to aspirate cerebrospinal fluid into the syringe. If fluid is drawn into the syringe or drips from the needle when the syringe is detached it must be assumed that the dura has been punctured and in these circumstances either a subarachnoid injection is made (see p. 138) or the whole procedure should be abandoned, for experience has shown that it is not safe merely to withdraw the needle slightly and proceed with the epidural injection. If all is well and the dura has not been punctured a syringe containing the local analgesic solution is attached to the needle and the injection made. If predominantly unilateral analgesia is required the sheep is maintained in lateral recumbency (the side to be desensitized being undermost) but if bilateral analgesia is desired the animal is turned on to its back as soon as the needle is removed. In either case it is an advantage to apply a 10° head-down tilt to the animal's body by raising the end of the table. The animal is maintained in position until analgesia is complete and the time taken for this will depend on the analgesic drug employed.

It has been found that a rather concentrated solution is required for epidural analgesia. If procaine hydrochloride is used, the strength must not be less than 3%. However, the drug of choice is undoubtedly lignocaine hydrochloride 1·5% with the addition of adrenaline from an ampoule to give a final concentration of 1:100,000 adrenaline. This gives excellent analgesia of about two hours' duration. The volume of lignocaine solution injected is, of course, dependent upon the size of the sheep and ranges from 8 to 15 ml.

The injection of this quantity of 1·5% lignocaine solution usually causes a slight fall in blood pressure due to paralysis of the splanchnic nerves and 5 mg of metaraminol bitartrate (Aramine) should be injected intramuscularly in one of the hind-legs as soon as the epidural injection has been completed. Occasionally (in about 5% of cases) the fall in blood pressure may be severe and the animal will show signs of distress due to hypotension. In these circumstances 5 to 10 mg of methoxamine hydrochloride (Vasoxine) should be given immediately by intravenous injection, in addition to the intramuscular dose. It is always a wise precaution to insert an indwelling intravenous needle such as a Mitchell needle into a vein before any spinal nerve block is performed so that difficulties of venepuncture do not delay the intravenous administration of the vasopressor drug.

Motor nerve fibres are not blocked by a 1·5% solution of lignocaine hydrochloride so an animal can still move its hind legs during an operation. Because the afferent sensory fibres are blocked, however, the reflex arc is not intact and the sheep is unable to stand for four to six hours from the time of injection. The phrenic nerves and the motor nerves to the intercostal muscles are also unaffected and respiration is not embarrassed even if the solution permeates high up into the cervical region.

The sheep should be allowed to lie quietly while recovering from the effects of the epidural block. The animal can maintain itself in sternal recumbency and any attempt to hasten it to rise may cause it to become excited. Damage to hip-joints or pelvic bones by forceful uncoordinated movements may occur if the animal is frightened or excited during the recovery period.

Continuous epidural block (see page 127) may be produced by repeated injections given through a fine nylon cathether introduced with a Tuohy needle (Fig. 68).

Subarachnoid Analgesia

It is probable that there are no indications for the deliberate induction of a subarachnoid or 'true spinal' nerve block in sheep for on all occasions when it might be used an epidural block is to be preferred. Subarachnoid block is, therefore, only likely to be induced when the dura is accidentally punctured during an attempt to perform an epidural block.

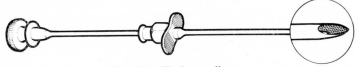

FIG. 68.—Tuohy needle.

The specific gravity of the fluid injected into the subarachnoid space, coupled with the posture of the animal, has a most important bearing on the spread of analgesia. It has been found that cinchocaine as Heavy Nupercaine (i.e. 1 in 200 Nupercaine in 6% glucose) is a satisfactory agent for use in sheep. This solution is hyperbaric and sinks to the most dependent part of the meningeal sac. Its spread within the subarachnoid space is shown in Fig. 69 and it is important to note that the natural curvature of the spine plays an important part in the distribution of the solution when this is injected in the lumbar region and allowed to spread under the influence of gravity. Diffusion of the drug into the cerebrospinal fluid usually plays only a small part in the spread of analgesia.

If the dura is accidentally punctured and it is decided to carry on and perform a subarachnoid block then 1·5 to 2 ml of Heavy Nupercaine are injected through the needle and the needle withdrawn. For a unilateral block the sheep is maintained in lateral recumbency so that the nerve roots on the underside of the animal become impregnated with the drug, while for a bilateral block the sheep is placed on its back as soon as possible after the needle has been removed. Spread of analgesia towards the head or tail is obtained by tilting the table so that the sheep's body is either inclined head down or head up. The extent of analgesia is tested from time to time by pinching the skin with a pair of forceps or towel clips and when the desired area of analgesia is attained the table top is returned to the horizontal position. Analgesia persists for about 3 hours and the sheep is able to stand after a further 2 to 3 hours have elapsed. If Heavy Nupercaine solution is not available 2 or 3 ml of 3% lignocaine hydrochloride solution may be injected, but the spread of analgesia is not so easily controlled and the duration of the block is much less.

Subarachnoid or 'spinal' block appears to cause a more profound fall in blood pressure than is encountered with an epidural block and vasopressor drugs such as methoxamine should be given as a routine. After a dural

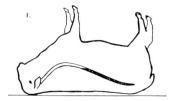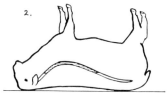

FIG. 69.—Spread of solution in subarachnoid space when injected in the lumbar region.
(1) Hyperbaric solution, i.e. specific gravity of solution greater than specific gravity of cerebrospinal fluid. (2) Hypobaric solution, i.e. specific gravity of cerebrospinal fluid.

SUBARACHNOID COMPARED WITH EPIDURAL ANALGESIA

Epidural	Subarachnoid
1. Meningitis unlikely.	1. Meningitis a possibility.
2. No post-operative malaise.	2. Post-operative malaise.
3. Usually only a slight fall in blood pressure.	3. Fall in blood pressure often severe.
4. Spread to medulla impossible.	4. Spread to medulla possible.

puncture, whether or not this has been followed by a spinal block, most sheep exhibit signs which may well indicate that they are suffering from a headache. They grind their teeth, avoid bright light and press their heads against walls or cold water buckets. Headache is a well recognized sequel to spinal puncture in man.

Lumbar Epidural Analgesia in the Pig

In the pig the spinal cord ends at the junction of the fifth and sixth lumbar vertebrae and the spinal meninges continue, around the phylum terminale, as far as the middle of the sacrum. At the lumbosacral space the sac is comparatively small, and it is improbable that needle introduced at this point will penetrate into the subarachnoid space. The lumbosacral aperture is large. Its dimensions in an adult are approximately 1·5 cm in the antero-posterior direction and 3 cm transversely. The depth of the canal is about 1 cm.

The site for insertion of the needle is located as follows: the anterior border of the ilium on each side is found with the fingers. A line joining them crosses the spinous process of the last lumbar segment. The needle is inserted in the midline immediately behind this spine and directed downwards and backwards at an angle of 20° with the vertical. The depth to which the needle must penetrate in pigs of from 30 to 70 kg (65 to 150 lb) will vary from 5 to 9 cm. The landmarks described are readily detected in animals of smaller size

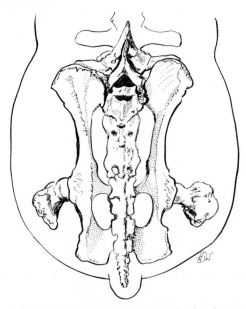

Fig. 70.—The lumbosacral space in the pig.

but they may be entirely masked by the overlying tissues in larger ones. In these a point 15 cm in front of the base of the tail serves as a fairly accurate guide. Provided the needle is introduced in approximately the correct position and direction, the size of the lumbosacral space makes its detection comparatively easy. Eighteen gauge needles are used; for pigs between 30 and 50 kg (65 to 110 lb) one 8 cm long, and for animals of 70 kg (150 lb) and above, 12 cm.

Before inserting the epidural needle an insensitive skin weal should be produced. The animal is restrained either on its breast or side. The latter is preferable, for by it sudden movement can be better controlled. As soon as the injection is made, the animal should be allowed to pass on to its breast again during the period of development of analgesia, otherwise that of the upper side may be incomplete. Owing to difficulties in restraining the animal, it is generally necessary to make the injection comparatively rapidly. Penetration of the canal is generally associated with sudden movement, for which attendants must be prepared.

Indications and Dosage

Epidural analgesia has been used for the castration of pigs of 40 to 50 kg (90 to 100 lb), injecting 10 ml of 2% procaine solution with adrenaline. Complete desensitization of the scrotum, testes and spermatic cord was present in ten minutes, and there was a partial motor paralysis of the hindlimbs. Recovery was complete at the end of the second hour. Frank recommends a similar dosage (1 ml/10 lb body weight). A point to be considered in the pig is—up to what weight should this computation be employed, for in adults fat often represents a considerable proportion of body weight; 100 kg (220 lb) is suggested as the upper limit, with a maximum dose of 20 ml.

When 2% lignocaine solution without adrenaline is used analgesia lasts for up to 90 minutes after full development of the block (Hopcroft, 1965).

Other indications are obstetrical manipulations, return of the prolapsed rectum and amputation of the prolapsed uterus.

Lumbar Epidural Analgesia in the Dog

In the dog the spinal cord ends at the junction of the sixth and seventh lumbar vertebrae, and the meninges continue to the middle of the sacrum. Cuille and Chelle (1931), who first studied the practical application of this form of analgesia in the dog, originally made the injection at the sacrococcygeal space but found that the technique was difficult. They subsequently discarded it in favour of lumbosacral puncture, which is easier to effect and has not special disadvantages. Brook (1935), who has studied the sacral meningeal cul-de-sac in the dog, points out that its dimensions at the lumbosacral space are so small it is improbable that it will be penetrated by a needle inserted at this point, and thus it may be taken that the injection is always extradural. The greater splanchnic nerve arises from the twelfth thoracic ganglion and a serious fall in blood pressure may occur if the anaesthetic solution extends in front of the first lumbar segment. To reduce this danger Brook advises that the animal be restrained on its back during the onset of analgesia so that the central spinal nerve roots which contain the vasomotor fibres are less profoundly affected than the dorsal roots containing the sensory fibres.

Location of the Site

The iliac prominences on either side are located. An imaginary line joining them crosses the spinous process of the last lumbar segment. The site for insertion of the needle is in the midline immediately behind this process. The interarcual ligament lies at a depth of 2 to 4 cm from the skin and the approximate dimensions of the space in a 14 kg dog are: anteroposteriorly, 0·4 cm, and laterally, 0·7 cm.

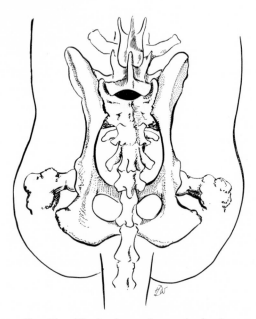

FIG. 71.—The lumbosacral space in the dog.

Solutions Used

Frank (1928) recommends a 2% procaine hydrochloride solution with 1 in 200,000 adrenaline hydrochloride. Brook (1935) in his work used Parsetic (2·25% procaine with adrenaline). Smiley (1932), using Tutocaine, had uncertain results with a 1% solution but found 2% reliable. He points out that, using Tutocaine, analgesia is present in 3 to 4 minutes and persists for 35 to 40 minutes, while with procaine the onset is delayed 10 to 15 minutes, but duration is longer (1 to 1½ hours, Spreull, 1958). Recently 1% lignocaine has been used.

Technique of Injection

The dog is probably best restrained firmly on its right side with its back adjacent to the edge of the table. (Some anaesthetists make the injection with the dog in the standing position or restrained on its breast. Sudden forceful movement, however, cannot effectively be prevented when the animal's limbs are beneath it.)

An insensitive skin weal is made just behind the last lumbar spine by the injection of a little of the local analgesic solution, using a short, fine needle. For the epidural injection a 21 gauge needle 34 to 5 cm long is employed. Its point should be cut at an angle of 45°. It is introduced directly in the midline, immediately behind the last lumbar spine, and pressed downwards and slightly backwards (assuming the animal to be in the normal position), taking care that its direction does not deviate to one side. Penetration of the inter-arcual ligament imparts a distinct 'popping' sensation to the finger. Should

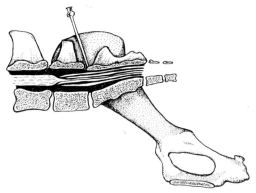

Fig. 72.—Epidural analgesia in the dog.
The site and direction for insertion of the needle.

bone rather than ligament be encountered, it indicates that the direction of the needle has been wrong and that its point has struck an articular process or the roof of the first sacral segment. If this occurs the needle is slightly withdrawn and a search made for the space by redirecting it a little backwards, forwards or to one side. As has already been mentioned, there is a remote possibility that the meningeal cul-de-sac will be penetrated, in which case cerebro-spinal fluid will escape from the needle. The needle should be gradually withdrawn until the flow ceases. Spreull stresses the necessity for ensuring that the needle point lies in the epidural and not in the subarachnoid space before injection is commenced, and states that one cannot be certain unless a test for negative pressure is made by slightly withdrawing the syringe plunger. That the canal has been entered is indicated by the complete absence of resistance to the injection. In the majority of animals no difficulty will be experienced in locating the space, but in very fat dogs it may be impossible to palpate either the iliac tuberosities or the last lumbar spine, and in these failure may attend efforts to induce spinal analgesia. Again, with highly nervous animals, movement during injection may cause failure. Smiley stresses, and other workers agree, that the injection must be made slowly, otherwise vomiting and possibly convulsions may occur. Ten to fifteen seconds should elapse during injection. The local analgesic solution should be warmed by placing ampoules in hot water before use.

Dosage and Indications

In the dog interference with motor power of the hind-limbs is of no consequence, and thus the classification block into anterior and posterior does not arise. The indications for surgical interference about the tail and perineum are less in the dog than are those about the posterior abdominal and inguinal regions, and thus the degree of epidural analgesia induced is generally of the anterior type. For abdominal interferences, the setting of hind-limb fractures, etc., Frank recommends a dosage of 1 ml per 5 lb body weight (0·5ml/kg). Brook, for the performance of posterior laparotomies such as hysterectomy or cystotomy, advises a similar dosage, expressing it as follows: For operations demanding analgesia to a little in front of the umbilicus the following is recommended:

Breed (adult)						Dosage (ml)
Pekingese	.	.	.	.	.	. 2 to 3
Fox terrier	.	.	.	.	.	7
Airedale	.	.	.	.	.	9
Larger breeds	.	.	.	.	.	11 (increased with care)

Complications

The complication most likely to occur is hypotension. Smiley records a case in which the animal died 10 minutes after completion of hysterectomy for pyometra. He states: 'Opinion was divided as to whether the causative factor was surgical shock and heart failure or a complication arising from anaesthesia or anaesthetic.' Benesch states that epidural injection in the dog is not without danger of shock if large quantities are injected rapidly. The methods of combat are similar to those outlined for cattle (page 123). The dose of methoxamine, by intravenous or intramuscular injection, is up to 5 mg. It must be born in mind that the neural canal at the lumbosacral space is almost completely occupied by the nerves comprising the cauda equinum and it is by no means impossible that some permanent injury may result from epidural injection. Again, the greatest care must be taken that all apparatus and local analgesic solution shall be sterile, otherwise the canal may become a focus of sepsis.

Discussion

Epidural analgesia in the dog was first introduced at a time when the general anaesthetic in common use was chloroform by inhalation and there was no doubt that the risks associated with it were less than with chloroform. The great advance which the introduction of the barbiturate anaesthetics represented caused the method to fall into disuse.

Within the last few years the method has again come into prominence, particularly for abdominal operations and for fracture treatment about the hind-limbs. Harthoorn and Brass (1954) working in the Hannover School report favourably on the method in a series of cases widely representative of abdominal surgery. They used 2% procaine hydrochloride solution without adrenaline following the dosage recommended by Frey (1957) relative to body-length, and as a standard for a dog of 55 to 60 cm (occiput–tail root measurement) injected 1 ml for each 10 cm into the lumbosacral space. Smaller dogs were given slightly less and larger dogs rather more than this dose. For operations involving the stomach they recommend that the dose be increased by $\frac{1}{2}$ to 1 ml, for although the standard dose was adequate for incision of the abdominal wall, sensation was sometimes evinced when traction was exerted on the mesogastrium. Except in acutely toxaemic cases, morphine was used for premedication. In general, analgesia was entirely satisfactory for operations of up to 40 minutes' duration. In two cases in which abdominal interference was prolonged beyond this time, returning sensation necessitated the induction of general anaesthesia. In one case motor paralysis without loss of sensation developed. No deaths ascribable to the method occurred nor were there any late ill-effects. Joshua (1956) has also reported experience of the method in dogs of all types and size and she confirms the absence of ill-effects either locally or generally; she acknowledges, however, technical failure in a small proportion of cases. 1% lignocaine hydrochloride solution with 1/100 000 adrenaline was used in a dosage range of 1·5 to 11 ml, according to the size of the dog, for operations behind the umbilicus.

Among the advantages of the method over general anaesthesia are: the absence of respiratory worries when dealing with the brachicephalic breeds, the completeness of muscle relaxation, the absence of straining when traction is applied to the peritoneum and the absence of depression of the foetuses in Caesarean section. Evers (1968), however, recorded a 2% maternal mortality when using epidural block for Caesarean section.

REFERENCES

ARTHUR, G. H. (1956). *Vet. Rec.* **68**, 254
BROOK, G. B. (1930). *Vet. Rec.* **10**, 30
——— (1935). *Vet. Rec.* **15**, 549, 576, 597, 659
BUCHOLZ, J. (1948). *Diss. Giessen Tierärztl. Umschau.* **3**, 149
CUILLE, J. and CHELLE, P. (1931). *Rev. gen. Med. Vet.* **40**, 393
EVERS, W. H. (1968). *Vet. Med. small Anim. Clin.* **63**, 1121

146   VETERINARY ANAESTHESIA AND ANALGESIA

FRANK, E. R. (1928). *J. Am. vet. med. Ass.* **72**, 336.
—— (1931). *Vet. Rec.* **11**, 867
FREY, H. A. (1951). Cited by Harthoorn and Brass (1954)
HARTHOORN, A. M. and BRASS, W. (1954). *Vet. Rec.* **66**, 117
HOPCROFT, S. C. (1965). *Brit. J. Anaesth.* **37**, 982
JOSHUA, J. O. (1956), *Vet. Rec.* **68**, 801
MAGDA, I. I., SHALDUGA, N. E. and VOSKOVOINIKOV, M. (1952). *Veterinariya*, **29**, 47
SMILEY, H. D. (1932). *J. Am. vet. med. Ass.* **80**, 565
SPREULL, J. S. A. (1958). *Vet. Rec.* **70**, 981
ST. CLAIR, L. E. and HARDENBROOK, J. H. (1956) *J. Am. vet. med. Ass.* **129**, 405

9

Premedication

Pre-anaesthetic medication or 'premedication' helps both the anaesthetist and the animal, for it makes the induction and maintenance of anaesthesia easier for the anaesthetist while at the same time rendering the experience safer and more comfortable for the patient. It implies the administration, usually before but sometimes immediately after the induction of anaesthesia, of both sedative drugs and agents which inhibit not only the flow of saliva but also secretion from the glands of the tracheobronchial tree. This medication is valuable in overcoming the apprehension, fear and resistance to anaesthesia (provoked by strange attendants, strange surroundings and the necessary preparations for surgery) which are often only too apparent in many animals when sedatives have not been given. By controlling this emotional disturbance and thus minimizing the release of catecholamines, suitable premedication smooths the whole course of anaesthesia and ensures a quiet emergence from the anaesthetic state.

The degree of activity of the central nervous system at the time when anaesthesia is induced determines the amount of anaesthetic which has to be administered to produce surgical anaesthesia. This activity is lowered by wasting diseases, senility and surgical shock and increased by fear, pain, fever and conditions such as thyrotoxicosis. Sedatives, tranquillizers and analgesics are used in premedication to decrease the irritability of the central nervous system and thereby enhance the effects of the anaesthetic agents. In general, the depressant effects of the drugs used in premedication summate with those of the anaesthetic and unless this is clearly understood overdosage may occur. Many sedative drugs depress respiration, and if given in large doses before the administration of an anaesthetic which also produces respiratory depression (e.g. thiopentone sodium or halothane), respiratory failure may occur before surgical anaesthesia is attained. Premedication must, therefore, be regarded as an integral part of the whole anaesthetic technique, and never considered as an isolated event.

In the past, premedication has often been given simply to ensure a quiet recovery from anaesthesia. However, it may well also prolong the recovery period, and this is not always acceptable. A prolonged recovery may cause serious difficulties in equine surgery and is most undesirable in ruminants. The provision of a padded, dimly-lit area where an animal can recover undisturbed by stimuli from the environment is a better way of ensuring that recovery will be free from excitement, and premedication should only be used for this purpose when this provision cannot be made.

Premedication may be given by any one or more of the five routes of drug administration. The choice is governed both by the nature of the drug to be used and the time which is available. If there is plenty of time before anaesthesia is to be induced then the drugs may be given by mouth or into the rectum. (The rectal route is not, however, very satisfactory and is only used when for some reason the others are impracticable.) If about an hour is available then subcutaneous or intramuscular injection can be used, but if only 5 to 10 minutes will elapse before anaesthesia is induced then the intravenous route must be employed. It is always as well to ensure that the preliminary medication exerts its full effects before the administration of a general anaesthetic is begun; otherwise respiratory depression and respiratory failure may occur even during light anaesthesia.

In all animals, when pain is present, an analgesic drug should be incorporated in the premedication, and in animals other than ruminants and horses the addition of a 'drying agent' such as atropine or hyoscine is beneficial in minimizing secretions in the respiratory passages. In ruminants these 'drying agents' do not stop the flow of saliva; they seem to have the property of making the secretions more viscid and, thus, more difficult to remove from the respiratory tract. Opinion is divided as to their usefulness in horses. Because copious salivation and bronchial secretion is not a problem (irritant agents such as ether are seldom, if ever, employed), some anaesthetists never administer drying agents to horses. Others argue that their inclusion in the premedication may be of value in blocking the muscarinic effects of depolarizing muscle relaxants commonly used in equine anaesthesia.

The last decade has seen the introduction and development of a technique named 'neuroleptanalgesia'. Briefly, this technique involves the use of analgesic drugs to produce sufficient depression of the central nervous system to enable surgical operations to be performed without the patient being aware of pain. Most analgesics produce effects other than analgesia, and since most of these (e.g. nausea, vomiting, respiratory depression) are undesirable, a second agent is incorporated into the technique to counteract them. The so called 'neuroleptic' drugs used in this technique are tranquillizers which possess the ability to antagonize the emetic activity of morphine-like analgesics.

New powerful morphine-like analgesics have widened the scope of the technique, but there is nothing new in combining analgesia with sedation; many veterinarians have for many years used combinations of narcotics and tranquillizers to make animals more manageable. The introduction of the ugly word 'neuroleptanalgesia' to describe this well-recognized technique cannot be welcomed, for it is a term which has defied definition in the English language.

When the newer powerful analgesics were first introduced into veterinary practice as part of neuroleptanalgesia the aim was to produce surgically useful levels of central nervous depression by these drugs alone (Marsboom and Mortelmans, 1964). However, for a variety of reasons, these attempts proved to be either undesirable or unsuccessful, and so neuroleptanalgesia came to be supplemented by the administration of anaesthetic agents to provide conditions under which surgery could be performed (Soma and Shields, 1964). With the passage of the years the dosage levels of the drugs decreased, while anaesthetic supplementation increased, so that now 'neuroleptanalgesia' appears to refer to rather heavy premedication in which the very powerful analgesics play a prominent part. Thus, it seems logical to discuss neuro-leptanalgesia under the heading of 'premedication' rather than as an alternative to the older methods of general anaesthesia.

Drugs Employed

Atropine, hyoscine, sedative narcotics, tranquillizers and analgesics all have a place in premedication. The choice of drug and the dosage to be used in any particular case gives the anaesthetist an opportunity to demonstrate artistry as well as science.

Atropine

The most important of the alkaloids obtained from *Atropa belladonna* (deadly nightshade), atropine is used in anaesthesia as its water-soluble sulphate.

The metabolism of atropine is not the same in all species of animal. When administered to dogs, atropine disappears very rapidly from the bloodstream. Part of the dose is excreted unchanged in the urine, part appears in the urine as tropine and the remainder is apparently broken down in the body to as yet unidentified products. In cats atropine is hydrolysed by either of two ester-ases which occur in large quantities in the liver and kidneys. These esterases are also found in rabbits and rats, but their presence has not been demon-strated in other animals.

Atropine inhibits transmission of post-ganglionic cholinergic nerve impulses to effector cells. Inhibition is not equally effective all over the body, and atropine has less effect upon the urinary bladder and intestines than upon the heart and salivary glands. It is used in premedication as an antisialogogue, and to antagonize the unwanted muscarinic action of anticholinesterases when these are required for their nicotinic effects at the motor endplates of striated muscle.

Certain cerebral and medullary centres are stimulated and subsequently depressed by high doses of atropine. Death from atropine poisoning results from respiratory failure due to depression of the respiratory centre. Small doses given by subcutaneous or very slow intravenous injection produce an initial powerful vagal stimulation with obvious cardiac slowing.

The main action of atropine is on the heart rate, which it usually increases by inhibiting the cardiac vagus peripherally; the initial slowing due to central action is only seen before the onset of the peripheral inhibition. Blood pressure is usually unchanged, but if already depressed by vagal activity due to reflex or drug action (e.g. halothane) it will be raised by the administration of atropine.

The minute volume of respiration is slightly increased due to central stimulation. Bronchial musculature is relaxed and bronchial secretions are reduced. Both anatomical and physiological dead-space are increased by atropine (Nunn and Bergman, 1964). The report by Tomlin, Conway and Payne (1964), that the administration of atropine was associated with hypoxaemia in the pre-operative, operative and post-operative periods in man, has not been confirmed by more recent studies (Scott and Taylor, 1964; Taylor, Scott and Donald, 1964). Studies in dogs at the Cambridge School and elsewhere have shown no hypoxaemia attributable to atropine administration.

Mydriasis results from the local or systemic administration of atropine and thus it is probable that atropine should not be given to animals suffering from glaucoma. The mydriasis may interfere with the ocular signs of anaesthesia (see page 199).

In pigs, dogs and cats atropine may be given by subcutaneous injection 20 to 40 minutes before the administration of anaesthetic agents or depolarizing muscle relaxants which provoke secretory activity in salivary and bronchial glands. (For a more rapid effect atropine may, of course, be given by intramuscular or intravenous injection.) The dose of atropine for pigs and dogs ranges, according to the size of animal, from 1·8 to 0·3 mg while 0·3 mg is adequate for the largest of cats. The exact dose is largely determined by the fact that atropine sulphate for injection is still supplied (at least in the United Kingdom) in a solution containing 0·6 mg/ml—a legacy from earlier times when doses were measured in grains. Atropine should not be given to ruminants, for clinically acceptable doses make their copious secretions more viscid and, therefore, more difficult to remove from the mouth and respiratory tract. When ether is to be administered to a horse, the animal may be premedicated with up to 60 mg of atropine sulphate.

To neutralize the muscarinic effects of the anticholinesterases, such as neostigmine, in cats, dogs and pigs, 0·6 to 1·2 mg of atropine sulphate are usually given slowly intravenously 2 to 5 minutes before these agents are injected. In horses doses of 10 mg appear to be adequate for this purpose. Kemp and Morton (1962) have shown that, at least in man, atropine and neostigmine may safely be given together.

Hyoscine

Hyoscine (Scopolamine) is an alkaloid resembling atropine, found in the same group of plants but usually obtained from the shrub henbane (*Hyoscyamus niger*). The peripheral actions of hyoscine resemble those of atropine. It blocks the action of acetylcholine liberated at parasympathetic post-ganglionic nerve endings and, in fact, at any site where this exhibits muscarine-like effects.

When given by subcutaneous injection it tends to cause a decrease in heart rate by central stimulant activity; when given by intravenous injection it usually causes an increase in heart rate. In man, hyoscine is known to produce amnesia and is used to control motion sickness, though its exact mode of action is uncertain.

In horses, hyoscine may produce considerable excitement and, in general, it may be said that although hyoscine is used in man as a depressant of nervous activity it is not suitable for this purpose in animals. It has been used as the hydrobromide for premedication in dogs in doses of 0·2 to 0·4 mg and it is often used in combination with papaveretum (Omnopon–Scopolamine, Roche). The standard preparation contains 20 mg of papaveretum with 0·4 mg of hyoscine per ml of solution.

Morphine

Morphine is the principal alkaloid found in opium (the partially dried latex obtained from the unripe capsule of *Papaver somniferum*). It is probably the most powerful naturally occurring analgesic drug. As the alkaloid itself is practically insoluble in water, it is used as one of its soluble salts—usually the sulphate or hydrochloride. A phenanthrene derivative, it was first isolated by Serturner in 1803 but its synthesis is comparatively recent. There is no commercial production except by extraction from opium because its synthesis is difficult.

After subcutaneous injection the onset of the drug's action occurs in 5 to 10 minutes and the maximum effects are seen after 45 to 60 minutes. The actions of morphine in normal, healthy, pain-free animals have been well described by Alexander (1960). It depresses the higher functions of the brain, stimulates then depresses medullary functions, and stimulates spinal reflexes. In birds, rabbits and dogs it is said to act as a depressant producing sleep in addition to analgesia and, in large doses, coma. In the cat, all but small doses cause what Alexander describes as 'delirium' and what others have described as 'maniacal excitement'. In normal horses, cattle and pigs its effect is said to be unreliable, sometimes producing narcosis and sometimes excitement. In dogs it may produce a pin-point pupil by excitation of the nucleus of the oculo-motor nerve, as it does in man. In other species of animal it may cause sufficient excitement to dilate the pupil.

The stimulant effect on the vagal centre increases gastro-intestinal activity. The tone of the visceral muscle is raised, especially that of the pyloric, ileo-colic and anal sphincters. Segmenting contractions increase and truly propulsive movements diminish. The delay of intestinal contents in the large bowel allows an increased absorption of water to occur and, finally, the normal defaecation reflex is inhibited more easily than usual because the distended rectum no longer produces the usual discomfort. In species of animal with a developed vomiting centre morphine first stimulates then suppresses vomiting. When vomiting occurs it is not necessarily associated with the usual unpleasant emotional reactions even when violent and repeated, so that animals do not appear distressed. Morphine also produces retention of urine, distension of the bladder causing less central effect.

Effects upon the respiratory system are mainly through the central nervous system. Although the central depression decreases respiratory activity, respiration becoming slow and deep, it is most important to note that the analgesic effect of morphine vastly improves respiration where this has been fast, shallow and inefficient due to pleural pain or trauma. Similarly, where the lungs are oedematous, as in left ventricular failure, central depression by morphine prevents the Hering–Breuer reflex from initiating expiration before a useful inspiratory volume has been achieved. Morphine crosses the placenta and reaches the foetus, depressing its respiratory centre and making the initiation of breathing difficult after birth. Analgesic doses of morphine do not affect normal uterine contractions at parturition.

Therapeutic doses have negligible effects upon the heart rate and blood pressure, but larger doses slow the heart by depressing conduction in the myocardium and stimulation of the vagal centre.

Although the most profound actions of morphine are on the central nervous system only small traces are detectable there. About nine-tenths of a dose are eliminated, mainly by the kidneys, and mostly in a conjugated form.

Some is excreted in the faeces and more is destroyed in the liver. Traces are found in sweat and milk.

Much of the confusion concerning the actions of morphine in animals which is readily discernable on any study of the veterinary literature is, today, explicable. In the past, the recommendations of pharmacologists were accepted rather uncritically by clinicians with the result that doses administered to sick animals tended to be much too high. Careful observations have now convinced clinicians that therapeutic, analgesic doses of morphine are much smaller than was formerly believed. Moreover, although it has long been known in man that morphine produces euphoria in the presence of pain, but discomfort, anxiety, fear and apprehension in normal individuals, this has only just been recognized as being equally true in animals. In general, when given in appropriate doses to relieve pain, morphine has a sedative, calming effect in all species of animal. Most of the discrepancies concerning the actions of morphine in domestic animals as found in the veterinary literature can, therefore, be accounted for by the fact that pharmacologists have reported its effects in normal animals while clinicians have recorded its use (often in excessive doses) in animals suffering pain.

The analgesic effect of morphine reaches its peak about 20 minutes after intravenous injection and about $1\frac{1}{2}$ hours after intramuscular or subcutaneous injection. Duration of action is about 4 hours. The best effects are obtained when dosage precedes the onset of painful stimuli and thus morphine should be given in the anaesthetic recovery period before consciousness is regained. Morphine appears to relieve pain in at least three ways: by raising the threshold of appreciation of pain; by inducing sleep which in itself raises the pain threshold; and by inducing hypercapnia which produces a further rise in the pain threshold. Reduction in body temperature, due to lowered muscular activity, increased heat loss through peripheral vasodilatation and decreased metabolic rate, may also be a contributory factor.

The dose of morphine for horses and cattle is up to 60 mg for very large animals; pigs may be given up to 20 mg, dogs up to 10 mg and cats 0·1 mg/kg. Morphine is conjugated less readily in cats than in dogs, but the duration of action is still of the order of 4 hours (Davis and Donnelly, 1968).

Papaveretum

Papaveretum, better known as Omnopon (Roche), is often used in dogs instead of morphine. It is a preparation which contains all the alkaloids of opium and seems to cause less nausea and vomiting than morphine itself. Large dogs may be given 20 mg of Omnopon for anaesthetic premedication and this dose contains 10 mg of morphine. The preparation known as Omnopon–Scopolamine (Roche) is also convenient for premedication (see page 151).

One ampoule of this preparation given by intramuscular injection together with 3 to 5 mg of acepromazine has been found to make even the largest and most vicious of dogs easy to handle with safety.

Pethidine

Pethidine (meperidine) hydrochloride, ethyl-1-methyl-4-phenylpiperidine-4-carboxylate hydrochloride, combines spasmolytic properties comparable with those of atropine and papaverine with a central analgesic action similar to that of morphine. It has little hypnotic effect and relieves pain without interfering with muscular activity, muscle coordination or special sense responses. Therapeutic doses have very little effect on blood pressure and the cough centre is not depressed although there is some degree of respiratory depression. Pethidine is rapidly destroyed in the liver and very few toxic reactions have been reported after normal doses, but there is evidence that in ruminants and dogs the injection of the drug may cause the release of histamine.

There is little species variation in response to its depressant action, and unless an emetic action is particularly desired, pethidine can replace morphine in pre-operative medication. When administered by injection, it acts in 10 to 15 minutes and its effects last for 3 to 4 hours. About 100 mg of pethidine are equivalent, in terms of pain relief, to 10 mg of morphine. Horses and cattle are given up to 1 g; pigs up to 0·5 g; dogs up to 150 mg; cats up to 10 g. If these doses are exceeded undesirable respiratory depression may be produced. It was at one time believed that this respiratory depression could be overcome by giving pethidine together with a small amount of a specific antagonist such as levallorphan. A preparation of this nature was known as Pethilorfan (Roche), each millilitre of this solution containing 50 mg pethidine and 0·625 mg of Lorfan (levallorphan tartrate). However, it is now considered that the antagonist also reduces the analgesic activity of the pethidine. The same degree of analgesia as produced by a given dose of Pethilorfan can be achieved with a smaller dose of pethidine alone without any more respiratory depression than that produced by the Pethilorfan dose. The inclusion of an antidote in this manner is, therefore, of no advantage.

Diethylthiambutene

Diethylthiambutene hydrochloride (Themalon) is the name given to 3-diethylamino-1:1 dithienylbut-1-ene hydrochloride, a white crystalline solid marketed in 50 mg tablets. These tablets are dissolved in water to give a solution of 25 to 100 mg/ml which is given by subcutaneous or intravenous injection.

The drug is only used in dogs and in these animals it has analgesic and hypnotic properties similar to those of morphine. Owen (1955), in clinical studies on dogs of various breeds, ages and weights, adopted a standard dosage of 2·2 mg/kg by subcutaneous injection and 4·4 mg/kg by intravenous injection. The depths of narcosis induced using both routes of administration varied in individual animals from light to deep.

Administration of the drug usually causes increased salivation (which often cannot be readily controlled by the usual doses of atropine) and defaecation. Intravenous injection may provoke struggling, high-pitched barking and convulsive movements of legs. A most striking feature is the length of time for which the respiratory depressant effects produced by the drug appear to persist. Induction of anaesthesia with very small quantities of anaesthetic agent any time up to four or five days after the administration of diethylthiambutene may result in respiratory failure.

Undesirable side-effects following normal doses are not uncommon. Some dogs are said to be 'hypersensitive', convulsions or tetany occurring when the drug is given by intravenous injection. A period of depression with nausea and vomiting is seen in some animals following apparent recovery from the larger doses, especially when these have been given by subcutaneous injection. Nalorphine (N-allylnormorphine) has been used as an antagonist to diethylthiambutene, and dogs which have been deeply narcotized with this drug can be restored to consciousness by the injection of suitable quantities of Nalorphine. However, these dogs remain in a very sleepy condition for a further 48 to 72 hours after the administration of the antagonist and some relapse into the unconscious state for many hours.

In horses, cattle and cats, diethylthiambutene gives rise to undesirable effects such as muscle spasms, muscle tremors and narcotic excitement.

Methadone

Methadone (Amidon, Adanon, Dolophine, Diasone, Miadone, Physeptone, Polamidon, Polamivet) is another synthetic substance which has many of the properties of morphine including the production of addiction in man. Although a good analgesic it also produces respiratory depression.

This compound has been widely used on the Continent of Europe, usually in conjunction with a phenothiazine ataractic (see page 163), but it has not been used to any extent in veterinary practice in the United Kingdom. The preparation used on the Continent, Polamivet, contains 2·5 mg of the laevorotatory isomer of methadone, together with 0·125 mg of the atropine-like compound diphenylpiperidino-ethylacetamide hydrochloride, per millilitre of solution. The dose for the horse is 0·1 mg/kg; dogs may be given up to 0·25 mg/kg.

Pentazocine

Pentazocine, 2'-hydroxy-5, 9-dimethyl-2-2(3, 3-dimethylallyl)-6-7-benzomorphan, is an analgesic discovered during investigation of a new group of narcotic antagonists based on the benzmorphan nucleus (Archer and Keats, 1962). These investigations were stimulated by the unexpected finding that nalorphine (N-allylnormorphine), which had been introduced into medicine as a morphine antagonist, was comparable to morphine as an analgesic, yet did not produce addiction in man. Pentazocine was the most promising compound discovered, and it was found that, although only weakly antagonistic to morphine, it was as effective as morphine in controlling severe pain. In man Swerdlow and Dalal (1966) and Dundee, Clarke, Loan and Hamilton (1967) found 20 mg pentazocine to be as effective as 10 mg of morphine. The WHO Expert Committee on Dependence-producing Drugs officially recommended in 1966 that narcotics control and restrictions as applied to opiates were not needed either internationally or nationally for pentazocine.

The freedom from restriction in use may well make pentazocine a most valuable analgesic for veterinary use. So far it has not been very widely used, but, in dogs, parenteral doses of up to 30 mg given every 4 hours have produced no untoward effects. It is still too early to assess the effectiveness of the drug in the relief of pain in animals. In experimentally induced pain in horses pentazocine has been shown to produce analgesia lasting 15 to 90 minutes with increasing doses of 0·5 to 4·0 mg/kg; doses in excess of 4·0 mg/kg resulted in ataxia and muscle tremors (Lowe, 1969). This compound is also said to be effective when given by mouth.

The Strong Analgesics

In recent years some very potent analgesic drugs have been introduced into medical and veterinary practice, often as part of neuroleptanalgesia.

Etorphine (M99)

This is a recently introduced, very potent derivative of morphine which is, apparently, effective in a dose of about 0·5 mg per 500 kg. It appears to have all the properties of morphine, its sole advantage being its great potency. Because the effective dose can be dissolved in a very small volume of solvent, it has been widely used by dart injection to immobilize wild game. In anaesthetic practice its very potency makes it a difficult drug to handle, while its property of producing stimulation before depression of the central nervous system is highly undesirable, especially in equidae. In an attempt to overcome this initial excitement etorphine is now marketed in combination with a phenothiazine tranquillizer (see page 163) and both small animal and large animal packs are available (Immobilon). Small animal Immobilon contains 0·074 mg etorphine hydrochloride together with 18 mg methotrimeprazine/ml of solution, while each millilitre of large animal Immobilon contains 2·45 mg etorphine hydrochloride and 10 mg acetylpromazine maleate. Like all opiates, etorphine can be antagonized by related compounds. A specific antagonist, diprenorphine, has been synthesized and is available in a small animal and a large animal preparation (Revivon). The Revivon solutions have been designed to balance the Immobilon preparations, small animal Revivon containing 0·272 mg and large animal Revivon 3·0 mg diprenorphine hydrochloride/ml of solution.

Horses are given 0·5 ml/50 kg of large animal Immobilon by intramuscular injection, or 0·25 to 0·5 ml/50 kg intravenously. Cattle receive 0·5 ml/50 kg by either route, sheep 0·25 ml/50 kg and pigs 0·5 ml/50 kg by intramuscular injection. Intravenous injection in horses is claimed to minimize the initial excitement phase. In all these animals awakening is achieved by the intra-venous injection of a like volume of large animal Revivon. The volume of Revivon injected must always be the same as the total amount of Immobilon used irrespective of the injection route used for the Immobilon.

Dogs are given 0·1 ml/kg intramuscularly, or 0·05 ml/kg intravenously, of the small animal Immobilon, and awakened by the intravenous injection of a like volume of the small animal preparation of Revivon.

It is likely that Immobilon and Revivon will prove useful in dogs and pigs because in these animals combinations of opiates and phenothiazine tran-quillizers have been employed for many years with generally satisfactory results. As yet, however, even in these species, little is known of the effects of Immobilon and Revivon in clinical cases where systemic disease may compli-cate the picture.

In horses the method of 'knockdown' followed by pharmacological reversal with recovery in a matter of a few minutes is very attractive. There is no doubt that if Immobilon and Revivon can be shown to be devoid of harmful effects these drugs may make a major contribution to equine anaesthesia and restraint. However, to date essential information concerning their effect on blood pressure, cardiac output, respiration and the activity of the gut and bladder is lacking. Moreover, the initial excitement, even if brief and easily managed in small experimental ponies, may prove to be a serious disadvantage in large, less easily controlled horses. Yet another very undesirable feature has recently come to light—etorphine, being excreted in the bile, recycles from the intestine and produces prolonged excitatory effects which appear several hours after apparent recovery. Unless these are expected and troublesome precautions are taken, horses

may inflict severe damage on themselves during this second excitement
period.

Phenoperidine (R1406)

This is a typical morphine-like analgesic which is about 50 times more
potent, but shorter-acting than pethidine. It has not been widely used in
veterinary medicine.

Phentanyl (R4263, Sublimaze, Fentanyl)

This is a 4-acylanilino-piperidine compound, shorter-acting than phenoperidine and about 1000 times as potent as pethidine. It has been used to
produce complete surgical anaesthesia in dogs (Marsboom, Verstraete, Thienpont and Mattheeuws, 1964), but is usually given with an ataractic ('neuroleptic') in neuroleptanalgesia.

The pharmacology of phentanyl, N-(1-phenethyl-4-piperidinyl) proprion-
anilide dihydrogen citrate, has been described by Yelnosky and Gordocks
(1963) and Marsboom and Mortelmans (1964). It reduces sensitivity to pain
in all animals and causes respiratory depression which can be counteracted
with nalorphine. In dogs, rats and primates it induces sedation and myosis,
but in horses, mice and cats it is said to produce excitement and mydriasis.

Phentanyl was used with haloanisone (see page 168) for neuroleptanalgesia
in dogs by Marsboom *et al.* in 1964 as a 1:50 mixture (Haloanisone Comp.).
Given at a dosage level of 0·1 mg/kg of phentanyl with 5 mg/kg of haloanisone
by slow intravenous injection it produced a period of surgical anaesthesia
after short and mild excitement. Recovery was slow, the time varying from
2 to 10 hours before recovery of full consciousness. These workers compared
the results of this technique with what appears to have been badly administered thiopentone–halothane anaesthesia and concluded that the neuroleptanalgesia was safer, with minimum toxicity, and impressive cardiovascular
stability.

Soma and Shields (1964) found that in dogs it was necessary to give atropine to prevent bradycardia caused by the intra-muscular injection of a 1:50
phentanyl–dehydrobenzperidol (Droperidol, see page 183) mixture (Innovar–
Vet). The analgesia, sedation and immobility produced by this mixture were
sufficient for diagnostic procedures and minor surgical intervention. Complete unconsciousness was not produced and the dogs could respond to auditory stimuli. The respiratory effects of the combination were variable, with
both hyperpnoea and respiratory depression occurring. They concluded that
the advantages of their mixture were ease of administration; wide safety

margin; quiet post-operative state; reversibility with narcotic antagonists (such as nalorphine); and tolerance by animals in poor physical condition. Its disadvantages were listed as variable response in certain breeds; the spontaneous movements which can occur; the need, on occasion, to employ nitrous oxide or local analgesia in addition; and the possibility of respiratory depression.

Phentanyl has also been used in the United Kingdom for neuroleptanalgesia in dogs. The preparation used was a combination of phentanyl (0·315 mg/ml) with haloanisone (Hypnorm). Diarrhoea has been reported to follow the administration of this mixture in over 25% of cases.

Mitchell (1966) studied the effects of phentanyl with haloanisone (0·2 mg: 10 mg/ml) and phentanyl with dehydrobenzperidol (0·05 mg: 2·5 mg/ml) in pigs. He concluded that neither mixture produced better sedation than dehydrobenzperidol given alone.

In primates and lower monkeys the results of neuroleptanalgesic techniques are more impressive (Marsboom, Mortelmans, Vercruysse and Thienpont, 1962; Marsboom, Mortelmans and Vercruysse, 1963). It would appear that in these animals the technique may have distinct advantages over the more conventional methods of general anaesthesia, especially when skilled assistance is not available.

Phencyclidine

Phencyclidine (Sernyl, Sernylan) is phenylcyclohexyl-piperidine, a compound which acts primarily on the central nervous system either by stimulation or depression, the overall effect produced varying considerably according to the species of animal concerned, and the dose rate used. It has been used in man (Griefenstein, De Vault, Yoshitake and Gaweski, 1958; Johnstone, Evans and Baigel, 1959; Collins, Gorospe and Rovenstine, 1960) and its pharmacology has been reported by Chen, Ensor, Russell and Bohner (1959). Several workers have reported its use in monkeys (Chen and Weston, 1960; Rutty and Thurley, 1962; Spalding and Heyman, 1962). In the veterinary field it has been used in goats (Wilkins, 1961), chicken (Wright and Jordan, 1963) and wild game animals (Harthoorn, 1962). However, because its effects in animals other than primates and lower monkeys have given cause for concern, it is today not recommended for general use in veterinary practice. Nevertheless, many still consider it a useful sedative for pigs.

Tavernor (1963, 1964) has given detailed accounts of the effects produced by the intramuscular injection of 2 mg/kg in pigs. This dose produces some excessive salivation which may be controlled by atropine, slight incoordination after 1 to 2 minutes and recumbency after 5 to 10 minutes. Recovery is quiet and animals are normal again within 5 to 6 hours of administration. A positive effect is achieved at lower dosage levels and pigs can be handled with ease after the intramuscular injection of 0·25 mg/kg. Tavernor had 3 deaths in 110 pigs, one being due to an overdose of halothane during anaesthesia subsequent to apparently satisfactory premedication. Another pig died after a total dose of 6 mg/kg (4 mg/kg intramuscularly followed by 2 mg/kg intravenously 20 minutes later) and one further pig (which had received 2 mg/kg) died during subsequent halothane/oxygen anaesthesia from respiratory difficulties.

In 1964 general practitioners working under field conditions reported that, in a small proportion of pigs, side-effects such as prolonged recumbency and hyperexcitability had been noted. It is possible that these side-effects may be due to the so-called 'salt-poisoning syndrome' (Scott-Cameron, 1964). The administration of phencyclidine to pigs which are on the border line as far as water intake is concerned, coupled with increased water excretion due to the excitement caused by handling and injection may, it is suggested, trigger off symptoms of 'salt-poisoning'.

It seems probable that many of the undesirable effects of phencyclidine in pigs result from the intramuscular injection of relatively large doses. Large doses are given because of the difficulty of ensuring that, in pigs, solutions really are injected into muscle, rather than into fatty tissue. Absorption from fatty tissues is slow and uncertain so that the effects of any dose deposited into fat may be disappointing. These poor results are then attributed to underdosage and on subsequent occasions a higher dose is given.

At the Cambridge School smaller doses of phencyclidine together with atropine have been given to hundreds of pigs by intravenous injection and untoward reactions have not been countered. Large sows are given up to 0·5 mg/kg with 2·4 mg of atropine sulphate into an ear vein. Sedation is almost immediately apparent after the intravenous injection; most pigs become recumbent and unable to stand within 5 to 10 minutes; and recovery is usually complete within 2 to 3 hours of injection. The degree of analgesia obtained is quite remarkable. Large sows suffering from fractures of limb bones have submitted very quietly to radiological examination and manipulation of the injured limbs while still apparently aware of their surroundings and still able to make vigorous, though uncoordinated, movements. A series of over 200 boars weighing between 110 and 180 kg have received 0·2 mg/kg of phencyclidine with 1·2 to 1·8 mg of atropine sulphate by injection into an ear vein prior to halothane/oxygen anaesthesia. The sedation produced was a little variable but it was always sufficient for anaesthesia to be induced without difficulty and was never so deep as to cause concern for the animals' welfare. Respiratory depression was not observed either before or during anaesthesia.

Tiletamine Hydrochloride

Tiletamine hydrochloride (CI-634), known chemically as 2-(ethylamino)-2-(2-thienyl) cyclohexanone hydrochloride, is a new cataleptic agent for cats. It is similar to phencyclidine hydrochloride and to another compound, ketamine hydrochloride, which is used in man.

The pharmacology of tiletamine has been reported by Chen and Ensor (1968) and the compound has been subjected to numerous clinical trials. Given by intramuscular injection in doses of 0·5 to 1·0 mg/kg it produces salivation (which is easily controlled with atropine), lacrimation, mydriasis and ataxia. Recovery, as indicated by ability to walk without ataxia, occurs within 1 to $1\frac{1}{2}$ hours. At this dosage level the threshold to external stimuli is increased, there is no loss of consciousness or analgesia of the skin. Doses of 5 to 10 mg/kg produce observable sedation after 3 minutes. Loss of consciousness is not apparent at the lower end of the dosage scale but unconsciousness seems to be produced by doses of 10 mg/kg. Response to stimulation is generally absent and recovery occurs in from 2 to 8 hours. High doses of 20 to 30 mg/kg given by intramuscular injection produce deep depression bordering on general anaesthesia which lasts 1 to 2 hours. The swallowing, pedal and palpebral reflexes are not abolished and muscle relaxation is absent. Recovery after these high doses occupies 8 to 12 hours or even longer. Even very high doses of the drug have little effect on the cardiovascular system.

Although introduced for clinical trial as an anaesthetic agent for cats, it seems unlikely that tiletamine will be accepted as such in veterinary practice. At the high doses required to abolish response to stimulation, the respiratory depression produced, together with the lack of muscle relaxation and long recovery period, are serious disadvantages (Garmer, 1969). Another disadvantage of the preparation made available for trials is that its intramuscular injection causes pain. However, if another formulation which does not give rise to pain on injection can be made, tiletamine may prove to be a useful agent for immobilization and premedication of cats.

Xylazine

Xylazine (Rompun, Bayer, Va 1470) is a new sedative agent, 2-(2,6 dimethylphenylamino) 5-6 dihydro-4H-1,3-thiazine, first synthesized in 1962. Its pharmacological properties have been investigated in animals and in man (Wirth, Hoffmeister and Krieskott, 1965; Kroneberg, Oberdorf, Hoffmeister and Wirth, 1966; Oberdorf, Hoffmeister and Kroneberg, 1967) and it has been subjected to clinical trials in Western Germany, the United Kingdom and the United States of America. It was supplied for trial as clear, colourless, 2% and 10% solutions for intravenous and intramuscular injection.

6

Although xylazine may be given to all domestic animals it would appear to have no place in the management of canine, feline or porcine patients. In dogs and cats better sedation can be produced with other agents and in pigs its effects are too fleeting to be of any practical value. It is in the management of horses, cattle, sheep and goats that this compound appears to hold great promise. Although not devoid of undesirable attributes it possesses certain properties which make it a better sedative for horses than any other compound in current use. In cattle, sheep and goats it can be used to produce depression of the central nervous system ranging from mild sedation to deep basal narcosis.

In horses, intramuscular injection of a 10% solution is well tolerated and 2 to 3 mg/kg produce deep sedation which develops over 10 to 15 minutes following the injection. Deep sedation lasts 15 to 20 minutes and recovery is complete within 1 to 2 hours of injection. Xylazine may also be given by slow intravenous injection in doses of 0·5 mg/kg, producing an almost immediate effect of deep sedation lasting 15 to 20 minutes, followed by complete recovery within 30 minutes of the time of administration. The deep sedation produced by xylazine is characterized by lowering of the head, drooping of the eyelids and lower lip and a marked reluctance to move. In the male, the penis protrudes from the prepuce but this is not a marked feature of the drug's action. While it is possible to arouse the sedated animal, this arousal is never associated with excitement as it can be in animals under phenothiazine derivative-type sedation. Horses do not 'go down' after these doses of xylazine and there is no noticeable analgesia. The intramuscular injection of the drug produces only negligible effects on the cardiovascular and respiratory systems, but intravenous injection causes an immediate, transient rise in arterial blood pressure, bradycardia and a fall in cardiac output (Clarke and Hall, 1969). Most horses given xylazine sweat around the ears and poll region, and seem particularly sensitive to noise during the recovery period although evidence of excitement during the recovery period has never been recorded.

Cattle are much more sensitive to xylazine. The intramuscular injection of 0·05 to 0·1 mg/kg is sufficient to produce deep sedation in most animals and they lie down within 10 to 20 minutes after the injection. Deep sedation lasts 30 to 35 minutes and recovery is usually complete in 2 to 3 hours. Intravenous injection of these doses produces much more profound sedation which closely resembles deep narcosis induced with chloral hydrate (see page 179). In cattle, xylazine produces a rise in blood sugar and it is said to be contra-indicated in the last trimester of pregnancy because premature birth has been reported after its administration to heavily pregnant cows. Although the ability to eructate, cough and swallow is retained during the period of sedation, cattle must be closely watched during the recovery period. It has been found that some animals will get to their feet, walk around and appear fully conscious, then relapse in lateral recumbency and become tympanitic. These recumbent animals must be disturbed so as to provoke eructation. Fortunately, this danger period does not last for more than 2 to 3 hours.

Some reports indicate that xylazine produces analgesia in cattle, and surgical operations have been performed under the sedation produced by this compound on its own. Others have reported an absence of demonstrable analgesia, and have stated that for surgery supplementation with a general anaesthetic or the use of local analgesia was essential to prevent movement in response to painful stimulation.

The use of xylazine for premedication has apparently been followed by less respiratory depression during anaesthesia than is encountered after premedication with acepromazine (see page 167). Recovery after anaesthesia has not been as quiet as after acepromazine premedication, presumably because of the relatively shorter duration of action of xylazine.

Xylazine has been given to several mares to produce sedation at the time of service, and at regular intervals through the subsequent pregnancies right up to parturition. None aborted and all foals born were normal in every respect.

Sheep are more resistant, and goats more susceptible, than cattle to the effects of xylazine, but this compound promises to be a useful sedative for both these species of animal.

Ataractics

An ataractic drug is one which produces sedation without at the same time causing drowsiness. (Ataraxy is defined in the *Shorter Oxford Dictionary* as 'stoical indifference' or as 'freedom from disturbance of mind'.) Such sedatives are popularly known as 'tranquillizers'. This group of drugs includes the Rauwolfia derivatives such as reserpine, the phenothiazine derivatives, the diphenylmethyl compounds, the butyrophenones and the benzodiazepam derivatives. Of these various compounds only the phenothiazine derivatives and the butyrophenones have been used to any extent for premedication in veterinary anaesthesia.

The ataractic drugs derived from phenothiazine have a wide range of pharmacological actions. As a group, it may be said that in general they produce central sedative effects coupled with a variety of peripheral effects such as antihistamine or anti-adrenaline activity. The degrees of activity in the different pharmacological actions vary, sometimes markedly, from one compound to another. For example, chlorpromazine is characterized by a clinically useful sedative action, a marked anti-adrenaline activity and a very weak antihistamine action, while promethazine has a similar central sedative activity, but is a valuable antihistaminic and has very little anti-adrenaline action. So far it has not been possible to correlate in detail these variations in pharmacological activity with variations in chemical structure.

It appears that the central sedative action of these compounds is exerted at subcortical levels, probably on the brain stem arousal mechanism (reticular activating system). It is known that an afferent stimulus capable of causing arousal takes two routes to the brain. One is through the classical sensory system to the appropriate part of the sensory cortex and the other through the central part of the brain in a neuronal mesh called the 'reticular system', and entry to this path is by means of collaterals from the main sensory tracts. This secondary system prepares, or alerts, the brain to receive and appreciate stimuli which arrive by the classical route at specific areas in the sensory cortex, and in the absence of this alerting process stimuli reaching the cortex by the classical route cannot enter into full consciousness. Thus, by their depressant action, the ataractic drugs reduce alertness and therefore the extent to which afferent stimuli are perceived and their implications appreciated. This ensures a tranquil mental state free from disturbance of mood, and the anaesthetics which act primarily on the cortical system become effective in lower concentration. Also by lowering alertness they make pain more endurable.

The consequences of a specific depression of the reticular system are many and varied. Beside the potentiation of the effects of anaesthetics there are other actions such as antiemetic, antipyretic, hypothermic and hypotensive actions.

Promethazine Hydrochloride (Phenergan)

This is 10-2'-dimethylaminopropyl-phenothiazine hydrochloride. Solutions of this drug are irritant to the tissues and should be injected deeply in a large muscle mass 40 to 60 minutes before anaesthesia. In emergencies the drug can be given, after dilution with isotonic saline, by very slow intravenous injection. Rapid intravenous injection causes a profound fall in blood pressure which may be fatal in shocked animals.

Chlorpromazine Hydrochloride (Largactil, Thorazine)

This is 2-chloro-10-3'-dimethylaminopropyl-phenothiazine hydrochloride, and has been used most extensively in veterinary practice. Its central sedative action is marked and in domestic animals it blocks conditioned responses but does not interfere with responses to unconditioned stimuli such as needle pricks and painful manipulations. It has potent anti-emetic, anti-adrenaline and vagolytic properties. Since it causes vasodilatation it should be used with caution in animals suffering from shock, but if given prior to operation it will counteract any tendency to tissue hypoxia and help to prevent the onset of shock.

Chlorpromazine has a wide safety margin and animals will recover from the effects of very large doses, but it should be used with caution where there is severe depression of the heart or central nervous system or where there are extensive liver or lung lesions. The liver is probably the main site for detoxication of the drug and the action of chlorpromazine is enhanced in animals suffering from liver damage. Detoxication is not rapid and even in healthy animals its effects may still be apparent 24 to 47 hours after the administration of a single intramuscular dose.

For premedication of horses, doses should not exceed 0·4 mg/kg by intramuscular injection, because larger doses may give rise to what appears to be a state of panic due to muscle weakness caused by the drug, and the animal's response may be alarming and difficult to control. The rate of absorption into the bloodstream from the site of intramuscular injection appears to be very irregular, but premedication with chlorpromazine will ensure that a horse will recover quietly from anaesthesia, even though a sedative effect may not be readily obvious before anaesthesia is induced.

Cattle should not be given chlorpromazine before the administration of a general anaesthetic for the drug will cause a most inconvenient delayed recovery. It is, however, of some use when an operation is to be performed under some type of local analgesia. Cattle may be given 1 mg/kg by intramuscular injection about one hour before the injection of the local analgesic; this dose should not be exceeded if the operation is to be performed on the standing animal.

Pigs are easily restrained for intravenous injections if chlorpromazine is given in a dose of approximately 1 mg/kg 40 to 60 minutes before venepuncture is attempted. Under the influence of chlorpromazine they do not squeal when handled and are much less likely to try to dislodge the venepuncture needle by head-shaking. Chlorpromazine itself may be given to pigs by the intravenous route but only very dilute solutions should be given if thrombosis of the vein is to be avoided. When given by intravenous injection the drug should be allowed 10 to 20 minutes to produce its full effects. Intravenous injection may be followed by hyperpnoea which lasts for about 15 minutes, but the reason for this is unknown.

Chlorpromazine was used very extensively for premedication in dogs both by intravenous and intramuscular injection, in doses up to 1 mg/kg. After intramuscular injection the full effects are not seen for 60 to 90 minutes, while after intravenous injection there is a time lag of about 10 to 15 minutes before maximum activity is manifest. Chlorpromazine premedication ensures an absence of narcotic excitement during recovery from barbiturate anaesthesia and almost completely eliminates post-anaesthetic vomiting after cyclopropane. It may be used in obstetrical cases for it does not appear to depress the respiratory centre of the puppy or suppress labour in the bitch.

In cats, chlorpromazine is an effective tranquillizing agent and may be used in doses of up to 1 mg/kg for premedication. Normal care should be observed in approaching and handling cats which have received chlorpromazine and, as always, forcible restraint should be avoided.

Promazine Hydrochloride (Sparine)

This is 10,3'-dimethylaminopropyl phenothiazine hydrochloride. Its actions are very similar to those of chlorpromazine and it has been used as an ataractic in all the domestic animals. As is the case with all the phenothiazine derivatives, no rigid dose can be prescribed due to considerable variation in response. However, for premedication the drug is usually employed in doses of up to 1 mg/kg by intramuscular injection. Horses under the influence of promazine appear to be hypersensitive to noise and may react violently to such disturbances as the rattle of bucket handles. A fearful horse can be quickly roused from promazine sedation when sensitive areas are interfered with and its response may be no less vigorous than would have been the case without the drug.

Trimeprazine (Vallergan)

This is 10-(3-dimethylamino-2-methylpropyl) phenothiazine tartrate. In general it may be said to be more effective than chlorpromazine, but less effective than promethazine, as a central sedative. Its effects are not so long lasting as those of chlorpromazine—they are never apparent on the next day.

In horses, doses of 0·5 mg/kg given for premedication by intramuscular injection ensure a quiet recovery from anaesthesia without causing any marked increase in recovery time. In cattle intramuscular doses of up to 500 mg are useful for sedation when operations are to be performed under local analgesia. In pigs, dogs and cats the drug is used in doses of about 1 mg/kg.

Perphenazine (Fentazine)

1-(2-Hydroxyethyl)-4-3-(2-chloro-10-phenthiazinyl-1-propyl) piperazine has been used in doses of 0·2 mg/kg for sedation in pigs, cattle, dogs and cats.

Pecazine (Mepazine, Pacatal, Paxital)

This is 10-(N-methyl-3-piperidylmethyl)-phenothiazine. It is supplied in tablet form for oral administration or in aqueous solution for parenteral use. The tablets contain the active ingredient in the form of its hydrochloride monohydrate; the solution is of the acetate dihydrate. In man it is euphoriant whereas chlorpromazine dulls the emotions, but this difference is not apparent in animals. However, when given to dogs by intravenous injection it causes an increase in blood pressure while all the other phenothiazine derivatives produce some degree of hypotension when given by this route. The duration of action of pecazine appears to be about 12 hours. In dogs doses of 2 mg/kg produce useful pre-anaesthetic sedation and do not delay recovery from anaesthesia.

Propionylpromazine (Combelen)

N-(3-Dimethylamino)-3-propionyl-phenothiazine is a compound which has been widely used in Scandinavia and on the Continent of Europe. It has usually been used in combination with methadone (page 155) for the general sedation of all species of animal. In horses it is used in doses of 0·15 to 0·25 mg/kg and in dogs the dose ranges from 0·2 to 0·3 mg/kg.

Acepromazine (Acetylpromazine)

Acepromazine has been used extensively as a premedicant and general sedative in both small and large animals. Extensive trials indicate that while the drug is by no means without certain disadvantages common to all phenothiazine ataractics, it is probably the ataractic of choice for large and small animals.

Acepromazine is the 2-acetyl derivative of promazine with the chemical formula 2-acetyl-10-(3-dimethyloaminopropyl)-phenothiazine. It is prepared as the maleate compound—a yellow crystalline solid melting at about 136°C.

Like the other phenothiazine derivatives it is a central nervous system depressant with associated activity on the autonomic nervous system. It possesses anti-emetic, anticonvulsant, hypothermic, hypotensive and anti-spasmodic properties and is the most potent of the whole group of compounds used in veterinary practice, the effective parenteral dose being very small. Because of the high potency and consequent low dosage rate, acepromazine is unlikely to give rise to undesirable side-effects. During toxicity trials dogs have received doses of over 3 mg/kg by intramuscular injection without untoward effect. Such doses represent 12 to 24 times the recommended level for clinical use.

Acepromazine, like all phenothiazine derivatives, appears to produce an optimal effect at a certain dosage rate. This dose can then be increased without markedly increasing the degree of sedation until the animal either lapses into profound depression or reaches a stage of excitement. An obvious effect can be produced in all species of domestic animals using acepromazine at a dose of 0·5 mg/kg by intramuscular injection. A dose as high as 1 mg/kg produces very little more sedation, but the onset of action is more rapid and the duration of sedation is increased. Usually the lower dose rates are adequate and produce an effect sufficiently quickly while, at the same time, reducing the chance of unpleasant or unwanted effects, such as excitement, to a minimum. Slightly increased doses may be advisable, however, in animals of known violent or excitable nature.

The parenteral dose of acepromazine for horses, cattle, sheep and pigs is of the order of 0·03 to 0·1 mg/kg by intramuscular injection. For dogs and cats the intramuscular dose is between 0·1 and 0·2 mg/kg and the oral dose lies between 1 and 3 mg/kg.

Haloperidol (R1625, Serenace)

This is a butyrophenone tranquillizer with a relatively long duration of action. Although one of the first butyrophenone derivatives to be introduced into veterinary practice it was never widely used.

Dehydrobenzperidol (R4749, Droperidol, Droleptan)

This is 4′-fluoro-4-(N-4″(N-benzimidazolone)-3,4-tetrahydropiperidino)-butyro-phenone hydrate. It is about 20 times as potent as the much longer acting haloperidol and is the most potent anti-emetic known. It is said to antagonize the respiratory depressant effect of morphine-like compounds by increasing the sensitivity of the respiratory centre to carbon dioxide, and to be almost devoid of such side-effects as the production of extrapyramidal symptoms (Marsboom and Mortelmans, 1964).

Mitchell (1966) reported that dehydrobenzperidol produced useful sedation in pigs when administered by intramuscular injection. Doses of 0·1 to 0·4 mg/kg produced sedation in 5 to 15 minutes and recovery in 2 to 5 hours depending on the dose used and the state of health of the recipient. Defaecation was observed during the onset of the drug's action. Induction of anaesthesia with halothane was greatly facilitated. He concluded that dehydrobenzperidol has a definite place in porcine sedation and no advantage appeared to result from combination with phentanyl (see page 159) and indeed it seemed that this agent decreased the efficiency of dehydrobenzperidol as a sedative. These observations have been confirmed to some extent by Lamberth (1968) who found dehydrobenzperidol to be a useful sedative for weaner pigs.

Soma and Shields (1964) combined dehydrobenzperidol with phentanyl for neurolpetanalgesia in dogs (see page 158).

Haloanisone (R2028, Fluanisone)

This is 4′-fluoro-4-(1-[4-(2methoxy)-phenyl]-piperazino)-butyrophenone. Mitchell (1966) found that a combination of 50 parts of this compound with 1 part of phentanyl had no advantage over dehydrobenzperidol as a sedative for pigs. Marsboom *et al.* (1964) gave haloanisone 5 mg/kg and phentanyl 0·1 mg/kg to produce neuroleptanalgesia in dogs. Results were claimed to be good, especially when the drugs were given simultaneously. They comment that the method is contra-indicated in Caesarian section because it may cause fatal respiratory depression of the puppies.

Azaperone (R1929, Suicalm, Stresnil)

4′-Fluor-4-[4-(2 pyridyl)-1-piperazinyl] butyrophenone is a tranquillizer for pigs which has undergone extensive trials in Belgium and the United Kingdom. Doses of 0·5 mg/kg are said to prevent excitement, while 1·5 to 3·0 mg/kg by intramuscular injection prevent aggressiveness and fighting which may occur on mixing litters (Symoens and Van den Brande, 1969). Doses of 4 to 8 mg/kg produce deep sedation together with clinically insignificant reductions in cardiac output and heart rate (Marsboom and Symoens, 1968). Clarke (1969) reported a consistent small fall in blood pressure after intramuscular doses of 0·3 to 3·5 mg/kg.

Excitement is known to occur if an animal is disturbed during the first 15 minutes after injection and thus animals should be allowed at least 15 to 20 minutes to become sedated before being handled. Once sedated, pigs are easily restrained for the induction of general anaesthesia and azaperone premedication appears to antagonize the respiratory depressant effects of most anaesthetic agents.

REFERENCES

ALEXANDER, F. (1960). *An Introduction to Veterinary Pharmacology.* Edinburgh: Livingstone
ARCHER, S. and KEATS, A. S. (1962). *Science, N.Y.* **137**, 541
CHEN, G. M. and ENSOR, C. R. (1968). *Am. J. vet. Res.* **29**, 863
———— RUSSELL, D. and BOHNER, B. (1959). *J. Pharmac. exp. Ther.* **128**, 241
———— and WESTON, J. K. (1960). *Anaesth. Analg.* **39**, 132
CLARKE, K. W. (1969). *Vet. Rec.* **85**, 649
———— and HALL, L. W. (1969). *Vet. Rec.* **85**, 512
COLLINS, V. J., GOROSPE, C. A. and ROVENSTINE, E. A. (1960). *Curr. Res. Anesth.* **39**, 132
DAVIS, L. E. and DONNELLY, E. J. (1968). *J. Am. vet. med. Ass.* **153**, 1161
DUNDEE, J. W., CLARKE, R. S. J., LOAN, W. B. and HAMILTON, R. C. (1967). *Br. J. Anaesth.* **39**, 88
GARMER, L. N. (1969). *Res. vet. Sci.* **10**, 382
GRIEFENSTEIN, F. E., DE VAULT, M., YOSHITAKE, J. and GAWESKI, J. E. (1958). *Anesth. Analg.* **37**, 283.
HARTHOORN, A. M. (1962). *Vet. Rec.* **74**, 410
JOHNSTONE, M., EVANS, V. and BAIGAL, S. (1959). *Br. J. Anaesth.* **31**, 433
KEMP, S. W., and MORTON, H. J. V. (1962). *Anaesthesia,* **17**, 170
KRONEBERG, G., OBERDORF, A. F. HOFFMEISTER, F. and WIRTH, W. (1966). *Naturwissenschaften,* **53**, 502
LAMBERTH, J. L. (1968). *Aust. vet. J.* **44**, 333
LOWE, J. E. (1969). Personal communication
MARSBOOM, R. and MORTELMANS, J. (1964). *Small Animal Anaesthesia.* Oxford: Pergamon
———— ———— and VERCRUYSSE, J. (1963). *Vet Rec.* **75**, 132
———— ———— ———— and THIENPONT, D. (1962). *Nord. Vet. Med.* **14**, 95
———— and SYMOENS, J. (1968). *Tijdsch. Diergenskde,* **93**, 3
———— VERSTRAETE, A., THIENPONT, D. and MATTHEEUWS, D. (1964). *Br. vet. J.,* **120**, 466

MITCHELL, B. (1966). *Vet. Rec.* **79**, 651

NUNN, J. F. and BERGMAN, N. A. (1964). *Br. J. Anaesth.* **36**, 68

OBERDORF, A. F., HOFFMEISTER, F. and KRONBERG, G. (1967). *Arch. Pharmak. exp. Path.* **257**, 48

OWEN, L. N. (1955). *Vet. Rec.* **78**, 561

RUTTY, D. A. and THURLEY, D. C. (1962). *Vet. Rec.* **74**, 883

SCOTT, D. B. and TAYLOR, S. H. (1964). *Lancet*, **i**, 165

SCOTT-CAMERON, R. (1964). Personal communicotion

SOMA, L. R. and SHIELDS, D. R. (1964). *J. Am. vet. med. Ass.* **145**, 897

SPALDING, V. T. and HEYMANN, C. S. (1962). *Vet. Rec.* **74**, 158

SWERDLOW, M. and DALAL, A. (1966). *Anaesthetist*, 15, 43

SYMOENS, J. and VAN DEN BRANDE, M. (1969). *Vet. Rec.* **85**, 64

TAVERNOR, W. D. (1963). *Vet. Rec.* **75**, 1377

——— (1964). *Small Animal Anaesthesia.* Oxford: Pergamon

TAYLOR, S. H., SCOTT, D. B. and DONALD, K. W. (1964). *Lancet*, **i**, 841

TOMLIN, P. J., CONWAY, C. M. and PAYNE, J. P. (1964). *Lancet*, **i**, 14

WILKINS, J. H. (1961). *Vet. Rec.* **73**, 767

WIRTH, W., HOFFMEISTER, F. and KREISKOTT, H. (1965). *Neuropsychopharmacology*, **4**, 379

WRIGHT, A. and JORDAN, F. T. W. (1963). *Vet. Rec.* **75**, 471

YELNOSKY, J. and GORDOCKS, J. F. (1963). *Fedn Proc. Fedn Am. Socs exp. Biol.* Abstr. **164**, 22

Into the Stomach

On the Continent of Europe the drug is often offered in drinking water in quantities of 20 to 70 g after withholding water for 24 to 36 hours. Eberlein in Berlin found that 75% of horses so treated drank the solution. It may, however, be taken that a horse needs to be very thirsty before it will drink water containing chloral hydrate in a concentration of 2 oz in $2\frac{1}{2}$ gallons and quite apart from the undesirability of prolonged water-deprivation in animals in which general anaesthesia is about to be induced, the method presents many other and obvious inconveniences.

The difficulties and possible dangers associated with drenching require no reiteration. Because of its irritant properties the drug should only be given well diluted in water, in concentrations not greater than 1 in 20, to which may with advantage be added syrup, treacle or mucilage. The dosage is the same as that to be described for the stomach tube method but allowance should be made for wastage during administration.

The stomach tube method is to be preferred. The agent can be given in greater dilution, there is no wastage and there is no danger, provided that the tube has been introduced properly, that a subsequent drenching pneumonia will develop. At the same time individual subjects will be met in which the tube, when passed via the nostril, almost invariably enters the trachea. Again, the nasal haemorrhage it sometimes provokes may preclude the subsequent adoption of inhalation anaesthesia. In these cases, provided a suitable gag is available, the tube may be passed via the mouth. The method is not practicable in young untrained subjects.

The dosage employed will depend upon the depth of narcosis desired. In *light narcosis* the animal maintains the standing position but its reactions to simple external stimuli are reduced. There is some locomotor incoordination and the gait is unsteady. Skin sensation is not reduced. The application of hobbles is facilitated and the struggling associated with casting is reduced. In many subjects, when restrained in the recumbent position, a state of hypnosis supervenes and the performance of simple operations under local anaesthesia is greatly facilitated. Chloral hydrate narcosis is not advised for operations in the standing position, for occasionally an animal will be met in which interference provokes an exaggerated narcotic response. In *medium narcosis* the animal is unable to remain standing, but flounders and falls. It generally makes attempts to rise and flounders again; thus, once down, the animal should be immediately restrained, for when restrained it generally lies quietly. This degree of narcosis is also a useful aid to operation under local and regional anaesthesia. *Deep narcosis* is a state bordering on anaesthesia. The animal will go down when medium depth narcosis has supervened, but as narcosis is rapidly deepening it is improbable that there will be struggling. When narcosis attains its depth, respirations and pulse are not appreciably altered, but there is considerable muscular relaxation. Skin sensation is reduced, but not entirely lost and the application of painful stimuli provokes a sluggish and transient response. This depth of narcosis is to be aimed at when it is proposed to perform some extensive operation under inhalation anaesthesia.

DOSAGE TABLE

Per 50 kg (110 lb) body weight*

Route: Into the empty stomach by drench or stomach tube

	Grammes
Light narcosis	3–3·5
Medium narcosis	4–4·5
Deep narcosis	5–6

* For practical purposes the unit of weight (50 kg) may be taken as 1 cwt.

These doses represent for:	Light narcosis (g)	Medium narcosis (g)	Deep narcosis (g)
(a) Average hunter	35	50	65
(b) Average vanner	42	57	70
(c) Average heavy draught . . .	50	70	85

To ensure that the stomach is empty, food should be withheld for 24 hours before administration and if the animal has the habit of eating its bedding a muzzle should be applied. When the stomach tube is used the dose is dissolved in 6 to 8 litres of warm water.

These doses will give reasonably uniform results in healthy horses and are well within the safety limits. The onset of narcosis commences in five to 10 minutes and generally attains its maximum depth in 10 to 20 minutes.

It is a good practice to stand the animal near to the operating bed during administration and 5 minutes later to apply the hobbles. When the animal is seen to be swaying it is cast and secured.

By Intravenous Injection

The method of injection generally employed is that of gravitation into the jugular vein. As the rate of injection is comparatively slow, it is obvious that when carried out in the standing position the animal will 'go down' when a dose ranging between *medium* and *deep* has been given. Provided that no technical mishap occurs, and that the administration is carried out in a suitable place (as regards the animal 'going down'), the method has much to commend it, for there is no fear of overdosage. If it is the intention to complete the induction of general anaesthesia with chloral hydrate, it is necessary to continue administration after the animal has fallen and has been restrained, or to administer the whole of the injection after casting.

DOSAGE TABLE

Per 50 kg (110 lb) body weight

Route: Slow intravenous injection

		Grammes
Medium narcosis	. . . .	4–5
Deep narcosis	. . . .	5–6

These doses are similar to those recommended for administration into the stomach.

The great disadvantage of chloral hydrate as an agent to be administered by intravenous injection is that solutions of it are very irritant and thus it is essential that none shall infiltrate the wall of the vein or the perivascular connective tissue. The degree of irritation provoked is proportional to the concentration, and thus the greatest dilution compatible with technical expediency should be employed. At the same time, when administering the drug in the standing position by gravity, the volume of solution employed must not be so great that injection occupies too long a period, for there is a limit to the time during which most horses will stand still, and stillness during injection is most important if administration is to be carried out successfully. The optimum concentration is 1 in 10. When the dose selected is 60 g (a deep narcotic dose for the average hunter), the volume is 600 ml. With the apparatus recommended the injection of this volume by gravity occupies about 4 minutes and this is the optimum time in which to induce narcosis. Obviously the rate at which injection occurs will depend upon the diameter of the needle (or cannula) employed and the height at which the container of the solution is held. In the event of movement by the horse during injection, the possibility that the needle has left the vein and that the solution is infiltrating the perivenous tissue should immediately be suspected and steps taken to ascertain it. Should it be the case, injection must be stopped at once, so that the amount of perivascular infiltration shall be reduced to a minimum. Taking these precautions and using the concentrations recommended, it is improbable that the small amount of solution entering the tissues will cause a serious inflammatory reaction. When, however, injection is made by some method of pumping, or when, to reduce bulk, high concentrations are employed, there is a grave danger that any of the solution introduced into the connective tissue will set up severe local irritation, with possibly serious results such as acute local abscess formation, phlebitis, etc. (For the apparatus used, and the technique of injection see page 233.)

Estimation of the dose. The horse is weighed and the dose calculated. Under field conditions it is improbable that weighing facilities will be available, but the following average figures will be helpful.

							kg
Children's ponies	.	.	.	.	.	.	150–300
Donkeys	.	.	.	.	.	.	150–200
Thoroughbred: yearlings		.	.	.	.	.	300–350
two-year-old	.	.	.	.	.	.	300–400
three-year-old	.	.	.	.	.	.	400–450
adults	.	.	.	.	.	.	450–550
Hunters: mares	.	.	.	.	.	.	450–550
geldings	.	.	.	.	.	.	500–675
Cart: yearlings	.	.	.	.	.	.	350–450
two-year-old	.	.	.	.	.	.	450–525
Half-legged vanners	.	.	.	.	.	.	550–625
Heavy vanners	.	.	.	.	.	.	650–850

The weight of a horse may also be estimated with acceptable accuracy from the formula:

$$\text{Weight (kg)} = \frac{\text{Girth (inches)}^2 \times \text{Length (inches)}}{660}.$$

The girth is measured just behind the elbow and the length is from the point of the shoulder to the line of the ischial tuberosity. Both are more conveniently measured in inches than in centimetres, but if the metric scale is used these measurements may be converted to inches by dividing each by 2·5.

If administration of the drug is to be in the standing position, estimation of body weight is quite satisfactory provided sufficient solution is prepared, for horses generally fall when a constant depth of narcosis is attained, and if deeper narcosis is required an additional quantity of about one-fifth that already injected should be given.

Mode of administration. In considering the welfare and comfort of the animal, the first reaction is that the drug should be administered with the horse standing so that it eventually falls to the ground in a state of narcosis. Clearly this procedure is more humane than to cast forcibly the fully conscious animal. Furthermore, by it the risks associated with forcible casting are largely eliminated. But in practice the procedure adopted will be influenced by many considerations. 'Unbroken' or fractious animals may not remain still while injection is being made, yet to avoid with certainty undesirable local sequelae this is essential. Moreover, when dealing with large and vigorous animals it is important that a sufficient quantity shall be given to cause the animal to 'go down' in a state of deep narcosis for if less is given the horse may flounder and struggle violently thus subjecting both itself and those attending it to a risk of injury. Again, the place in which operation is to be performed must be considered. If space is confined and it is necessary for the horse to fall in a strictly limited area, it is better first to cast it. Although if the animal is quiet it is still possible to adopt the standing method, the hobbles being loosely applied before injection is commenced, or during its course, and the animal cast as it commences to fall. Conversely, animals will be met in which the application of casting tackle causes fear and struggling, and others may kick viciously when their hind-legs are interfered with. In these administration in the standing position is indicated. On the other hand, the technique of administration is more difficult in the standing position and errors are more likely to occur.

Duration of narcosis. An important point to be considered when using non-volatile narcotics in the horse is the duration of narcosis. When medium depth narcosis is induced with chloral hydrate, the animal will be able to

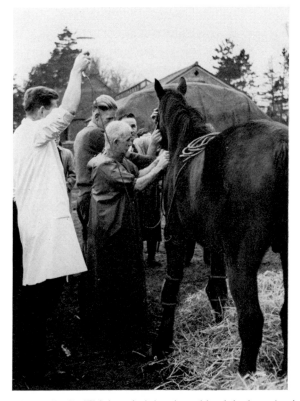

FIG. 73. Professor J. G. Wright administering chloral hydrate by intravenous injection under field conditions.

rise and maintain the standing position in from 30 to 45 minutes after administration. Even when chloroform has been used in addition, excretion of the latter is so rapid once administration ceases that the recovery time will not be appreciably lengthened. When deep narcosis is induced the period of recovery will be delayed for about 1 hour. If the drug is used for the induction of general anaesthesia it is improbable that the animal will be able to rise before $1\frac{1}{2}$ to 2 hours, or even longer, have elapsed. Under conditions of practice this is a matter of some consequence, for it is necessary that the animal shall be watched during this period and, if necessary, restrained, for occasionally the period of recovery is associated with narcotic excitement. *On no account should vigorous attempts be made to induce the animal to rise before it is reasonably certain that it will be able to do so effectively, otherwise floundering will occur and the animal may sustain injury.*

Over the years chloral hydrate narcosis has been used in some 600 equine surgical cases in the clinics of the Liverpool University Veterinary School and the experience gained in this series of cases has been recorded by Wright (1958, 1963).

His account reveals a very high standard of achievement and there can be little doubt that, properly used, chloral hydrate is a most satisfactory basal narcotic for horses. It must be noted, however, that the Liverpool workers consider that it is always safest to cast a horse before administering chloral hydrate by intravenous injection. Under the conditions which prevail in general practice today, expert casting teams are most unlikely to be available, and since inept casting techniques can be most hazardous it is possible that workers in the field may have difficulty in obtaining results as good as those of Wright and his colleagues. Moreover, the safe intravenous administration of the drug to standing horses requires a degree of competence greater than that necessary for simple venepuncture—the needle or cannula must not only be introduced into the vein, it also has to be maintained in position in the vein with certainty, for 3 to 4 minutes in an animal which may be anything but quiet during this period.

Administration per Rectum

Chloral hydrate is sometimes administered as a cerebral sedative and narcotic by rectal injection. The method is not as satisfactory as those already described and results are irregular. The rectum is first emptied by hand and a well-lubricated rubber tube (a stomach tube serves well) is inserted through the rectum into the terminal part of the colon. The solution is injected by gravity. It should be at body temperature, and the appropriate bulk is about 4 litres. If the solution is introduced into the rectum or is pumped into the colon, the distension caused generally provokes its expulsion. When other methods of administration are not practicable, this route may be adopted. The onset of narcosis is delayed, but is generally evident in about 30 minutes.

Cocu (1930) gives 50 to 60 g of chloral hydrate with morphine 0·5 g by rectal injection. He states that anaesthesia develops which lasts about 15 to 20 minutes.

Intraperitoneal Injection

The method is said to be both safe and simple. A concentration of 10% of chloral hydrate in normal saline solution is used, to which is added citrate in the proportion of 1 g to each 2 g of chloral. The onset of narcosis occurs in 20 to 30 minutes, and its duration is 1 to 3 hours.

Cattle

In general, chloral hydrate is the basal narcotic of choice for use in adult cattle. It is also used to induce light general anaesthesia. In calves the barbiturates are more often adopted. To obtain light to medium depth narcosis *in cows* the drug is generally administered as a drench in doses of 30 to 60 g as a 1 in 20 solution in water. Sedation attains its maximum depth in a period of 10 to 20 minutes. Used in this way the drug is a most valuable adjunct to operation under local or regional analgesia. This includes operations on the stomach and the digits, and also Caesarean section. For the induction of deep narcosis approaching the plane of light general anaesthesia, intravenous injection is employed. The dosage required is similar to that recommended for the horse, viz: 5 to 6 g/50 kg. The method of preparation of the solution and the technique of injection are the same as those described for horses.

As cows can generally be cast and restrained without difficulty, administration will generally be in this position with the head and neck extended. In these circumstances the external jugular vein can readily be distended by finger pressure and the use of choke cords is unnecessary. As was the case in the horse, the induction and recovery periods are quite quiet.

Bulls require special consideration. Young ones present no particular difficulty provided their temperament is such that they can be effectively restrained for safe drenching or precise intravenous injection. Heavy bulls, however, may present a difficult problem for the mere restraining of a very heavy animal in lateral recumbency may cause great respiratory embarrassment due to compression of the undermost lung and restriction of the diaphragm by pressure of the abdominal viscera; in fact breathing may cease unless the bull is quickly returned to the breast position or placed on its back. The precise intravenous injection of drugs in the standing position may not only be uncertain on account of difficulties in satisfactorily introducing the needle into the vein but sometimes impossible because of movement by the animal.

In many instances the temperament of the bull to be dealt with is such that large doses of chloral hydrate have to be given by the mouth in order to obtain sufficient sedation to allow of the application of casting tackle. The further administration of the drug by intravenous injection after casting gives rise to a danger of fatal overdosage consequent on continued absorption from the stomach. When, without any previous medication, chloral hydrate is given to a bull by intravenous injection at the usual rate, the dose required to induce deep narcosis is the same as for the big cow—about 5·5 g/50 kg. When the drug is given by the mouth a dose of 140 to 200 g (or even more) may be required to induce a degree of sedation whereby the animal may be handled and even after such a quantity the animal may still be able to stand.

A frequent demand in relation to adult bulls is the trimming of their over-grown hooves and it may help readers if the method employed in the Liverpool School, where considerable numbers are dealt with, is described. The first and essential requirement is a strong man with experience in the handling of bulls and of drenching them, together with three or four assistants. After applying the leading pole to the animal's ring, it is blindfolded. In many instances it is possible by force applied to the pole to maintain the bull's jaws in a position a little above the horizontal while lateral head movement is steadied by a man holding the horns. If it is impossible to raise the bull's head sufficiently high by these means alone, a rope tied around the base of the horns is passed over a beam and the head hauled up. The initial dose of chloral hydrate given to Ayrshire and Friesian bulls weighing about 800 kg is 140 g. This is slowly drenched in 5 litres of water. The bull is then left tethered for 20 minutes. If at the end of that time it allows itself to be approached and handled without significant objection, the casting and the operation are proceeded with. If, however, the animal still shows resentment, a further dose of 30 to 60 g is given. The bull is cast by Reuff's method and then hobbles are applied. *During the treatment of the hooves the bull is held on its back with supports to its sides.* Bulls have been kept in this position for as long as 1½ hours without harm resulting therefrom.

Finally, references should be made to the bull which is running free in a yard or a loose-box and which it is quite dangerous even to approach. In such cases it is advised that drinking water be withheld for 36 hours and that the animal then be offered water containing 90 to 120 g of chloral hydrate in 12 litres. It is generally taken and the degree of sedation is such that, with care, it can be approached and a leading pole applied.

Xylazine

Because it is a more convenient agent to use, xylazine (see page 161) will, it seems, replace chloral hydrate for the production of basal narcosis in cattle. It may be administered in small volumes of solution by both intramuscular and intravenous injection. Perivascular injection does not give rise to trouble because solutions are almost non-irritant to all tissues. Intramuscular doses of 0·2 to 0·3 mg/kg, and intravenous doses of 0·1 to 0·2 mg/kg produce basal narcosis of 30 to 50 minutes' duration and recovery is usually complete 2 to 3 hours later. It appears that the use of xylazine may be contra-indicated during the last trimester of pregnancy, but as yet no other contra-indications have been reported.

Pentobarbitone Sodium

Pentobarbitone sodium is the name given to sodium 5-ethyl-5-(1-methyl-butyl) barbiturate (Nembutal, Sagatal).

The main action of pentobarbitone sodium is to depress the central nervous system, and effects upon other systems of the body only become important as the toxic limitations to the use of the drug are approached. It depresses the cerebral cortex and, probably, the hypothalamus. Because it depresses the motor areas of the brain it is used to control convulsive seizures. It has only a weak analgesic action and relatively large doses must be administered before pain reception is affected by the drug. Like all barbiturates it is, in fact, primarily a hypnotic drug. Pentobarbitone sodium takes an appreciable time to cross the blood–brain barrier and when given by intravenous injection the rate of injection must be slow if the full effects produced by the drug are to be assessed as injection proceeds.

The drug depresses the respiratory centre and in pregnant animals it diffuses readily across the placenta into the foetal circulation inhibiting foetal respiratory movements. It appears to have no direct toxic action on the myocardium but it may cause a slight fall in blood pressure due to peripheral vasodilatation from depression of the vasomotor centre. The blood pressure may, however, rise due to hypercapnia consequent upon the respiratory depression produced by the drug. It has no direct action upon the kidney but may inhibit water diuresis probably by causing a release of antidiuretic hormone from the pituitary gland. Pentobarbitone sodium has no appreciable effect on the gastro-intestinal system or on liver function but large doses may cause further injury to an already damaged liver. The drug is destroyed primarily in the liver, although other tissues may also have the power of breaking it down and some of the dose administered to an animal is excreted in the urine.

It is marketed in capsules as a sterile 6·5% solution and, for euthanasia, in non-sterile solutions of about 20%.

The Horse

Pentobarbitone sodium should not be used as a basal narcotic in horses for the recovery rate is slow and recovery from narcosis is usually associated with marked excitement and struggling. However, small doses (15 to 20 ml of the 6·5% solution, i.e., 1 to 2·25 g) may be given to both horses and cattle to prolong basal narcosis which has been induced with chloral hydrate. The dose of pentobarbitone sodium is injected intravenously as soon as the chloral hydrate narcosis becomes inadequate and provided that the injection is made slowly no harmful effects occur. By this method the period of recumbency is much less than if additional doses of chloral hydrate are administered and recovery is not associated with struggling and excitement. More than one injection of pentobarbitone sodium may be given to supplement chloral hydrate narcosis and as much as 4 g has been given in this manner during the course of long operations.

The Ox

Since the introduction of this drug into veterinary surgery in 1931 reports have from time to time occurred regarding its use as a general anaesthetic in cattle. Toosey (1959) has recorded his satisfactory experiences with it, not only as a general anaesthetic but as a sedative and basal narcotic in a general cattle practice. Instead of the standard solution (6·5%) he used one of 20% in order to reduce the volume required. As a sedative for the control of nervous symptoms or for the restraint of nervous or excitable animals, the solution was injected slowly into the jugular or mammary vein until the desired depth of sedation was attained, which in most cases was the point at which the animal swayed slightly on its hind legs but was able to walk unaided. The dose was from 0·5 to 1 ml/50 kg (for a 500 kg cow this represents 1 to 2 g of pentobarbitone sodium). As a basal narcotic prior to the induction of general anaesthesia the injection was continued to the stage just short of the animal going down, the dose required being in the region of 3 g of the drug/500 kg body weight.

As in horses, small doses (15 to 20 ml of the 6·5% solution, i.e. 1 to 1·25 g) may be given to prolong basal narcosis which has been induced with chloral hydrate. The dose of pentobarbitone is injected intravenously as soon as the chloral hydrate depression becomes inadequate and provided that the injection is made slowly and to effect, no harmful effects occur. By this method the period of recumbency is much less than if additional doses of chloral hydrate are administered and recovery is not associated with struggling and excitement. More than one injection of pentobarbitone may be given in this manner during the course of long operations.

The Dog

Basal narcosis may be induced in dogs (and in pigs) by the slow intravenous injection of 20 to 25 mg/kg of pentobarbitone sodium. This dose produces unconsciousness, minimal respiratory depression, and has virtually no effect on the cardiovascular system. Basal narcosis produced by pentobarbitone sodium in this dosage range is often used for diagnostic cardiac catheterization studies where blood gas analysis is required.

Bromethol

Bromethol, $CBr_3CH(OH)_2$, is a white crystalline solid, soluble in water to 3.5% at $40°$ C. At higher temperatures it may split up into hydrobromic acid and dibromacetaldehyde and as these substances are irritant to body tissues, solutions of the drug should never be heated to above $40°$ C. Avertin, a 100% solution of bromethol in amylene hydrate, is a clear, colourless, syrupy liquid. It is now only of historical interest in veterinary anaesthesia.

REFERENCES

Cocu (1930). *Bull Acad. vet. France*, **3**, 141
Eberlein (1914). Cited by Frus, *Abstr. Vet. Rec.* **26**, 382
Humbert (1875). Quoted by Marcenac and Lemétayer (below)
Marcenac and Lemétayer (1930). *Bull. Acad. vet. France*, **3**, 141
Toosey, M. B. (1959). *Vet. Rec.* **71**, 24
Wright, J. G. (1958). *Vet. Rec.* **70**, 329
——— (1963). *17th World Congr., Hanover*

11

Introduction to General Anaesthesia

General anaesthesia is a state of unconsciousness produced by a process of controlled, reversible intoxication of the central nervous system, in which there is a lowered sensitivity to stimuli from the environment and a diminished motor response to such stimuli. Thus an anaesthetic agent may be defined as a substance which produces, in a controllable manner, both loss of consciousness and an absence of motor response to noxious stimuli.

General anaesthesia was first induced in animals by the inhalation of ether. Almost immediately after the publication of Morton's work on the administration of ether to human beings (1846) it was adopted for animals in the Royal Veterinary College, London. The introduction of chloroform as an anaesthetic in man by Sir James Simpson was followed by its application in the horse all over the United Kingdom.

General anaesthetics may be volatile or gaseous substances, which are inhaled into the lungs, or water-soluble non-volatile compounds, which are generally administered by intravenous injection but which may be given by the mouth, per rectum or by intraperitoneal or intramuscular injection. Intravenous injection presents certain advantages over other methods but unless the actions of the agents administered in this way are fully appreciated these advantages may be more than offset by hazards peculiar to this technique. Intravenous agents are popular in veterinary anaesthesia for all species of animal and this is undoubtedly partly due to the speed and pleasantness with which they produce unconsciousness. However, undue emphasis is often placed on this aspect and it must be appreciated that a well-administered inhalation induction of anaesthesia can be more pleasant for the patient than innumerable unsuccessful attempts at venepuncture. Moreover, almost all intravenous anaesthetics are irritant to the tissues and the deposition of small amounts of these substances at various places in all four limbs and around the jugular veins, together with haematomata, is too great a price to pay for the rapid loss of consciousness which most intravenous anaesthetics guarantee.

Volatile and gaseous anaesthetic agents introduced into the upper respiratory tract have to be transported to the brain before they will produce loss of consciousness and there are three steps involved in this process, each occupying an appreciable period of time. The first step is the transference of the gas or vapour from the upper respiratory tract to the lung alveoli and for this free external respiration is necessary. The gases inhaled will contain a certain proportion of the anaesthetic agent, but it is important to note that the volume of that inspiration, the 'tidal volume' (Fig. 74), is only a small fraction of the volume of air contained within the lungs and air passages so that a considerable dilution of the anaesthetic agent will take place. Only after several breaths will the concentration of anaesthetic vapour or gas in the alveoli approximate

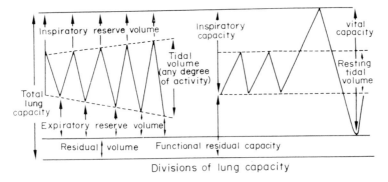

Divisions of lung capacity

FIG. 74.—Divisions of lung capacity.

to that in the inspired mixture. The actual depth of respiration or volume of the tidal air is an important factor in this process and deep breathing is more effective than shallow breathing. For example, in a dog where the tidal volume is 300 ml and the dead-space volume (volume of the conducting airways) is 100 ml the effective alveolar ventilation will be 300 ml minus 100 ml, i.e. 200 ml. If, in this dog, the tidal volume is reduced to 200 ml the effective alveolar ventilation becomes 200 ml minus the same 100 ml dead-space volume, i.e. 100 ml, so that in this dog a decrease of one-third in the tidal volume halves the alveolar ventilation. From this it might be concluded that when the tidal volume is decreased so that it equals the volume of the conducting airways, the alveolar ventilation becomes zero. However, this does not happen because the gases travel through the airways, not as a block with a square front, but rather with a spike or cone front. For this reason, some inspired gas does reach the alveoli even when the tidal volume is less than the volume of the dead-space. It has been shown that a small fraction of the inspired gas penetrates to the alveoli when the tidal volume is as little as half the volume of the conducting airways. Thus, the type of calculation given above is not strictly valid, especially when the tidal volume is extremely low, but it serves to illustrate the effectiveness of deep breathing.

Sedative drugs given to an animal as premedication before the administration of an inhalation anaesthetic usually cause a decrease in the tidal volume, and so interfere with the transport of the gas or vapour to the alveoli.

The second step, the absorption of the anaesthetic gas or vapour from the alveoli of the lung into the blood, depends on laws which govern the diffusion of gases through membranes. The flat cells of the alveolar epithelium and the endothelial cells of the capillaries constitute the membrane through which the anaesthetic agents will pass until they attain the same partial pressure on each side. The process of blood saturation is also influenced by the rate of blood flow through the lungs. Factors which accelerate this rate of flow will reduce the time in which a balanced gaseous tension between the alveolar air and blood is attained.

One other factor must be considered here. The dead-space comprises more than the volume of the conducting passages, a volume which is spoken of as the *anatomical dead-space*. That portion of the inspired gases which traverses the conducting passages and enters the alveoli is always called the alveolar ventilation but in some animals not all of this alveolar ventilation is equally effective in arterializing the mixed venous blood or in adding or subtracting anaesthetic agents to this blood. There may be areas of the lung which are ventilated but have no blood flowing through their capillary network. The inspired gases which enter these areas are wasted; the animal must expend energy to move this gas back and forth, but this achieves no respiratory function. This condition may also vary in degree—some alveoli may have blood flowing through them but have ventilation far in excess of that necessary for the equilibration of the blood, so that a proportion of the ventilation which enters these alveoli is also wasted. Such wasted gas is sometimes called *alveolar dead-space gas*. The volume of this alveolar dead-space gas, however, is not the volume of all the alveoli which either have no blood flow or excessive ventilation but only the volume of the inspired gas which enters these alveoli on each breath. It therefore fills no physical or anatomical space as does the gas in the conducting passages and cannot be included in the 'anatomical dead-space'. Together with the anatomical dead-space it is known as the *physiological dead-space*. Clearly, the physiological dead-space will be increased in pathological conditions of the lung and the presence of such conditions will interfere with the transport of anaesthetic gases and vapours to the blood.

The final step in the process, circulation by the blood and diffusion into the tissues, results in the distribution of the anaesthetic agent throughout the body. Neither this distribution nor the rate of absorption by cells is uniform;

they vary with the differences in the blood supply and lipoid content of the respective tissues. The brain is very vascular and has a high lipoid content and soon acquires a concentration of the anaesthetic equal to that in the blood. Cerebral function is thus depressed early in the process of induction of anaesthesia. If the anaesthetic is administered for only a short time, recovery of consciousness will be accelerated by the distribution of the drug from the brain to the other tissues of the body. On the other hand, if the administration is continued until the whole body is saturated with the drug, recovery of consciousness will be slower because of the absence of a tension gradient between the brain and the other tissues.

Because of their irritant nature the vapours of the volatile liquid anaesthetics such as chloroform and ether can only be inhaled when given in low concentrations so that the three phases of transference from the alveolar air to the tissues occupies an appreciable time. Gases such as nitrous oxide are not irritant to the respiratory tract; they can be administered in high concentrations so that their partial pressures in the lung aveoli soon become high and diffusion into the blood and body tissues is rapid.

Elimination of the anaesthetic from the body takes place by a reversal of this process. The partial pressure of the anaesthetic in the alveoli falls below that in the blood so that the tension gradient is reversed and the agent passes from the tissues to the blood, from the blood to the alveolar air and from there, by exhalation, to the atmosphere. During anaesthesia a small quantity of the anaesthetic is lost from the body through the skin and from any operation wound.

Drugs injected into a vein are distributed directly in the bloodstream to the brain and the other tissues of the body, while those given by the alimentary route (by mouth or by injection into the rectum) must first be absorbed into the blood and then pass through the liver before reaching the central nervous system. If the drugs administered by these routes are non-volatile (e.g. chloral hydrate and thiopentone sodium), their elimination from the body is not a reversal of the process of absorption; they are broken down, mostly in the liver, and are then excreted mainly by the kidneys. Volatile agents such as ether can be administered intravenously or by rectum, but they are always mainly excreted unchanged, principally through the lungs.

The Mode of Action of Anaesthetic Drugs

The mode of action of anaesthetic drugs in the tissues is not understood. They all interfere with cell metabolism to an extent which depends on the amount of anaesthetic present, the period of time during which the cell is exposed to the anaesthetic, and on the toxicity of the drug.

The work of Meyer (1899) and Overton (1901) resulted in the 'lipoid solubility theory of anaesthesia' and Meyer postulated that 'all chemically indifferent substances, which are soluble in fats or fatty substances, must exert a narcotic action on living protoplasm, in so far as they become distributed in it'. Olive oil was used as a standard to estimate the fat solubility of various narcotics and determine their oil/water partition coefficients, i.e. the ratio of solubility in fat/solubility in water. The prime determinant of uptake, distribution and elimination of anaesthetics is solubility (see page 326), but Meyer's generalization cannot be accepted. There are many drugs which have high oil/water coefficients yet do not produce narcosis, while morphine and other basic narcotics, which are almost insoluble in fats, produce a state of narcosis in living cells. It is thus clear that lipoid solubility is not an indispensable requisite for the production of narcosis.

Traube (1904) drew attention to the close relationship existing between (a) the ability of a narcotic to lower the surface tension of water and (b) its narcotic potency. It is true that, when a homologous series of narcotics is considered, the ability to lower the surface tension of water increases in parallel to the intensity of narcotic action of succcessive members of the series, but other properties such as molecular weight, boiling point and oil/water coefficient also vary in a like manner. Moreover, when dissimilar narcotics are compared the parallel between ability to lower surface tension and narcotic potency is by no means exact.

Any correlation of narcotic potency with lipoid solubility and/or surface tension phenomena does not explain narcosis or anaesthesia. Neither of these physical properties is essential for a drug to be able to combine with cell protoplasm and produce narcosis, but as factors assisting the uptake of narcotic drugs by cells, singly or together, it is likely they have a significant influence on drug fixation and so on narcotic action.

In 1961 Pauling and Miller independently announced their molecular theories of anaesthesia. The substance of Pauling's hypothesis is that simple molecules may be linked to one another by hydrogen bonding as the result of instantaneous dipole moment. Clathrates or lattices are formed, the cavities or interstices of which may be occupied by second molecules. For example, chloroform and water form a hydrate which reverts to its separate components at 2°C. The relatively inert gas, xenon, which at high pressures has anaesthetic properties, can stabilize the hydrate crystal giving a higher temperature of decomposition.

First proposed in 1959, Pauling's hydrate microcrystal theory was based on the behaviour of an alkylammonium salt with a clathrate structure resembling xenon hydrate. The resemblance of the salt to certain amino acid side-chains of proteins suggested that the proteins in brain tissue could form stable hydrates at body temperatures in the presence of an anaesthetic agent. Theoretically, the microcrystal so formed could interfere with ionic mobility, electrical charge, chemical reactions or enzymic activity that are in some way involved in consciousness. If this were so, anaesthetic activity should be proportional to the polarizability of the molecule which, in turn, influences the stability of the hydrate crystals. A significant correlation has, indeed, been found for several anaesthetics between the partial pressures which produce anaesthesia and the partial pressures necessary for the formation of hydrate crystals at $0°C$. Unfortunately, when corrected to $37°C$ and allowance made for the effects of salts in the interstitial fluid, the partial pressures are such as to preclude the use of most anaesthetic drugs or even to permit their vaporization at ambient temperatures.

Consideration of these points led Miller (1961) to propose that the water surrounding a gas molecule is in a more ordered state than water in bulk, and forms a so-called 'iceberg structure'. Such icebergs or ice clusters may exist in a dynamic condition in liquid water, not all gas molecules being surrounded by icebergs. Calculations show that at a given temperature the fraction of a surface (whether a membrane, polysaccharide, or other polymer) covered by water in a more highly organized state ('ice cover') in the several levels of anaesthesia is proportional to the partial pressure of the anaesthetic. The analogy of Pauling's theory is completed by Miller's suggestion that the ice cover possibly 'lowers conductance', 'stiffens up the lipoid membranes' or 'plugs up the pores of a membrane'. Although Miller doubts that micro-crystals are formed and stabilized by protein side-chains or that crystals could be formed at all, he suggests that gas-filled icebergs are equivalent to Pauling's microcrystals.

The production of anaesthesia by electrical currents applied to the brain may bear some relationship to the action of drugs. Indeed, it has been suggested that electrical influences on the brain could involve clathrate formation, thus linking electrical anaesthesia to Pauling's and Miller's hypotheses. The current status of electrical anaesthesia, however, shows little advance since Van Poznak reviewed it in 1963 and it is not easy to discern any contribution made by it towards an understanding of the mode of action of anaesthetics.

Featherstone and Muehlboecher (1963) suggested that protein molecules may play a role not only in the absorption, distribution and possibly the metabolism and excretion of anaesthetics, but in the mechanism of anaesthesia as well. It has been demonstrated (Featherstone, Muehlboecher, De Bon and Forsaith, 1961) that the solubility of cyclopropane in blood increases directly with the concentration of serum albumen, probably as a result of a reversible association of the anaesthetic with a protein—a theory propounded as long ago as 1904. Clearly, the effect of proteins relates primarily to the transport of an anaesthetic in the body, both binding and diffusibility being related to the pH of the fluid, the pK of the compound and the degree of dissociation, but at least consideration of these aspects diverts attention from preoccupation with lipoid molecules.

Reversible structural alterations of proteins has been induced by a number of anaesthetic compounds (Balasubramanian and Wetlaufer, 1966). Interaction of anaesthetics and protein molecules has also been demonstrated by X-ray crystallography (Schoeborn, 1968). Thus, it is possible that binding of the anaesthetic at specific sites on the protein molecule results in conformational changes of the protein. If such changes occur on the surface membrane of excitable cells some alteration in function might be expected.

There is much experimental evidence relating to the effects of anaesthetic agents on neuronal transmission, but the relevance of these studies to the phenomenon of clinical anaesthesia is most uncertain. For example, it has been shown that diethyl ether gradually depolarizes neurones and then maintains them in this inexcitable state so that they cannot return to their normal resting potential. However, these effects are only produced by environmental concentrations of ether far in excess of those attained around the neurones during deep surgical anaesthesia. Similar observations have been made for other anaesthetic agents. It has been shown that a blood level of 0·2 mM/litre of pentobarbitone produces surgical anaesthesia, whereas a concentration of 1·8 mM/litre is needed to produce anoxal block (McIlwain, 1961). All the available evidence, therefore, suggests that the anaesthetist produces the sequence of changes associated with developing surgical anaesthesia by pharmacological interference with intercommunication between neurones rather than by altering intraneuronal conduction. The essence of the anaesthetist's ability to regulate this deliberately induced distortion of function lies in the skill with which he can determine its course and regulate its progress. This must be done in the light of the influence not only of the anaesthetic agents but also of a multiplicity of factors that arise during surgical procedures which will distort still further the functions of the nervous system. The highly developed empirical art can only be converted to a science when some of the neurological aspects of anaesthesia are understood.

Neurological Principles in Anaesthesia

It is not possible in the space available to give a systematic account of all the facets of neurophysiology that are of importance in anaesthesia. For information on the basic physiology of neurones, action potential, excitation, the propagation of nerve impulses, synaptic transmission and the special physiology of the sensory, motor and visceral nervous systems, reference should be made to recent textbooks of neurophysiology. All that can be attempted here is a brief account of the mechanisms by which neurones in the body communicate with one another and an examination of the manner in which these mechanisms are affected by some of the agents employed in clinical anaesthesia—subjects of particular interest to anaesthetists.

Synaptic Transmission

Synaptic transmission is essentially the transfer of energy from one neurone to another, and occurs throughout the central nervous system and in the ganglia of the visceral nervous system wherever the terminations of an axon impinge on the dendrites or cell body of another neurone. The neuromuscular junction is a special type of peripheral synapse and is discussed later in this book (see page 387).

Synaptic transmission is still far from being completely understood, and may have differing consequences for the postsynaptic cell in that its activity may be either promoted or suppressed by the arrival of impulses in the presynaptic fibres. If the arrival of impulses in the presynaptic fibres increases the activity of the postsynaptic cell which, in appropriate circumstances, may then discharge impulses into its axon the process is known as 'synaptic facilitation'. On the other hand, if impulses arriving in the presynaptic fibres diminish the activity of the postsynaptic cell, even to the point of arresting its discharge in response to coincident activation from other (facilitatory) presynaptic fibres, the process is called 'synaptic inhibition'. Thus, at any moment of time, the excitability of a particular postsynaptic cell is governed by the integrated effect of combined facilitatory and inhibitory influences being brought to bear upon it. Facilitatory and inhibitory systems do not result from any particular structural property of the component nerve fibres, but from the special nature of the chemical and electrical events that result at the respective synaptic terminations on the arrival of impulses there. It seems possible that facilitation is associated with the depolarization of the postsynaptic regions while inhibition involves temporary hyperpolarization of the cell, during which its excitability is diminished. This hyperpolarization results from flow of current out of the postsynaptic cell in the subterminal regions into more remote regions of the cell (proximal axon, axon hillock and distal dendrites). The direction of current flow in relation to activated inhibitory terminals is thus the exact reverse of that created around facilitatory terminals, although the duration of current flow is similar in the two instances.

In both facilitation and inhibition the production of localized permeability changes which result in current flow is attributed to the action of chemical transmitter substances released from the presynaptic terminals. The transmitter substances responsible for inhibition are either different from those liberated during facilitation, or else are the same substances present in different concentrations. However, Dale's Law states that the transmitter agents released by a neurone are similar at all of its terminals, and that their action is identical at all synaptic junctions in which those terminals are involved. In other words, a neurone does not simultaneously produce facilitation at some of its terminals and inhibition at others.

The evidence available at present indicates that acetylcholine is an important, but not the only, facilitatory transmitter substance in the central nervous system. The nature of the inhibitory transmitter substance is quite unknown as yet, although there is probably more than one such substance. Suggestions have been made that in certain sites adrenaline, 5-hydroxy-tryptamine and even acetylcholine might act to produce inhibition, although producing facilitation at other sites. Another substance, γ-aminobutyric acid, has also been found to have an inhibitory effect on transmission through certain synaptic systems.

Synaptic transmission in the ganglia of the visceral nervous system is essentially similar to facilitatory transmission in the central nervous system, and the principal transmitter substance involved is known to be acetylcholine.

Most neurologically effective drugs used in anaesthesia exert their effects primarily by interfering with synaptic transmission. They produce changes in the response of the postsynaptic cell and not in the activity of the presynaptic terminals. Some raise the threshold of the postsynaptic cell so that it is no longer depolarized by the transmitter substance (non-depolarizing or anti-depolarizing agents), while others depolarize and maintain depolarization and hence inexcitability (depolarizing agents). Procaine is a non-depolarizing agent which, when administered systemically, blocks central synaptic transmission mainly through inhibitory systems. It therefore reduces the release of inhibitory transmitter substances on the final (effector) postsynaptic cell, preventing the generation therein of the inhibitory postsynaptic potential. Procaine thus produces an increased excitability of efferent systems for these are no longer restrained by inhibitory influences. Diethyl ether is a depolarizing agent. In low concentrations it seems to prevent transmission of activity through inhibitory systems, leading to central excitatory effects such as are seen during the induction of ether anaesthesia. In higher concentrations it blocks both inhibitory and facilitatory transmission non-selectively at synapses in the central nervous system. The mode of action of halothane is unknown, but it is probably a non-depolarizing agent. Barbiturates are non-depolarizing agents which appear to act mainly on facilitatory synaptic transmission; their blocking action is more effective in multisynaptic pathways and thus they block polysynaptic reflexes such as the flexor reflex before monosynaptic reflexes such as the knee-jerk. Morphine and atropine are both non-depolarizing agents. Morphine blocks transmission at cholinergic synapses and as most internuncial synapses are cholinergic it is upon the more complex internuncial relays (e.g. brain stem reticular system) that morphine exerts its principal effect. Further, as most inhibitory systems are multineuronal, morphine may produce central excitatory effects by selective depression of cholinergic transmission between interneurones in polysynaptic inhibitory systems.

Electrical Activity of the Brain

Throughout all animal species when aggregates of neurones are organized into functional units by mutual intercommunication, they produce rhythmical electrical activity that oscillates within fairly narrow frequency limits. The study of such activity of the brain constitutes the field of electro-encephalography. The dimensions of the electrical activity of the brain reflect the metabolic state of the millions of neurones of which it is comprised. Analysis of the records of such activity (electro-encephalograms) during an operation may, therefore, reveal to the anaesthetist not only the extent to which the patient's cerebral metabolism is specifically modified by the anaesthetic agents, but also the degree to which this pharmacological action is being influenced by the variations in circulatory, respiratory and general biochemical functions of the individual animal that arise during the course of surgical procedures.

In clinical practice cerebral electrical activity is recorded from electrodes held in contact with the scalp and arranged in relation to the underlying anatomical regions of the brain. The techniques of electro-encephalography (like those of anaesthesia) cannot be learnt from books; adequate skill can only be acquired by practical experience gained under the supervision of a properly qualified teacher. While a detailed analysis of the sequence of electro-encephalographic changes associated with anaesthesia in man is available, little information relating to animals has been reported and, therefore, the value of electro-encephalography in veterinary anaesthesia is largely unexplored.

The brain waves that are recorded from the surface of the head by clinical electro-encephalography are oscillations of electrical potential generated in the cerebral cortex and modified by the resistance of the tissues (meninges, skull and scalp) through which they pass. Each component wave is the integrated envelope of the synchronous discharges of a large number of cortical units. The potential oscillations are generated mainly in the dendrites of the cortical neurones and the degree of synchronization between different cortical units varies from time to time and with alterations in the prevailing environmental circumstances. Furthermore, the synchronization of these

7

cortical dendritic potentials is regulated from neurones located in the brain stem, from which axons ascend into the cerebral cortex to synapse with the cortical neurones.

In all 'higher' vertebrates, including man, there is a diffuse collection of neurones extending longitudinally throughout the brain stem that constitutes the 'reticular complex'. These cells, interrelated through multiple synapses, extend from the caudal end of the fourth ventricle upward into the thalamus and hypothalamus. They receive afferent connections by way of collateral branches from all ascending sensory tracts of the spinal cord and from the sensory roots of the cranial nerves. They project axons to cells in nearly all regions of the cerebral cortex, in what is known as the 'reticulocortical system' of fibres. In addition, the reticular nuclei project downwards into the spinal cord in the reticulospinal and propriospinal tracts. The cerebral cortex itself also projects downwards to the underlying brain stem reticular system.

The brain stem reticular system continuously activates, through its diffuse ascending projections, the neuronal networks of the entire cerebral cortex. The prevailing pattern of cerebral cortical activity, as well as awareness of environment (i.e. state of consciousness), is related to the intensity of this reticulocortical activation. Thus, the electrical activity recorded by the electro-encephalograph is affected by alterations in the brain stem reticular formation, and such changes are accompanied by alterations in awareness of the environment. If reticulocortical activation be increased, there is acceleration and desynchronization of the brain waves, augmented awareness of the environment and hyper-reactivity to sensory stimuli. Conversely, if reticulocortical activation be diminished, the reverse changes occur. There is progressive slowing of the brain wave frequencies, diminishing awareness of the environment and reduced reactivity to sensory stimuli. Such considerations are of great significance to the anaesthetist, for they reveal the neurological mechanism behind the many of the empirically observed features of general anaesthesia. The anaesthetist induces the succession of neurological phenomena that constitute the progressive stages of general anaesthesia by deliberately inducing, and carefully controlling, changes in reticulocortical activity.

It is important for the anaesthetist to realize that even in surgically anaesthetized animals volleys of impulses from peripheral sensory receptors, especially pain receptor systems, continue to bombard the primary sensory regions of the cerebral cortex through the thalamocortical relay paths. These paths are extremely resistant to depression by anaesthetics (Brazier, 1960, 1963). That pain is not appreciated by the anaesthetized animal is due simply to the suppression of the reticulocortical activating system. Injury of a sensory nerve still causes an impulse to be transmitted to the brain where, although not consciously perceived, it may produce such effects as hypotension and bronchospasm.

The Signs and Stages of Anaesthesia

In the past it has been customary to divide the transition from consciousness to complete surgical anaesthesia into a number of 'stages' or 'levels'. To speak of 'levels of anaesthesia' imputes some kind of spatial relationship to the anaesthetic process in that it implies the possibility of movement in a vertical direction from some level of anaesthesia to another, either higher or lower, level. The so-called 'classical signs' of anaesthesia, such as have been tabulated in earlier editions of this book and in most of the older textbooks of anaesthesia, are provided by the presence or absence of reflex responses in the anaesthetized subject to stimuli provided by the anaesthetist or surgeon. These changes in reflex function were given as indices of the extent of the supposedly vertical spatial distribution of the narcotic process within the central nervous system. Particular associations of signs were assumed to indicate that the narcotic process had descended further to a particular horizontal plane. Particular clinical signs of anaesthesia were, therefore, equated with particular anatomical 'levels' or 'planes' of depression of the central nervous system. These signs were often likened to a series of landmarks used to assess the progress made on a journey. Such empirical, traditional methods of assessing the progress of anaesthesia and the anatomical implications that go with these methods incorporate a fallacy, because they take no account of time—and the changing function in any biological system can only be assessed scientifically in terms of magnitude and time. A stage of anaesthesia is really a particular moment in a continuous temporal stream of neurological phenomena to be interpreted by the magnitude and quality of these phenomena that obtain at that moment. Thus, there can be no such thing as 'the maintenance of an even plane of anaesthesia over a period of time', and the anaesthetist must appreciate that the whole idea of levels of anaesthesia is a purely neurological conception, born towards the end of the last century. In trying to describe the progress of an anaesthetic in terms of a series of hypothetical levels, an attempt is being made to fit facts of contemporary experience into an artificial nineteenth-century model. This model may once have had the virtue of simplicity but its bears no relation to the realities of physiology and pharmacology as they are now understood in the latter part of the twentieth century.

As applied to general anaesthesia the hierarchical model of neurological organization assumes that the cerebral cortex, being the most recently acquired portion of the central nervous system and, therefore, responsible for the maintenance of consciousness, is the first part of the brain to be affected during the induction of anaesthesia. When its function is abolished, consciousness is lost and the 'lower' parts of the brain are released from the normal inhibiting influence of the cerebral cortex to become more active. Then, as anaesthesia deepens, various hypothetical centres are depressed in sequence from above down until only the neurones in the medulla and spinal cord continue to function and maintain life. The advances of neurology, particularly in the last 20 years, have made this concept quite untenable. When, however, the question is asked as to whether there is any place in modern anaesthetic practice and teaching for the old hierarchical model the answer must, it seems, be a qualified 'yes'. While it is clearly desirable to utilize acceptable quantitative measurements to assess the extent to which, and the rate at which, the function of the patient's brain is being distorted, the necessary apparatus is complicated and, especially in veterinary practice, seldom available. Clearly, it would be ideal if such measurements as the concentration of anaesthetic in the blood, or the alveolar tension of the anaesthetic (see page 327) were continuously available to the anaesthetist, but it is highly unlikely that such data will ever be forthcoming as a routine. In the absence of such measurements the anaesthetist is forced to safeguard the patient by relying on the older, well tested, empirical signs. Thus, the anaesthetist must still learn about, and look for, the various traditional signs and stages, but he must also be constantly aware that they are empirical and, as commonly taught, relate only to uncomplicated diethyl ether anaesthesia.

The transition from consciousness to complete surgical anaesthesia is, traditionally, divided into the four stages described below. They are most easily recognized when anaesthesia is produced by relatively slow-acting drugs such as diethyl ether and are not so well defined when quicker-acting drugs as halothane and thiopentone sodium are used.

Stage 1: Induction Stage or Stage of Voluntary Excitement

The animal is conscious and may make forcible efforts to avoid being anaesthetized. Breathing is entirely volitional and breath-holding may occur. Fear or apprehension causes an increase in the respiratory and pulse rates and dilatation of the pupils. Urine and faeces may be voided.

Stage 2: Stage of Involuntary Excitement

The animal loses consciousness abruptly on entering this stage of anaesthesia. Reflex response to stimuli is exaggerated and limb movements may become violent necessitating restraint of the animal. Dogs may whimper or howl, cats 'swear' and horses neigh. The degree of violence that may be exhibited is quite unpredictable, and bears no relationship to the temperament of the animal; some individuals pass quietly through this stage. Respiration is very irregular and breath-holding is an invariable accompaniment of struggling. The pharyngeal reflexes (swallowing and vomiting) are present in Stage 2 but become progressively depressed and disappear on entering Stage 3. The cough reflex is present and can be a source of great inconvenience to the anaesthetist but it is a welcome protective mechanism should vomiting occur.

It must be appreciated that Stage 1 and Stage 2 are always associated with difficulties for the anaesthetist and danger for the animal. The anaesthetist, therefore, aims to achieve Stage 3 as smoothly and as quickly as possible. Fortunately there are available narcotics such as morphine, chloral hydrate and the phenothiazine derivatives which, when given as premedicants help to achieve this goal.

Stage 3: Stage of Surgical Anaesthesia

This stage of surgical anaesthesia was divided into four planes by Guedel (1951) but more recent writers have considered that only three planes should be described, on the grounds that the fourth plane of Guedel indicates overdosage and should be included in the fourth stage of anaesthesia.

First Plane (Light) Anaesthesia

The advent of this plane is said to be indicated by the onset of regular automatic breathing and cessation of all limb movements. Inspection of the eyeballs will show them to be moving from side to side and as anaesthesia deepens these movements become more sluggish until finally the eyeballs become fixed. The animal is then considered to have entered the second plane. The palpebral, conjunctival and corneal reflexes disappear as anaesthesia deepens and are no longer present when the animal enters the second plane. In the dog and cat the pedal reflex (i.e. pulling away of the limb when the 'web' between the digits is pinched with the finger and thumb-nails) is brisk.

Many diagnostic investigations and minor operations such as the opening of abscesses can be performed in this plane of anaesthesia.

Second Plane (Medium) Anaesthesia

Little change should be noticed in the character of the respiration until the depth of anaesthesia approaches the next plane, when the rate increases and the amplitude decreases. The laryngeal reflex persists until the middle of the second plane is reached. In horses, cattle, sheep and pigs the eyeball is fixed and central but in dogs and cats the eyeball rotates downwards. Muscular relaxation becomes progressively more pronounced and in the dog and cat the pedal reflex becomes sluggish. This plane of anaesthesia is adequate for all except intra-abdominal surgery.

Third Plane (Deep) Anaesthesia

In this deep state of anaesthesia automatic breathing is still present but the respiratory rate increases while the depth of respiration decreases and a noticeable pause appears between inspiration and expiration. The thoracic component of the inspiratory act gradually disappears and any departure from regular automatic breathing rhythm is said to indicate that the animal has passed into the next stage of anaesthesia. In the dog and cat the eyeballs once again become central as the tone of the eye muscles is lost and the pedal reflex disappears.

THE REFLEXES IN THIRD STAGE ANAESTHESIA

Plane	Respiration	Reflexes		Relaxation
		Ocular	Laryngeal and pharyngeal	
1 (Light)	Regular, thoraco-abdominal	Eyeballs moving Palpebral, conjunctival and corneal—progressively depressed	Vomiting and swallowing absent Cough present	Limb muscles only
2 (Medium)	Regular, thoraco-abdominal, amplitude less	Eyeballs fixed (turned downwards in dog and cat) Corneal absent	Cough persists to middle of plane	Most (not abdominal) muscles
3 (Deep)	Regular, abdominal, minimal amplitude	Eyeball fixed and central in all animals Light persists to middle of plane	Cough absent	Abdominal muscles relaxed

Stage 4: Overdosage

In this stage paralysis of the thoracic muscles is complete and only diaphragmatic activity remains. During inspiration the contraction of the diaphragm causes the relaxed abdominal wall to bulge outwards while the flaccid walls of the thorax move inwards. Expiration causes the thoracic wall to return to its resting position. The movements of the diaphragm are jerky and respiration appears gasping in nature. The pulse becomes rapid and the pupils dilate while the eyeballs present a 'fish-eye' appearance due to cessation of lacrimal secretion.

If these warning signs are disregarded the animal's condition deteriorates rapidly. The gasping respirations become progressively less in amplitude and finally cease. Cyanosis appears and is soon replaced by the ashen-grey colour which indicates heart failure.

The Ocular Reflexes in Anaesthesia

At one time much importance was attached to the ocular reflexes but experience has shown that with one exception they are of little value. The one reliable sign is that of eyeball movement and fortunately for the animal this test involves inspection only and no touching of the delicate cornea and conjunctiva.

Agents such as morphine and atropine and variable conditions of lighting render the size of the pupillary opening an unreliable guide to the depth of anaesthesia. Also, different anaesthetic agents produce variable degrees of pupillary dilatation. Later on, when anaesthesia has become profound, the widely dilated pupil is confirmatory evidence of gross overdosage which, however, should have been diagnosed earlier from other warning signs. Such dilatation is due to paralysis of constrictor fibres of the iris and must be distinguished from simple reflex dilatation arising from emotional disturbances. Reflex dilatation usually passes off after Stage 3 is entered but it may persist longer.

The conjunctival and corneal reflexes (closure of the eyelids on gently touching the conjunctiva or cornea) generally persist until the second plane of the third stage is reached. In horses the corneal reflex may persist up to the point of respiratory failure.

The pupillary light reflex is elicited by closing the eyelids over both eyes for 10 to 20 seconds after which one eye is uncovered and a strong light shone into it. If the light reflex is present the exposed pupil will be seen to constrict. This reaction of the sphincter pupillae muscle fails about half way through the third plane of surgical anaesthesia. A preliminary dose of morphine tends to cause constriction of the pupils while atropine causes dilatation; to elicit the light reflex when these drugs have been used it may be necessary to keep the eyelids closed for a longer period than the 10 to 20 seconds usually allowed. The barbiturates produce an intense constriction of the pupils but the pupils dilate when the fourth stage of anaesthesia (the stage of overdosage) is reached.

Galla, Rocco and Vandam (1958) and Croft (1961) have suggested that the pupillary light reflex may be a useful indication of the level of consciousness when muscle relaxant drugs are incorporated in the anaesthetic technique and other reflex signs of anaesthesia are unobtainable. According to Croft, this reflex cannot be elicited in dogs until Stage 2 is reached in the recovery period. However, Croft's work was carried out in the laboratory. The level of anaesthesia in an animal during a surgical operation varies from minute to minute with the degree of surgical stimulation present at the time, and this complicates the interpretation of reflex tests.

Minimum Alveolar Anaesthetic Concentration

Recognition of the problems involved in establishing the stage of anaesthesia at any given moment with sufficient accuracy for its reproduction on another occasion has led Merkel and Eger (1963) to propose the concept of the minimum alveolar anaesthetic concentration (MAC). In animals or in man, MAC is defined as the alveolar concentration of an anaesthetic that prevents muscular movement in response to a painful stimulus in 50% of the test subjects. If adequate time is allowed for the anaesthetic in the brain to equilibrate with the anaesthetic in the blood, the alveolar partial pressure of the anaesthetic (which can be measured) is a reasonably accurate expression of the anaesthetic state. The stimulus, standardized as far as possible, usually consists of tail clamping in animals or surgical incision in man.

The measurement of MAC enables the relative potencies of anaesthetics to be compared, and with the MAC defined as $1 \cdot 0$, the stage of anaesthesia can be stated as the ratio of the alveolar concentration to the MAC. This reproducible method may be contrasted with the difficulty in using physiological parameters as an indication of the stage of anaesthesia, or the electro-encephalogram which varies according to the agent used.

Other methods are possible and de Jong, Freund and Robles (1968) have used depression of synaptic transmission for the same purpose. Any well defined response to a standard stimulus should be equally satisfactory provided the alveolar or arterial blood anaesthetic concentration is accurately measured.

REFERENCES

BALASUBRAMANIAN, D. and WETLAUFER, D. B. (1966). *Proc. natn. Acad. Sci. U.S.A.* 55, 762
BRAZIER, M. A. B. (1960). *Clin. Neurophysiol.*, Suppl. 13, 347
——— (1963). *Anesth. Analgesia Current Res.* 42, 748
CROFT, P. G. (1961). *J. small Anim. Pract.* 2, 206
DE JONG, R. H., FREUND, F. G. and ROBLES, R. (1968). *Anesthesiology*, 29, 1139
FEATHERSTONE, R. M. and MUEHLBOECHER, C. A. (1963). *Pharmac. Rev.* 15, 97
——— ——— DE BON, F. L. and FORSAITH, J. A. (1961). *Anesthesiology*, 22, 977
GALLA, S. J., ROCCO, A. G. and VANDAM, L. D. (1958). *Anesthesiology*, 19, 328
GEUDEL, A. E. (1951). *Inhalation Anaesthesia.* 2nd ed. New York: Macmillan
MCILWAIN, H. (1961). *Biochemistry and the Central Nervous System.* 2nd ed. London: Churchill
MERKEL, G. and EGER, E. I. II (1963). *Anesthesiology*, 24, 346
MEYER, H. H. (1899). *Archs exp. Path. Pharmak.* 42, 109
MILLER, S. L. (1961). *Proc. natn. Acad. Sci. U.S.A.* 47, 1515
OVERTON, E. (1901). *Studien über die Markose.* Jena.
PAULING, L. (1961). *Science, N.Y.* 134, 15
SCHOENBORN, B. P. (1968). *Fedn Proc. Fedn Am. Socs exp. Biol.* 27, 888
TRAUBE, J. (1904). *Pflügers Arch. ges. Physiol.* 105, 541
VAN POZNAK, A. (1963). *Anesthesiology*, 24, 101

12

The Anaesthetic Agents

The conditions under which veterinarians so often operate have in the past tended to encourage the use of intravenous rather than inhalation anaesthetics. More recently, however, the popularity of inhalation anaesthesia has increased, especially since the introduction of halothane, and the veterinary anaesthetist must now be competent to use both types of agent as and when indicated.

The Anaesthetic Drugs administered by Intravenous Injection

The intravenous anaesthetics are particularly useful for the induction of anaesthesia which is to be maintained by an inhalation technique, or where the operation to be performed is of relatively short duration and the induction dose can be relied on to give full anaesthesia for an adequate time. It is imperative that the person using them shall not only be skilled in the technique of intravenous injection but also familiar with the type of anaesthesia produced so that serious overdosage shall be avoided. With all the intravenous agents the clinical level of anaesthesia is very obviously related to the intensity of the surgical stimulus as well as to the degree of cerebral depression. An undisturbed animal may have depressed breathing and abdominal and masseteric relaxation, giving a picture of satisfactory surgical anaesthesia. On application of a surgical stimulus, however, the breathing may be stimulated, relaxation lost and there may be reflex movement of a limb. Herein lies one of the hazards of the use of intravenous agents as sole anaesthetics. If the above animal is now given sufficient of the intravenous agent to produce surgical anaesthesia in the presence of strong surgical stimulation, when this latter ceases a dangerous degree of respiratory depression may occur and prolonged unconsciousness may be expected. It must always be borne in mind that a significant difference between the majority of intravenous agents and those given by inhalation is that the action of the former is not quickly reversed after the cessation of administration.

Chloral hydrate was the first intravenous anaesthetic to be employed in animals and as early as 1875 Humbert described its effects in horses. The introduction of the barbiturate anaesthetics in the thirties was a great advance and it can with truth be said that the development of Nembutal (pentobarbitone sodium) anaesthesia revolutionized surgery in the dog. It is still widely used, particularly by veterinary surgeons working 'single-handed', and in laboratories. However, because its action is too prolonged for many purposes, other barbiturates have been tried in veterinary anaesthesia and of these thiopentone sodium has emerged as the 'standard' intravenous anaesthetic with which all others are compared.

If intravenous anaesthesia is to be controllable a rapid establishment of equilibrium between blood and brain is almost as essential as short duration of action. With some agents, however, there is an appreciable delay between injection and the onset of anaesthesia, with another similar delay before the full effects of the dose are observed. This delay may be caused by a 'blood–brain barrier', or the drug may be metabolized in the body to another compound which is capable of producing anaesthesia. Such a compound is obviously limited in its use, since rapid deepening of anaesthesia cannot be achieved.

Chloral Hydrate
See page 171.

Pentobarbitone Sodium
See page 181.

Thiopentone Sodium
In Great Britain thiopentone sodium (Pentothal, Intraval, Nesdonal, Trapanal) was introduced into veterinary practice as an anaesthetic agent by Wright, Sheppard and Sheppard in 1937 and since that time its use has been steadily increasing. However, the studies of its pharmacological action did not keep pace with the progress in the clinical field and only comparatively recently has any notable contribution to an understanding of its mode of action been made.

The original clinical trials showed that the drug produced only a relatively brief period of unconsciousness, and it came to be classed as an ultra-short-acting barbiturate. It was believed that the compound was detoxicated rapidly in the body and it is only recently that Brodie and his co-workers have shown this idea to be wrong. They followed the concentration of the drug in the urine and in various body tissues both in dogs and in man. It was found that the liver and plasma concentrations of thiopentone, which were high almost immediately after a single injection, soon fell rapidly. The muscle concentration, although high almost immediately after injection, continued to rise for some 20 minutes, then fell—the fall being fairly rapid during the first hour but becoming progressively slower in the next two or three hours. In contrast to this, the concentration in the body fat, which was negligible at first, increased rapidly during the first hour and then more slowly until a maximum was reached in from three to six hours. It was obvious that the concentration in the fat rose at the expense of that of the plasma and all other tissues. Although the brain concentration of thiopentone was below that of the blood plasma, both showed similar changes and therefore the depth of narcosis can be regarded as being related to the plasma concentration of the drug.

From these findings it is clear that the factors which govern the duration and depth of narcosis due to an injection of thiopentone are:

1. The amount of the drug injected.
2. The speed of injection.
3. The rate of distribution of the drug in the non-fatty tissues of the body.
4. The rate of uptake of thiopentone by the body fat.

The speed of injection and the quantity injected are related. For example, a small amount injected rapidly will produce a high plasma concentration and a parallel high brain level so that deep narcosis is induced rapidly. However, the drug soon becomes distributed throughout the non-fatty tissues of the body so that the plasma concentration and the brain concentration are reduced and there is a rapid decrease in the depth of narcosis. In contrast, a slow rate of injection of a larger quantity of the drug has the effect of maintaining the plasma level as the drug is distributed through the body tissues. This means that a larger amount of thiopentone will be necessary to obtain any given depth of narcosis and recovery will depend more on the uptake of the drug by the body fat, since the concentration of thiopentone in the non-fatty tissues will already be high at the end of injection.

Thiopentone appears to cross the blood–brain barrier with very great speed. The factor which limits the time of response following an injection is the circulation time from the site of injection to the brain. The absence of any appreciable blood–brain barrier makes the rapid injection of the drug very useful for the production of short periods of narcosis with rapid recovery as redistribution occurs. (It should be noted that pentobarbitone sodium takes a fairly long time to cross the blood–brain barrier. The maximum depth of narcosis is not reached until 3 to 5 minutes after injection. Thus a much slower rate of injection is necessary with pentobarbitone than with thiopentone.)

The rate of detoxication of thiopentone varies with the species of animal. It has been found that in dogs the plasma concentration drops at a rate of about 5% per hour once equilibrium has been reached between the concentrations in the plasma and in the fat. Since very little thiopentone is excreted unchanged in the urine, the fall in the plasma concentration must be due to breakdown of the drug by the body. This slow rate of detoxication means that narcosis will be very prolonged when anaesthesia is maintained by the repeated injection of fractional doses of the drug which saturate both the non-fatty and fatty tissues.

A period of apnoea usually follows the intravenous injection of thiopentone. This is probably due to the central depression caused by high plasma concentrations. The sensitivity of the respiratory centre to carbon dioxide is reduced progressively as narcosis deepens. As a result of the central depression the alveolar ventilation is diminished and this raises the carbon dioxide content of the arterial blood.

Thiopentone sodium causes a peculiar respiratory effect in horses. There is often a complete arrest of respiration for 20 to 30 seconds followed by 4 to 8 respiratory movements. These bursts of activity followed by inactivity may persist throughout anaesthesia (Longley, 1950; Waddington, 1950; Ford, 1951; Jones, Johnson and Heinze, 1960; Tyagi, Arnold, Usenik and Fletcher, 1964).

Carbon dioxide retention or the administration of this gas has the effect of reducing the plasma pH. Alteration of the plasma pH has a complex effect on the distribution of thiopentone in the body. Thiopentone is partially ionized and acts as a weak organic acid; the dissociation constant is such that a small change in pH will markedly affect the degree of ionization. If the plasma pH is lowered by carbon dioxide, the undissociated fraction of thiopentone is increased and since only this fraction is fat soluble, the decrease in pH results in an increase in the uptake of the drug by the fatty tissues. This lowers the plasma concentration and narcosis might be expected to lighten. However, this does not occur and Brodie has suggested that it is the undissociated fraction of the drug which is responsible for its pharmacological activity, for although the total plasma thiopentone is reduced, the concentration of the undissociated fraction remains roughly the same. A further mechanism may be implicated since thiopentone becomes bound on to the plasma protein and the degree of binding depends on the protein concentration and the pH of the plasma. Protein binding is reduced by a reduction in pH and since the pharmacological activity resides in the unbound fraction, narcosis might be expected to deepen when the plasma pH is reduced by carbon dioxide. To complicate the matter further, hyperventilation, which should have effects opposite to those of hypercapnia, has been shown to

reduce the amount of thiopentone necessary for the maintenance of anaesthesia. This, of course, is not necessarily contradictory since all three factors,
the uptake of thiopentone by the body fat, the degree of dissociation and the
degree of binding by the plasma proteins, affect the concentration of active
drug. It is unlikely that all three factors will be affected to the same degree
and in the same way by changes in the pH of the plasma.

There is considerable disagreement among research workers concerning
the effects of thiopentone on the cardiovascular system. This may well be due
to the varying methods used for determinations of such things as cardiac
output, differences of premedication, depth of narcosis and the degree of
carbon dioxide retention. It appears to be generally agreed, however, that the
rapid intravenous injection of the drug causes a fall in blood pressure. After
the initial fall the blood pressure returns to about the normal level. The drug
appears to have a direct depressant effect on the myocardium and in certain
circumstances may produce cardiac arrhythmias such as ventricular extrasystoles. It is doubtful whether the arrhythmias have any clinical significance,
since they do not seem to progress to fibrillation and usually pass off quite
spontaneously. In most instances only the electrocardiograph provides any
indication of their presence. Where myocardial damage is present, it is
unwise to use a very rapid rate of injection because this will submit the heart
to a very high initial concentration of the drug. Anaemia reduces the amount
of thiopentone necessary for any given level of narcosis but the reason for this
is unknown. In many types of anaemia the plasma proteins are reduced and
decreased protein binding could account for increased sensitivity to the drug.

After intravenous injection thiopentone rapidly reaches the central nervous
system and its effects become apparent within 15 to 30 seconds of injection.
Since the concentrations of the drug in the plasma and cerebrospinal fluid run
parallel, the depth of narcosis is dependent on, and varies with, the blood level.
However, this relationship is not a simple linear one, as acute tolerance to the
drug develops. The plasma concentration of the drug at which the animal
wakens increases as the duration of narcosis proceeds. Moreover, the depth
and duration of narcosis bear some relation to the initial dose. When a large
dose has been injected for the induction of narcosis, the animal will waken at a
higher plasma level than after a small dose. This acute tolerance is probably
the explanation for the clinical observation that recovery from the rapid
injection of a given dose of thiopentone is quicker than if the same amount is
given slowly. The initial concentration of the drug reaching the brain is
greater when the drug is injected quickly so that consciousness returns at a
higher plasma level than after a slower administration.

In clinical practice the intravenous injection of the drug is usually carried
out at such a rate that surgical anaesthesia is reached within 1 to 2 minutes and

the usual signs and stages of anaesthesia cannot be detected. In any case the clinical pattern of depression of the central nervous system by thiopentone differs from the classical picture in several respects. Apnoea sometimes occurs at a depth of anaesthesia which is insufficient to permit surgical intervention. The excitement stage is very rarely seen. The drug, like all barbiturates, has little, if any, analgesic action and reflex responses to stimuli are not abolished until an appreciably greater depth of anaesthesia is reached than is required with such agents as ether. With the barbiturates, more so than with any other drugs used in anaesthesia, the clinical level of narcosis is related to the surgical stimulus. For example, an animal which has received thiopentone may have depressed respiration, a relaxed jaw and relaxation of the abdominal muscles, corresponding to the second or third plane of third stage anaesthesia, yet if a towel clip is applied the respiratory volume increases, relaxation is lost and there may be reflex movement of a limb. The depth would now be assessed as being second stage or first plane of the third stage of clinical anaesthesia. Because of the lack of analgesic properties the signs and stages of thiopentone anaesthesia are more affected by premedication with analgesic drugs than is the case with other anaesthetic agents. This applies also to supplementation during anaesthesia with analgesics whether these be of the opiate type (pethidine) or analgesic mixtures of nitrous oxide and oxygen. They reduce or abolish reflex response to stimuli and enable operative procedures to be performed at plasma levels of thiopentone which would be insufficient if the drug were given alone.

There is an apparent increase in the sensitivity of the laryngeal and bronchial reflexes under light thiopentone narcosis. This is generally attributed vaguely to parasympathetic preponderance under thiopentone narcosis. It would be wrong, however, to assume that thiopentone itself produces laryngeal and bronchial spasm for these are reflex phenomena, usually evoked by stimulation of the sensory afferent nerves by small amounts of mucus, regurgitated gastric contents or by foreign bodies such as endotracheal tubes. They may also be initiated by stimuli from other parts of the body. During anaesthesia these reflexes are depressed centrally and it is probable that thiopentone does not affect the afferent side of the reflex pathway as much as other agents do so that deeper levels of depression are necessary for the suppression of these effects. Certainly, spasm is no more common in *deep* thiopentone anaesthesia than with other anaesthetic agents.

The incidence of hepatic damage after thiopentone anaesthesia is related to the dose administered. Hepatic dysfunction always follows the use of large doses. However, the presence of liver damage does not make the use of the drug unsafe so long as only minimal doses are employed. Gastric emptying time has been shown to be delayed during thiopentone anaesthesia. In dogs, the intravenous injection of 20 mg/kg may cause complete inactivity of the stomach and pylorus.

Like all anaesthetics, the drug may stimulate the supra-opticohypophyseal system so that antidiuretic hormone is released and oliguria produced. Uraemia increases the duration of thiopentone narcosis and the drug should be used with care, and in only minimal doses, in uraemic animals.

For many years thiopentone sodium has been used, in all but the larger farm animals, intravenously as a 5% solution, but today it is generally agreed that it is always safer to use a 2·5% solution (0·5 g in 20 ml). The intravenous injection of a 5% solution usually causes spasm and thrombosis of the vein, and subcutaneous injection produces tissue necrosis. The use of a 2·5% solution, on the other hand, does not cause venous thrombosis and ensures that accidental perivascular injection will not be followed by tissue necrosis. Moreover, it is a remarkable, and as yet unexplained fact that the use of a 2·5 rather than a 5% solution halves the total dose of the drug which has to be administered to any small animal patient. While there is no completely acceptable explanation for this it seems likely that acute tolerance may be involved. In large animals where injection is made into the jugular vein, high concentrations (10% or more) can be given without producing thrombosis for the very large blood flow through the vessel rapidly dilutes the drug as it is injected, but great care must be taken to prevent the accidental perivascular deposition of the solution.

The drug is available in 0·25, 0·5 and 1·0 g ampoules and 2·5 and 5·0 g multi-dose containers. It is usually supplied together with the appropriate quantities of sterile, pyrogen-free water to make a 2·5 or 5% solution. Solutions are not very stable and when ampoules are used only freshly prepared solutions should be administered. When prepared and stored in the multi-dose containers at room temperature the solution will remain fit for use for up to four or five days.

Thialbarbitone Sodium

This agent (Kemithal) is about half as potent an anaesthetic agent as thiopentone sodium but otherwise has very similar properties. There is some evidence that of the two drugs thialbarbitone is less depressant to the respiratory centre at any given level of narcosis, but the duration of anaesthesia and of the recovery period are much the same as with thiopentone.

The agent is a pale yellow hygroscopic powder freely soluble in water and is usually used as a 10% solution. Solutions should be freshly prepared.

Thiamylal

This drug (Surital) closely resembles thiopentone sodium in chemical structure except that while the latter is the ethyl derivative of the series, the former is the allyl compound. Thiamylal is rather more potent as an anaesthetic than is thiopentone and has less of a cumulative effect. It is claimed that in cats laryngeal spasm and apnoea are less likely to occur with thiamylal than with thiopentone, while in dogs it is said to give rise to less excitement during induction and recovery from anaesthesia. The drug causes greater salivation than does thiopentone and when using it premedication with atropine is almost essential.

Thiamylal is a yellow crystalline substance which dissolves in water to give a clear yellow solution with a pH of 10·3. These solutions are irritant when injected into the perivascular tissues.

The use of thiamylal as an intravenous anaesthetic has not progressed so quickly in Britain as in the United States of America. Since its action in dogs was first described by Reutner and Grulzit in 1948 there have been many favourable records of its use in America but it has apparently only been used in Britain since 1955 (Crawshaw, 1955).

Buthalitone

Buthalitone (Baytinal, Transithal) was originally introduced into anaesthesia with the claim that recovery was more rapid than after equipotent doses of thiopentone. It seemed, on clinical evidence, that thiopentone was twice as potent as buthalitone, but O'Mullane (1957) found that, at this ratio, buthalitone produced lighter levels of anaesthesia when judged by electro-encephalography. Thus, buthalitone may give a false impression of brevity of action because the depth of anaesthesia actually produced is not as great as it is with what are to be considered equipotent doses of thiopentone. In dogs, use of buthalitone is followed by high incidence of coughing and hiccup and this agent appears to have no place in veterinary anaesthesia.

Inactin

This agent, sodium 5-ethyl-5'-(1-methylpropyl)-2-thiobarbiturate, has apparently not been used in English-speaking countries, although it has been in widespread use in Germany for a number of years. It is a very satisfactory induction agent and, apart from being only about three-quarters as potent as thiopentone, the two drugs seem indistinguishable.

Methitural

By introducing a methyl-thioethyl group in the side chain it was hoped to accelerate the breakdown of the narcotic and, at the same time, to liberate methionine which would protect the liver from the harmful effects of the barbiturate (Zima, von Werder and Hotovy, 1954). Claims for the brevity of action of this compound (Thiogenal, Neraval) have not stood up to careful clinical examination.

Methohexitone Sodium

Methohexitone sodium (Brietal Sodium, Brevital) is sodium a-dl-l-methyl-5-allyl-5-(1-methyl-2-pentynyl) barbiturate. It differs from thiopentone, thialbarbitone and thiamylal sodium in that it contains no sulphur in the molecule and has two positions of unsaturation (one acetylenic, one olefinic) in the 5-position radicals. The structural formula is shown below:

$$C_2H_5—C{\equiv}C—\overset{CH_3}{\underset{\star}{\overset{|}{C}H}} \qquad \overset{O}{\overset{||}{C}}—N—CH_3$$

CH₃   O

C₂H₅—C≡C—CH   C—N—CH₃
           ★   \ /
            C   C—O Na
          / ★ \
CH₂=CH—CH₂   C—N
               ||
               O

* Denotes centres of asymmetry

Methohexitone sodium is stable in aqueous solutions kept at room temperature (25°C) for at least six weeks.

There are important differences between this agent and other intravenous anaesthetic agents. The significant features characteristic of methohexitone sodium are (1) potency two or three times greater than that of thiopentone sodium, (2) shorter duration of effect, and (3) more rapid recovery to full alertness, even after prolonged anaesthesia. It is the only drug for which there is convincing evidence of a more rapid recovery than from the 'standard' barbiturate, thiopentone.

In mice, rats, dogs, cats and monkeys methohexitone sodium has been shown to be an ultra-short-acting intravenous anaesthetic that is about twice as potent (on a weight basis) as the commonly used thiobarbiturates. Its action is characterized by a rapid and smooth induction, satisfactory surgical anaesthesia and quick recovery. The total duration of the mean anaesthetic dose rarely exceeds 30 minutes. Unfortunately, in animals the recovery period is often complicated by muscle tremors or even frank convulsions. These undesirable features are not seen if the animal is allowed to recover quite undisturbed, or if pethidine or the phenothiazine derivatives are used for premedication. Muscle tremors may also be seen in the induction period unless a rapid induction technique is practised.

The short duration of action depends both on the marked fat solubility which limits the duration of action of thiobarbiturates and also on a rapid rate of breakdown in the liver.

Methohexitone sodium is best administered to small animals as a 1% solution (10 mg/ml) but when large doses necessitate it, a 2·5% (25 mg/ml) solution may be used. In large animals more concentrated solutions of up to 6% are more convenient to handle. Owing to differences of pH solutions of methohexitone sodium should not be mixed with acid solutions such as atropine sulphate, tubocurarine and suxamethonium chlorides.

Rapid induction techniques usually produce temporary respiratory arrest. This is treated by maintaining the pulmonary ventilation until spontaneous respiration is resumed 30 to 60 seconds later. It is said that laryngospasm occurs less frequently with this than with the other intravenous anaesthetics. Rapid injection may produce transient hypotension but the blood pressure soon returns to normal levels. Fowler and Stevenson (1961, 1964) and Fabry (1963) have reported the use of methohexitone in small animal practice. There are few reports of its use in large animal patients. Tavernor (1962) has used this agent in horses, and Robertshaw (1964) demonstrated its value both as an induction agent and as a short-term anaesthetic for calves. Monahan (1964) has recorded the experiences of the Cambridge School with metho-hexitone sodium as an induction agent in 20 horses, 9 cows and 1 bull.

There is a place in veterinary anaesthesia for an agent which can produce rapid anaesthesia, but which is safe and from which recovery is rapid and complete. Methohexitone sodium fulfils these requirements, although the occurrence of muscle tremors in animals recovering from its effects indicates that it is not the perfect agent. However, methohexitone seems to have an advantage over the thiobarbiturates, in that recovery may be completed earlier as the animal is more alert and coordinated on regaining consciousness.

Steroids

In 1941 Selye reported that certain steriods had an anaesthetic action but it was not until 1955 that Laubach, P'An and Rudel selected hydroxydione as the most likely to be of clinical use. Hydroxydione (Viadril, Presuren) is 21-hydroxypregnane-3,20-dione sodium hemisuccinate. It is a water-soluble crystalline substance, aqueous solutions having a pH of 8 to 10, and has been used clinically in 0·5 to 2·5% solutions. It appears to be devoid of oestrogenic or androgenic properties.

Hydroxydione has been used in veterinary anaesthesia and appears suitable only for the dog (Fritsch, 1959; Stevenson, 1959), when given in doses of 50 to 100 mg/kg. The lethal dose is of the order of 400 mg/kg. The most striking difference between the action of hydroxydione and thiopentone is the delayed onset of unconsciousness after injection, and there is an equal or even longer delay between the injection of a large dose of the drug and the appearance of unwanted side-effects. Failure to realize this may account for the variations in reports of its effects on respiration and blood pressure. About 10 minutes may elapse between the administration of a dose which will eventually stop breathing and the occurrence of apnoea. Tachycardia and hypotension also accompany deep narcosis, and the time taken for the maximum depressant effects on the cardiovascular system to occur is greater than that for its action on respiration. Recovery is slow and this applies to recovery from its untoward side-effects. The duration of anaesthesia depends on the quantity of the drug injected. After 50 mg/kg it is about 20 minutes and after 100 mg/kg about 1 hour.

Hydroxydione is partly eliminated by the kidneys and 10 to 20% of the dose administered is excreted in the urine over a 3-day period. The drug is undoubtedly inactivated in some way in the body since bilateral nephrectomy has no effect on the duration or nature of its action. No toxic effect on the liver or kidneys has been demonstrated.

One of the most troublesome side-effects of hydroxydione is its irritant action on the endothelial lining of blood vessels. Thrombophlebitis is an almost invariable sequel to intravenous injection no matter what strength solutions are used or what precautions are taken. After accidental perivenous injection a painful inflammation occurs at the site.

This agent may be used in cats and in these animals its effects are similar to those in dogs. In horses hydroxydione appears to produce unexpectedly severe respiratory depression and anaesthesia is liable to be followed by a prolonged, often violent, recovery. In general the agent is too expensive for use in farm animals, but it has been given to both cattle and pigs without untoward effects. It is not possible to compare hydroxydione with the barbiturates because of its slow action. Minute to minute control of dosage is impossible, and if the drug is to be given in fractional doses it will take 20 to 30 minutes to induce anaesthesia with hydroxydione alone.

Phenoxyacetic Amines

Three drugs in this group of eugenol derivatives have been subjected to clinical trial in man and one has undergone extensive investigation, but there appear to be no records of similar investigations in veterinary anaesthesia. None of these drugs is sufficiently soluble in water to make the use of an aqueous solution feasible in anaesthetic practice. One, known as G29505 or Estil, is 2-methoxy-4-allyl-phenoxyacetic acid-N,N-diethyl amide, and this has been dissolved in a variety of inorganic solvents, the best apparently being 4% lecithin with 5% glucose.

G29505 appears to be about equipotent with thiopentone as an induction agent and the onset of anaesthesia is rapid. The striking feature of anaesthesia produced by G29505 is said to be the rapidity with which complete orientation occurs after recovery of consciousness. It may well be that this compound will prove to be useful in veterinary anaesthesia.

Propanidid

Propanidid (Epontol) is available as a 5% solution which can be diluted with water or saline as required. The 5% solution is rather viscid and requires a wide-bore needle for injection. With adequate dosage, loss of consciousness occurs as quickly as with thiopentone. Following the rapid intravenous injection of a calculated dose there is a period of hyperventilation immediately after consciousness is lost. The duration of action is very brief indeed. Propanidid causes much less venous thrombosis than any of the various solutions of G29505 or hydroxydione.

Trials in veterinary anaesthesia have had disappointing results. Doses of 15 mg/kg given to very small ponies by extremely rapid intravenous injection have produced anaesthesia sufficient for castration followed by complete recovery in less than 10 minutes. Because of the extremely short duration of action it has been found to be physically impossible to administer the drug fast enough to produce anaesthesia in larger horses, and violent excitement has followed the administration of sub-anaesthetic doses. In dogs, propanidid produces severe hypotension and respiratory depression.

Chloralose

Chloralose is prepared by heating equal quantities of glucose and chloral hydrate under controlled conditions so that two isomers are produced. Only the α-chloralose has narcotic properties: β-chloralose can produce muscular pain. The α-chloralose is available commercially as a white, crystalline powder and it is used as a 1% solution in water or saline. The solution is prepared fresh immediately before use by heating to 60°C. Heating to above this temperature results in decomposition and precipitation occurs on standing.

Anaesthesia with chloralose resembles that with chloral hydrate, but it is longer lasting. An intravenous dose of 80 to 100 mg/kg causes loss of consciousness but spontaneous muscular activity is common. The blood pressure is elevated and the activity of the autonomic nervous system is believed to be unaffected. The heart rate is often greatly increased and respiratory depression does not occur until very large doses are given. In the body chloralose is broken down to chloral and glucose and the safety margin is relatively wide.

Chloralose is still extensively used in physiological and pharmacological experiments and is given by intravenous injection. Because large volumes of solution have to be given before consciousness is lost, anaesthesia is often induced with some other agent such as ethyl chloride, ether, or methohexitone. The peak narcotic action of chloralose is seen some 15 to 20 minutes after injection. It is particularly useful for long, non-survival experiments which do not involve extensive surgical preparation.

Chloralose anaesthesia has no place in veterinary practice. Its disadvantages here are its relative insolubility, the long and comparatively shallow anaesthesia and the slow recovery which is accompanied by struggling.

Urethane

Urethane, the ethyl ester of carbaminic acid, produces a long period of light anaesthesia and is, therefore, like chloralose, used mainly for physiological and pharmacological experiments. Although it may be administered by other routes it is usually given by intravenous injection as a 10 to 20% solution in water. Urethane is believed to be carcinogenic and laboratory workers having contact with this compound are advised to handle it with care. It is often given with chloralose to suppress the muscular activity which occurs when chloralose is used alone. It is said that urethane has little effect on respiration and blood pressure.

Urethane has no place in veterinary anaesthesia.

The Anaesthetic Drugs administered by Inhalation

Chloroform

Chloroform is a heavy, sweet-smelling liquid, which is neither inflammable nor explosive. Its boiling point is 61°C. The vapour is non-irritating, and it is easy and not unpleasant to inhale. The liquid, however, is irritating to both skin and mucous membranes, and may cause burns of these tissues if spilt on them. It is decomposed by prolonged exposure to light and air and, therefore, should be stored in a cool place in amber-coloured bottles. Chloroform which has been in the anaesthetic machine for some time, or through which anaesthetic gases have been passed, should be discarded. Although chloroform is decomposed by alkalis, it may be used in anaesthetic circuits with soda lime without decomposition so long as the soda lime is of good quality and does not generate much heat.

Chloroform is a most powerful anaesthetic, a concentration of 0·035% in the blood causing anaesthesia, while 0·06% is fatal. To anaesthetize an animal in a reasonable time (10 to 12 minutes) concentrations of chloroform vapour in air or 1·5 to 2% are necessary. Such concentrations in the inspired air would, if persisted with, cause respiratory failure in a short time and thus, once the stage of anaesthesia is attained, it becomes necessary to reduce progressively the concentration inhaled. In addition to its action as an anaesthetic it has numerous side actions, which must be discussed when considering its use.

Dangers and Difficulties

The effects of chloroform on the circulatory system are complex, because the heart itself, the medullary centres and the peripheral blood vessels are concerned. In the early stages of induction slowing of the heart occurs, due, it is believed, to reflex vagal stimulation. One of the dangers associated with the agent is that cardiac failure may occur during the stage of induction and in animals there is usually an increase in the heart rate due to struggling. Once anaesthesia has been attained, the pulse becomes slower than normal but remains regular. There is always some dilatation of the heart and decrease in the force of its contraction. During the early stages of induction the vaso-motor centre is reflexly stimulated and this, together with the increase in the heart rate, causes blood pressure to rise. During anaesthesia the centre is depressed, the peripheral blood vessels dilate and blood pressure falls. In addition to this central effect the walls of the blood vessels themselves are affected and this is a contributory factor in the fall in blood pressure.

The respiratory centre is influenced both directly and indirectly. In the early stages respirations are accelerated due to struggling; they are also deep in character. During anaesthesia the susceptibility of the centre to carbon dioxide stimulation is depressed and breathing becomes slow and shallow. In addition the centre is directly affected by the general fall in blood pressure.

Body temperature progressively falls during anaesthesia. This is in part due to peripheral vasodilatation causing an increased heat loss, and in part to the reduction in heat production due to absence of movement and reduction of muscle tone.

In addition to its effects on the myocardium, chloroform has a toxic effect on the liver and kidneys, causing cloudy swelling and even acute fatty change in the cells. When severe these changes give rise to delayed poisoning the symptoms of which develop some 24 to 48 hours after administration. It is characterized by acute acidosis, with severe vomiting (in the dog and cat), acetonuria, albumenuria, mild pyrexia and icterus, and frequently terminates fatally with severe hyperpyrexia. The absence of symptoms is not evidence that the liver has been uninfluenced, for it is a remarkable fact that this organ is capable of undergoing extensive necrosis without any obvious abnormality of health becoming apparent.

While the placenta does not provide a barrier against the passage of chloro-form into the foetal blood, foetuses delivered from animals under medium depth chloroform anaesthesia are quite active and breathe well. It will be recalled that most of Simpson's work with chloroform was carried out on parturient women.

No statistics are available indicating the percentage of deaths which occurs in animals due to chloroform. In the horse, death during anaesthesia is a comparatively rare incident. This is no doubt due in part to the fact that the majority of equine anaesthetizations are of a transient nature, but cases are encountered in which post-anaesthetic pneumonia develops. This complication is more likely to occur after prolonged administration or when the animal's air supply has been seriously curtailed by the method of administration. In cattle, death during anaesthesia is also reputed to be rare, but in this species it is seldom that chloroform is administered beyond the stage of light anaesthesia. The incidence of post-anaesthetic pneumonia is reputed to be higher in this species than in the horse. Sheep and goats are generally regarded as responding badly to chloroform and animals which survive the period of anaesthesia often develop pneumonia inside a few days. The pig is a better subject and has no special susceptibility provided that care is taken in administration. In the days when chloroform was used in dogs and cats mortality was high. In fact it is said that when performing operations requiring continuous anaesthesia for periods of half an hour or longer the death rate was a high as 10%. This, of course, was before the introduction of modern methods of anaesthesia which utilize an intravenous barbiturate for induction and the toxicity of chloroform when used simply as a maintenance agent for dogs and cats may not be so bad.

Cardiac failure may occur during the induction period or it may occur later, particularly if the course of anaesthesia has been irregular. Not infrequently, an animal in a state of vigorous excitement collapses suddenly; the heart ceases to beat and after a few gasping movements respiratory function ceases also. A number of explanations for this accident have been given. Embley believed it to be due to excessive vagal activity. Levy's explanation that it results from ventricular fibrillation is more generally accepted. This may be due to the direct toxic action of chloroform consequent upon the high concentrations reaching the myocardium via the blood in the coronary arteries. There is experimental evidence to show that adrenaline can cause ventricular fibrillation in the presence of chloroform. From the clinical viewpoint it is clear that care must be taken not to 'push' the anaesthetic too vigorously during the first and second stages of anaesthesia, for there is no doubt that struggling and breath-holding predispose to this accident.

Respiratory failure may also occur during the course of anaesthesia. As anaesthesia becomes profound, reflexes disappear, respirations become shallow and slow and finally stop. The cause is overdosage and the heart may cease to beat simultaneously with respiratory failure or it may continue to beat weakly for several minues and finally stop from anoxia.

The record of chloroform undoubtedly contains accounts of many disasters and it is possible that if it had been subjected, at the time of its introduction into anaesthesia, to the full battery of tests which are applied to potential anaesthetics today, it would never have been accepted for clinical use. It is therefore of interest to note that Waters (1951) in his re-appraisal of chloroform in humans concluded that it has a place in anaesthesia, provided that care is taken in its administration. He emphasized the need to avoid hypoxia, which is a known factor in the potentiation of chloroform's toxicity on the liver and felt that accurate control and knowledge of inspired chloroform vapour concentration was highly desirable. Cases of gross cardiac conduction defects, hypotension and cardiac arrest which occurred in his series of cases were attributable to either hypoxia or accidental overdosage.

Trials involving brief administration of chloroform in women (Imray, Kennedy and Kilpatrick, 1964) and longer administration in horses (Hall, unpublished observations), in which Water's recommendations were carried out, failed to reveal any significant increase in serum glutamic pyruvic transaminase levels 24 hours after anaesthesia. It is possible that other more sensitive tests of liver function might have revealed liver damage due to chloroform for Reichart, Wiquist and Yllner (1960) demonstrated significantly increased levels of activity of serum ornithine carbamyl transferase, glutamic oxaloacetic transaminase* and glutamic pyruvic transaminase* in women after chloroform anaesthesia. However, Reichart et al. were studying parturient women given chloroform by the open drop method during the second stage of labour. The patients in their trial are likely to have been depleted of liver glycogen, the concentration of chloroform administered was unknown and there may have been a degree of hypoxia or hypercapnia involved due to the method of administration.

Probably all anaesthetists would agree that chloroform is more dangerous than any of the other anaesthetics in common use but, nevertheless, in certain circumstances in veterinary practice the advantages of using it may outweigh the dangers involved.

Diethyl Ether

Diethyl ether, commonly called 'ether', is a transparent, colourless liquid which boils at 35°C. It is much lighter than chloroform but its vapour is twice as heavy as air. It is highly inflammable and mixtures of its vapour in air or oxygen in certain proportions are explosive. The heavy vapour tends to pool on the floor and unless ventilation is good the possibility of explosions occurring is great. The vapour mixture may easily be exploded by sparks of static electricity or by sparks arising from faulty connections in electrical switches and apparatus. Ether should, of course, never be used in the vicinity

---

* By international agreement, glutamic oxaloacetic transaminase is now known as 'aspartate transaminase' and glutamic pyruvic transaminase as 'alanine transaminase'.

of gas fires or other open flames but it must also be remembered that explosions have been caused by the vapour mixture rolling along the floor into an adjoining room and being ignited there. Ether should not be administered in any place in which electrical equipment such as X-ray apparatus or diathermy is to be used, and in these places the ether bottle should be removed from the anaesthetic machine; it is not sufficient merely to empty it and replace it on the machine.

Ether is decomposed by air, light and heat; the liquid should, therefore, be stored in amber-coloured bottles in a cool dark place. Liquid ether can cause burns of the skin and mucous membranes if it is accidentally spilt over these tissues and if it is aspirated into the respiratory passages it may cause death. Irrespective of the method of administration ether is almost entirely eliminated from the body through the lungs. Ether is said to be very 'irritant' to the mouth, pharynx, larynx and respiratory tract because when inhaled it stimulates the secretion of saliva and mucus. 'Irritant' is not strictly correct for it does not cause those irritant effects on the respiratory mucosa which are produced by true irritant gases such as mustard gas. A pre-operative injection of an antisialogogue (e.g. atropine) usually prevents excessive secretion of saliva and mucus consequent upon the administration of ether. Any attempt to make an animal inhale strong concentrations of ether vapour causes coughing and breath-holding so the induction of anaesthesia with ether is both difficult for the anaesthetist and unpleasant for the animal. Basal anaesthetic agents are often employed in order to provide a smooth and rapid induction of anaesthesia. Unless an animal is very deeply anaesthetized ether cannot be introduced in the middle of an operation without provoking coughing, breath-holding or laryngeal spasm. If ether is to be given, it should be added to the inhaled atmosphere as early as possible during the administration of the anaesthetic so as to accustom the mucous membrane to its presence.

On the central nervous system ether exerts an initial effect of excitement which may be responsible for the occurrence of delirium during the induction of anaesthesia. After this initial stimulation the brain is depressed. The medullary centres are not paralysed, except by the administration of a dose which is many times greater than that necessary to produce surgical anaesthesia. The margin between the anaesthetic and toxic doses is very wide and for this reason ether is one of the safest anaesthetic agents. Failure of the respiration always precedes cardiac failure and since the effects of ether upon the heart are very slight resuscitation after respiratory arrest in deep anaesthesia is simple.

The inhalation of ether causes an initial increase in the force and frequency of the pulse. The cardiac output changes are the result of the antagonism between the direct myocardial depressant effect of ether and the inotropic effects of reflexly released adrenaline and noradrenaline. The safety of ether lies in the elevated levels of circulating catecholamines found during anaesthesia; in their absence the depressant effects of ether are not combated. As anaesthesia continues the pulse returns to its normal force and rhythm. The blood pressure shows an initial transient rise. After this it reverts to normal but in the deeper planes of anaesthesia it falls slightly due both to depression of the vasomotor centre and to depression of the tone of smooth muscle in the vessel walls. There is no correlation between the increases in circulating adrenaline and noradrenaline levels and the depth of anaesthetic. It seems that the circulating effects of ether are not quantitatively antagonized by the reflex release of catecholamines. It has been shown that ether increases the sensitivity of the carotid sinus and aortic and baroreceptors (Robertson, Swan and Whitteridge, 1956) and blocks transmission through sympathetic ganglia (Norman and Lofstrom, 1955). These actions may be responsible for the decreased peripheral resistance and the reduced sympathetic response to the fall in arterial pressure during the deeper levels of ether anaesthesia.

Respiratory movements are increased in light ether anaesthesia and are decreased as anaesthesia deepens. The intercostal muscles become progressively less active as anaesthesia progresses and the diaphragm tends to show increasing movement to compensate for this. In third plane anaesthesia the diaphragmatic movements may become short, jerky and rapid and may interfere with the performance of intra-abdominal operations.

In ether anaesthesia the spleen contracts while the intestines become dilated and atonic. The blood sugar level rises due to the mobilization of liver glycogen under the influence of the increased secretion of adrenaline. Liver function and the secretion of bile are decreased during ether anaesthesia and kidney function is also depressed. The liver and kidneys usually recover their normal function within 24 hours of the cessation of anaesthesia. The inhalation of ether causes a fall in the pH of the blood and in the plasma bicarbonate— i.e. acidosis occurs and ketone bodies may appear in the urine. Delayed poisoning is not seen after ether anaesthesia.

It is generally agreed that using the usual open and semi-open methods of administration it is impossible to achieve concentrations of ether vapour in the inspired air sufficiently high to induce or maintain anaesthesia in horses or adult cattle, the MAC of ether (see page 200) being 1·92%. However, ether may be given to these animals by semi-closed or closed absorption methods (when the vaporizer bottle is included in the breathing circuit) to maintain anaesthesia once this state has been induced with chloral hydrate, pentobarbitone sodium or thiopentone sodium. Auto-inhalation methods may also be used to maintain anaesthesia induced with these agents. Ether may be given to all other domestic animals by open, semi-open, closed or semi-closed methods both to induce and to maintain anaesthesia.

Ether possesses many disadvantages. Its inhalation provokes the secretion of mucus and saliva. Induction of anaesthesia with ether, as has already been stated, is unpleasant for the animal and difficult for the anaesthetist. It cannot be introduced easily in the middle of an operation without provoking inconvenient reflex effects. Post-operative nausea is pronounced and animals will not eat for several hours after they have been subjected to ether anaesthesia. On the other hand, ether has been in continuous use for over 100 years and millions of operations must have been performed on animals under ether anaesthesia. The number of deaths directly attributable to ether, apart from accidents (e.g. explosions and fires) and errors of technique, is very small indeed. There can be no doubt that ether is still the safest general anaesthetic agent available for most veterinary patients.

Ethyl Chloride

Ethyl chloride has a boiling point of 12·5°C so that at ordinary room temperatures it is a vapour. Nevertheless, it is easily compressed to form a clear, colourless liquid and it is supplied for anaesthetic purposes in this form in glass tubes which have spring loaded metal spraying nozzles. The vapour is heavier than air, has an ethereal smell and is capable of explosion when mixed with air or oxygen.

Ethyl chloride is non-irritant to the respiratory mucosa and animals do not object to its ethereal odour. Induction of anaesthesia is rapid but overdosage is easy due to the physical properties of the drug. Sudden circulatory failure due to overdosage is not uncommon during the induction of anaesthesia with ethyl chloride. Because the drug is so potent and simple to administer the greatest possible care should be exercised in its use. Once a rhythmical respiratory movement has commenced ethyl chloride should be abandoned: if necessary anaesthesia can be maintained with ether—a much safer agent.

The drug is sometimes used for local analgesia. A fine spray is allowed to fall on the operation area. The liquid vaporizes and as it does so it cools the skin to about −20°C and the surrounding water vapour freezes so that fine ice crystals are formed over the wound. Incision of the skin is painless but as the thaw sets in pain may become very severe.

Trichloroethylene

Trichloroethylene is a heavy, colourless liquid with a smell which is similar to that of chloroform but not so sweet. Its specific gravity is 1·46 and its boiling point is high (87°C) so that its volatility at room temperatures is low. Trilene, the trade name for the preparation which is used in anaesthesia in

Great Britain, consists of purified trichloroethylene, thymol (as a stabilizing agent) 1:10,000 and waxoline blue (dyestuff) 1:200,000. The dye is added to distinguish it from chloroform.

In its effects trichloroethylene resembles chloroform but it is much less potent and less toxic. The ratio between the anaesthetic and minimal lethal dose is high.

It causes little or no irritation to the upper air passages and is simple to administer. Induction is smooth but full surgical relaxation cannot be obtained with safety for tachypnoea and cardiac irregularities appear before relaxation becomes apparent. It produces a very high degree of analgesia and the main use of trichloroethylene in veterinary anaesthesia is to reinforce the analgesic properties of nitrous oxide.

Due to its low volatility open methods of administration are unsatisfactory and it is usually given in a semi-closed circuit with a mixture of nitrous oxide and oxygen. In the presence of soda lime its use is contra-indicated for in an absorber it may be broken down to such toxic products as hydrochloric acid, dichloracetylene, phosgene and carbon monoxide.

Trichloroethylene is the only inhalation agent which is broken down to any extent in the body. Butler (1949) studied its breakdown in dogs and isolated small amounts of trichloroethanol from the plasma and large amounts in conjugated form from the urine after anaesthesia. Trichloroacetic acid has also been found as a breakdown product in the urine. It seems that trichloroethylene is, initially, converted to chloral hydrate, which is the immediate precursor of both trichlorethanol and trichloroacetic acid. A fairly accurate assessment of the amount of vapour absorbed can be obtained by measurement of metabolite excreted in the urine. The majority of the trichloroacetic acid is excreted within the first three days, but it may persist in the body for more than a week, depending on the daily urine volume.

The main advantage of trichloroethylene is that it is non-explosive and non-inflammable in the concentrations used in anaesthesia.

Halothane

Halothane (Fluothane) is a fluorinated hydrocarbon, $CF_3CHClBr$. It is a heavy liquid with a specific gravity of 1·86 (chloroform 1·49, ether 0·7), and a boiling point of 50·2°C (chloroform 61·26°, ether 34·6°). It has a characteristic but not unpleasant odour. It is not inflammable and its vapour mixed with air or oxygen is not explosive. It decomposes slowly with the formation of volatile acids when exposed to light but this is overcome by storage in amber-coloured bottles and the addition of a small quantity of thymol. It is quite stable when in contact with soda lime and thus may be used in closed circuit methods of anaesthetization.

The pharmacology of the halothane in small animals was first described by Raventós (1956) following his studies in the Imperial Chemical Industries biological laboratories, and later by Burn, Epstein, Feigan and Paton (1957) of the University of Oxford. Many other studies have followed and a great deal of information has now accumulated. Indeed, it is probable that halothane has been subjected to more investigational studies than any other anaesthetic agent. In the veterinary field Fisher and Jennings (1961) studied its respiratory effects in cattle, horses, sheep and dogs, and Vasko (1962) has reported the effects of halothane on cardiac action and blood pressure in horses.

With vapour concentrations of from 2 to 4% in the inspired air induction of anaesthesia in all domestic animals is smooth and rapid. Anaesthesia can be maintained with concentrations of 0·8 to 2·0% of halothane in the inspired air, the MAC (see page 200) being 0·765%. Raventós found halothane to be about twice as potent as chloroform and four times as potent as ether. On the other hand its safety factor or therapeutic ratio (3·5) was shown to be twice that of chloroform or ether. Recovery from anaesthesia is rapid and free from excitement. When no other agents are administered animals are able to walk normally in 15 to 30 minutes after periods of anaesthesia lasting up to 6 hours. Blood concentrations are around 14 mg % during the maintenance of anaesthesia and fall rapidly during recovery so that levels of 4 to 6 mg % have been recorded 15 minutes after discontinuance of anaesthesia.

The respiratory passages are not irritated by halothane, and the formation of secretions is inhibited. The bronchi and bronchioles are relaxed. Respiration is depressed, leading to a decrease in the tidal volume. The arterial carbon dioxide tension is directly related to the alveolar concentration of halothane when this is above 0·7% (Merkel and Eger, 1963). Surgical stimulation during light levels of anaesthesia may give rise to shallow, very rapid breathing.

The administration of halothane causes the blood pressure to fall and the pulse to slow. During light anaesthesia the blood pressure slowly recovers and after about thirty minutes it usually has returned to normal. Raventós attributes the cardiovascular effects to ganglionic block, but Burn et al. consider that halothane has a direct depressant effect on the myocardium and a central depressant effect on the vasomotor centres. Burn and his co-workers recognize the ganglion block effect, but suggest that it plays little part in the production of hypotension. Halothane has about 70% of the activity of chloroform in reducing cardiac output, and increases the sensitivity of the myocardium to adrenaline. Bradycardia appears to be due to the preservation of activity in the vagus nerves. In animals the hypotension is associated with obvious cutaneous vasodilatation; in white pigs, for example, the skin becomes noticeably warm, dry and pink.

Usually a perfectly normal electrocardiogram persists throughout halothane anaesthesia, but ventricular extrasystoles and bigeminal rhythm have been reported as occurring in dogs. In cats A–V dissociation with interference and extrasystoles may occur; the circumstances under which these irregularities arise has been investigated by Purchase (1964).

Halothane has a minimal neuromuscular blocking effect, but increases that of non-depolarizing relaxants, while antagonizing the effect of drugs which act by depolarization (Graham, 1958). By its action of relaxing smooth muscle halothane may interfere with the normal involution of the uterus after Caesarean hysterotomy and be responsible for post-partum haemorrhage.

Shivering is often seen during recovery from halothane anaesthesia. The reason is unknown; it does not seem to be related to body or environmental temperature, and it has been observed in all species of domestic animals. Usually it is of no importance, but by increasing oxygen demands it may be harmful to animals suffering from respiratory and/or cardiovascular diseases which limit oxygen uptake when they are breathing air.

It is almost certain that halothane has minimal effects on the liver and kidneys. Raventós described a mild dilatation of the proximal convoluted tubules of the kidney after the use of halothane which was not associated with alteration of renal function. Recently it has been suggested that halothane may be associated with disturbances of liver function in man giving rise to jaundice. Most of these reports have originated in the United States and it is possible that coincidental virus hepatitis has been responsible for the lesions described (Vickers and Dinnick, 1964) since the incidence of virus hepatitis is higher in America than it is in Great Britain. The possibility that one administration of halothane may sensitize the hepatic cells so that trouble arises subseqently when halothane is employed on a later occasion cannot, however, be ignored. Comfort may be derived from the fact that in any case the incidence of this alleged complication is very small indeed. There have also been reports of liver damage following halothane anaesthesia in animals, but sound evidence has not been produced to support these claims.

A feature to be noted is that the sensitivity of the myocardium to adrenaline, with the provocation of ventricular fibrillation, is increased by halothane to a degree greater than that by chloroform and to a lesser degree than by cyclopropane.

Many authors have emphasized the dangers of using such a potent drug as halothane in a closed system with the vaporizer in the breathing circuit. Newman (1958) has attacked this conception on the grounds that 'the danger of a rapidly mounting halothane concentration is not due to rebreathing but to a rate of administration excessive for that particular situation'. Marrett (1959) working with a fully closed system found that despite maximal rebreathing the halothane concentration in the system did not rise appreciably even when the anaesthetic lasted for more than an hour, unless the vaporizer was set to deliver a high percentage of halothane. This suggests that within the limits absorption of halothane by the body tissues (mainly the fat) equals the rate at which fresh halothane vapour is added to the circuit, thus keeping the blood level constant. More evidence on this point in animals is required.

Most ether vaporizers incorporated in circle absorption systems (see page 257) are unsuitable for use with halothane as there is extreme difficulty in obtaining a constant vapour concentration. Moreover, many of these container bottles have a large area for vaporization immediately above the level of the liquid; the sudden release of this vapour into the inspired gases may lead to the inhalation of a dangerous concentration of halothane. This complication may be overcome by discarding the 'built-in' bottle and using a small vaporizer (e.g. Rowbotham's apparatus) placed in the expiratory limb of the circuit so that before vapour can reach the animal it must first be diluted by the gases in the reservoir bag.

Now more than 13 years since its introduction into veterinary anaesthesia (Hall, 1957) it has become widely accepted and by now most of its critics have, at least, modified their views. A danger may now lie in its unrestricted use by the inexperienced anaesthetist in the belief that 'nothing ever goes wrong'.

It is clear from its popularity that there are frequently advantages to be gained by using halothane in preference to other agents. Ease of induction and maintenance, relatively prompt recovery, non-inflammability and the low incidence of sickness and inappetence after anaesthesia figure prominently here, and contribute in no small measure to the safety and comfort of the patient.

Ether–halothane Azeotrope

Halothane and ether form an azeotropic mixture (31·7% by volume diethyl ether and 68·3% halothane). This mixture has a boiling point of 51·5°C and the proportions of the constituents remain constant throughout the administration. Mixing with halothane in this way does not eliminate the explosion hazard which is normally associated with ether, but the lower limits of flammability of the mixture are said to be greater than the concentrations required for surgical anaesthesia. Although it has been claimed that the addition of ether modifies the cardiovascular and respiratory depressant effects of halothane (Hudon, Jaques and Boivin, 1958), Black and Love (1961) reported that the arterial pressure in children was depressed to a much greater extent by the azeotrope than by its constituents. It seems likely that the small concentrations of ether contained in the azeotrope are incapable of invoking compensatory increases in catecholamines and that, in the absence of an active sympathoadrenal response, the direct effect of ether on the myocardium and blood vessels predominates. The ganglionic blocking activity of halothane may also lower arterial pressure during anaesthesia with the azeotrope. The mixture seems on theoretical grounds to be an illogical one, and it has not gained wide acceptance, although it has been used in veterinary anaesthesia to some extent (Hime, 1963).

Methoxyflurane

Methoxyflurane (Penthrane, Metofane) is a halogenated ethyl methyl ether with the chemical name 2,2-dichloro-1,1-difluoroethyl methyl ether. Its structural formula is

$$\begin{array}{ccc} Cl & F & H \\ \diagdown & | & | \\ H-C-C-O-C-H \\ \diagup & | & | \\ Cl & F & H \end{array}$$

It is a clear colourless liquid which boils at 104·65°C at 760 mm of mercury pressure and freezes at $-35°C$. Although the boiling point is slightly higher than that of water it volatilizes more readily as a result of a low latent heat of vaporization (49 cal/g). It is non-explosive and non-inflammable in air or oxygen at the temperatures and conditions encountered in anaesthesia.

Methoxyflurane is chemically stable and is not decomposed by air, light, moisture or alkali such as soda lime. It may, however, slowly form a brownish discoloration due to the antioxidant used in the formulation but this does not affect the anaesthetic properties. Contact with copper, brass, or bronze may also cause discoloration but without apparent effect on safety or toxicity. The odour of methoxyflurane has been described as 'fruity' and is well accepted and tolerated by animals.

The saturated vapour pressure of methoxyflurane is only 25 mm of mercury at 20°C. Since the concentration of vapour obtainable during the administration of anaesthesia is limited by the vapour pressure and the efficiency of the vaporizer, the maximum obtainable concentration of methoxyflurane vapour at 23°C is less than 4%. Because of this the agent is not satisfactory as an induction agent and it is therefore recommended that animals should receive a minimal intravenous dose of a short-acting barbiturate, followed by the maximum obtainable concentration of methoxyflurane to complete the induction of anaesthesia.

Blood concentrations and tissue levels during and after surgical anaesthesia in dogs have been studied by Chenworth, Robertson, Erley and Golhke (1962). The MAC (see page 200) is 0·16%. The compound persists in the blood even after apparent complete recovery 24 hours after anaesthesia. This persistence is due to the marked affinity of methoxyflurane for fat depots, and the presence of low levels of the agent in the bloodstream is believed to account, in part, for the smooth post-anaesthetic emergence.

The maximum vapour concentration obtainable is only mildly irritating to inhale so that stimulation of secretions in the respiratory tract is minimal. In contrast to ether, but like halothane, methoxyflurane depresses respiration to a degree proportional to the depth of anaesthesia. As a result of the low vapour pressure, respiratory depression and rate of uptake by the tissues, it is extremely difficult to produce respiratory arrest in dogs and cats allowed to breathe spontaneously.

Methoxyflurane resembles ether in its effects on the circulatory system. Heart rate and rhythm are not altered until anaesthesia becomes very deep, when the rate becomes very slow. The blood pressure is remarkably stable during anaesthesia. Although early studies suggested that the agent did not sensitize the myocardium to adrenaline, later investigations demonstrated that large doses of adrenaline could produce atrioventricular block and arrhythmias. Bagwell and Woods (1962) reported cardiovascular depression in dogs, but the sympathetic nervous system was not blocked by methoxy-flurane.

The effect of methoxyflurane on the liver has been studied by North, Knox, Vartanian and Stephen (1961), Dobkin and Fedoruk (1961), Cale and Parks (1962) and Jumes and Siebecker (1960). Cephalin cholesterol flocculation becomes positive during anaesthesia but returns to normal within three weeks. Dogs anaesthetized for 1 hour each week for 30 consecutive weeks showed no evidence of liver damage. Gross overdosage for 5 hours only caused minimal hepatic changes—no fatty infiltration or necrosis was observed. Dogs exposed to 1% methoxyflurane vapour for 3 hours on 5 different occasions showed variable microscopic changes in the liver. There was little or no cellular damage but some fatty infiltration in the centrilobular areas. Two of these dogs showed an increase in BSP retention 48 hours after their last exposure to the vapour.

Chenworth et al. have shown that the urine contains only minute traces of methoxyflurane. Disturbances of renal function after anaesthesia have not been observed. Histological studies of kidneys of dogs subjected to overdosage with methoxyflurane have shown only minimal changes and no evidence of necrosis.

Methoxyflurane does not affect the blood picture and Dobkin and Fedoruk (1961) found no significant alteration in the haematocrit during anaesthesia.

In veterinary anaesthesia the use of methoxyflurane has been reported by Jones, Stockton and Tigert (1962), Douglas, Jennings, Longstreeth and Weaver (1964) and Hall (1964). It is apparent that it is really only suitable

8

for the maintenance of anaesthesia in small animal patients, although when used in the appropriate apparatus it will anaesthetize cattle and horses.

Nitrous Oxide

Nitrous oxide is a colourless gas with a faint, rather pleasant smell. It is not inflammable or explosive but it will support the combustion of other agents, even in the absence of free oxygen. It is one and a half times as heavy as air and liquefies when compressed into cylinders at 40 atmospheres pressure. The amount of nitrous oxide present in a cylinder can be measured only by weighing since the pressure of the gaseous nitrous oxide above the liquid level remains constant as long as any liquid remains. Thus, a pressure gauge screwed into the cylinder outlet will register a constant pressure until all the liquid nitrous oxide has been vaporized and after this the reading drops rapidly to zero as the gas leaves the cylinder. Some type of pressure reducing valve must be attached to the cylinder before the rate or flow of the gas can be accurately adjusted or measured.

Nitrous oxide is not irritant to the respiratory mucosa and because it is non-toxic it can be administered for very long periods without producing ill-effects. It is now generally accepted that the gas has a true, though weak, narcotic action on the cerebral cells, but its exact mode of action is still uncertain. It does not enter into chemical combination in any body tissue and the earlier belief that its action is due to the exclusion of oxygen is no longer held. Although the anaesthetic effect may be enhanced by introducing an asphyxial element into its administration such a procedure is most detrimental to the animal.

Because the gas is such a weak anaesthetic, it can be used in a satisfactory manner only in animals which have received adequate premedication and in which consciousness has already been abolished by the use of an intravenous agent such as thiopentone sodium. Even in these animals the best results are obtained only when careful attention is paid to the finer points of the administration of the gas. Great care must be taken to see that the highest possible partial pressure of nitrous oxide is presented to the lungs together with 20 to 25% of oxygen. Dead space must be kept to the minimum by the use of an endotracheal tube; leakage of air into the apparatus must be avoided, and rebreathing eliminated as far as possible by the use of high gas flow rates in the usual semi-closed circuits or by the incorporation of a non-return valve close to the animal. Because of the large gas flow rates necessary for large animal patients, and because of the cost of the necessary apparatus, its use represents a very expensive method of anaesthesia for horses and cattle.

The phenomenon known as 'diffusion hypoxia' sometimes occurs immediately following anaesthesia with nitrous oxide and oxygen when the gas is being rapidly eliminated from the lungs. Nitrous oxide may form 10% or more of the volume of the expired gas, and the outward diffusion of nitrous oxide into the alveoli lowers the partial pressure of oxygen in the lungs to dangerously low levels. The hypoxia so produced may cause cardiac arrest in elderly animals or in those suffering from pulmonary or cardiovascular disease. It is important to administer an oxygen-enriched atmosphere for some 10 minutes after the termination of a long nitrous oxide–oxygen anaesthetic.

The disadvantages of nitrous oxide are its lack of potency, its inability to produce muscle relaxation, its narrow margin of anaesthesia, its cost, the necessity for expensive, elaborate apparatus, and, in the hands of the unskilled, its tendency to be associated with asphyxia.

Nevertheless, when used with skill and discretion nitrous oxide has many advantages. It is non-explosive, non-toxic (in the absence of hypoxia), provides a rapid recovery and post-operative complications do not occur. For many operations, which do not stimulate sensitive structures, and in which muscular relaxation is not required, it approaches the ideal agent for the maintenance of anaesthesia. For others, its action may be supplemented with some more powerful agent, used carefully and at the correct times during the operation. The supplementary agent may be given as required and much less of this more toxic drug is thus administered than would be required if nitrous oxide were not being used. At the same time the presence of the supplement allows a higher oxygen concentration to be given thus avoiding all dangers of hypoxia. The agents commonly used to supplement nitrous oxide–oxygen anaesthesia are thiopentone sodium, pethidine, ether, halothane, methoxyflurane and trichloroethylene. The nitrous oxide, being a relatively insoluble agent, has a rather high initial uptake which augments the inspiratory flow of the anaesthetic mixture and consequently facilitates the uptake of soluble agents such as ether, halothane and methoxyflurane—the 'second gas effect' (Epstein, Rackow, Salanitre and Wolf, 1964; Stoelting and Eger, 1969).

Cyclopropane

Cyclopropane (C_3H_6) is a colourless gas with a characteristic odour; it is one-and-a-half times as heavy as air, and liquefies at 15°C under a pressure of 75 lb/sq in. It is stored in cylinders made of light alloy and no reducing valve is necessary as with other gaseous anaesthetics. It is as inflammable as ether, and mixtures of cyclopropane with air or oxygen are explosive. It is soluble in lipoid tissues and as an anaesthetic agent the gas is potent and quick acting. When an animal inhales a fixed concentration of the gas, the cyclopropane contents of the venous and arterial blood become almost equal in 15 minutes. It is as quickly eliminated and recovery, even after prolonged administration, is often disconcertingly abrupt. It is effective in a concentration of 15 to 20% with oxygen, and thus adequate oxygenation is possible in all circumstances. Inhalation of about 8% produces light anaesthesia, 20 to 25% good moderately deep anaesthesia, and over 35 to 40% respiratory failure. During induction the stage of excitement is often well defined and this is a disadvantage in large animals. Intravenous injection of a barbiturate for induction prevents this excitement, but if an excessive dose is given the respiration is depressed so that it may be difficult to obtain adequate anaesthesia.

The gas is non-irritating to mucous membranes, and although difficult to inhale in strong concentrations, it is not unpleasant in weak concentrations; ruminants, in particular, seldom object to breathing it.

Cyclopropane does not produce any marked metabolic acidosis, but because it is always depressant to the respiration its administration is always accompanied by some degree of respiratory acidosis. Indeed the gas is so depressant to the medullary centre that apnoea may be produced even before muscular relaxation is obtained. Respiratory acidosis can only be avoided by artificial ventilation of the lungs.

Cyclopropane has a pronounced effect on the cardiovascular system. The most constant effect is increased haemorrhage at operation sites. This haemorrhage is often very pronounced and is due to vasodilatation combined with increased blood flow. Doubtless some of this effect is caused by hypercapnia resulting from respiratory depression and can be avoided by manual or mechanical assistance of the pulmonary ventilation. Even when the carbon dioxide content of the blood is kept at, or below, normal levels, however, capillary oozing is increased. The increased bleeding seems to be confined to the skin and subcutaneous tissues, is particularly noticeable in obese animals, and constitutes one of the most objectional features of cyclopropane anaesthesia.

The studies of Price and his co-workers (1963, 1965, 1969) indicate that cyclopropane selectively depresses the depressor areas of the medullary vasomotor centres but to a certain extent spares the excitatory pressor areas. In cats it was found that preganglionic cervical sympathetic discharge frequency increased during cyclopropane anaesthesia. On the other hand, Markee, Wang and Wang (1966), in a similar experimental study, found that the medullary pressor component was more sensitive than the depressor area to the depressant action of cyclopropane and that the gas had a direct action on vascular smooth muscle. The controversy is yet to be resolved.

Cardiac arrhythmia is common under cyclopropane anaesthesia but, in practice, seems to be without significance as long as the circulation remains efficient as judged by the 'arteriolar-capillary refill time'. (This is the time taken for the colour to return to a given area of the buccal mucous membrane after it has been made ischaemic by pressure.) In any case, most of the arrhythmias encountered under cyclopropane anaesthesia disappear if the pulmonary ventilation is augmented in such a manner as to lower the carbon dioxide content of the arterial blood. Cyclopropane renders the myocardium particularly susceptible to the stimulant effect of adrenaline, to a more marked degree than does chloroform. The administration of atropine by intravenous injection during cyclopropane anaesthesia may be followed by severe and dangerous arrhythmias (Jones, Deutsch and Turndorf, 1961). The appearance or the exacerbation of ventricular irregularities following the reduction of an elevated arterial carbon dioxide tension during cyclopropane anaesthesia has been reported by Lurie and his associates (1958), and the likelihood of this increases with higher rates of fall of carbon dioxide tension and with higher concentrations of cyclopropane.

Cyclopropane has the property of increasing the activity of the vagus nerves and in ruminants this may be manifested by laryngospasm or even broncho-spasm. Contractions of the uterus are not inhibited, and the concentration of the gas in the blood of the foetus becomes almost equal to that in the blood of the mother after about 15 minutes. Since it is quickly eliminated from the foetus once respiration is established after birth, this is usually of little signi-ficance. Indeed, cyclopropane is very suitable for obstetrical cases because it is possible to administer a high concentration of oxygen along with it and this protects the foetus from anoxia.

The gas has very little adverse effect on the liver, even after preliminary chloroform poisoning, and this may be due to the high oxygen concentrations which may be used with cyclopropane. Renal blood flow and glomerular filtration rate are decreased during cyclopropane anaesthesia but return to normal when it is terminated. During light anaesthesia the intestine is usually active, and the activity of the rumen continues, but these movements are abolished in deeper anaesthesia. Post-anaesthetic vomiting is frequently encountered in dogs after cyclopropane anaesthesia.

Because of its high cost, the explosion risk, and because it is often necessary to assist respiration by rhythmical manual pressure on the breathing bag, it is usual though not essential to administer it by the closed circuit carbon dioxide absorption method. The explosion risk is a very real one and attempts have been made to overcome it by mixing helium with the respired gases. A mixture of 40% cyclopropane, 30% oxygen and 30% helium is non-explosive and non-inflammable, and its use in dogs, cats, calves, sheep and goats has been explored by Warren (1960).

The administration of cyclopropane to domestic animals, including the dog, for physiological experiments, was developed by Professor R. A. Gregory of Liverpool, and since 1950 it has been extensively employed in veterinary hospitals in Great Britain. It is particularly indicated for the production of short periods of anaesthesia when a rapid recovery is required in dogs and cats, and for most surgical interventions in small ruminants.

REFERENCES

BAGWELL, E. E. and WOODS, E. F. (1962). *Fedn Proc. Fedn Am. Socs exp. Biol.* **20**, 313
BLACK, G. W. and LOVE, S. H. S. (1961). *Anaesthesia*, **16**, 324
BRODIE, B. B. (1952). *Fedn Proc. Fedn Am. Socs exp. Biol.* **11**, 632
——— MARK, L. C., PAPPER, E. M., LIEF, P. A., BERNSTEIN, E. and ROVENSTINE, E. A. (1950). *J. Pharmac. exp. Ther.* **98**, 85
——— BERNSTEIN, E. and MARK, L. C. (1952). *J. clin. Invest.* **105**, 421
——— BURN, J. J., LIEF, P. A. and PAPPER, E. M. (1952). *Curr. Res., Anesth. Analg.* **31**, 145
BURN, J. H., EPSTEIN, H. G., FEIGAN, G. A. and PATON, W. D. M. (1957). *Br. med. J.* ii, 479
BUTLER, T. C. (1949). *J. Pharmac.* **97**, 84
CALE, J. O. and PARKS, C. R. (1962). *Anesthesiology*, **23**, 248
CHENWORTH, M. B., ROBERTSON, D. N., ERLEY, D. S. and GOLHKE, M. S. (1962). *Anesthesiology*, **23**, 101
CRAWSHAW, H. A. (1955). *Vet. Rec.* **67**, 266
CROFT, P. G. (1961). *J. small anim. Pract.* **2**, 206
DOBKIN, A. B. and FEDORUK, S. (1961). *Anesthesiology*, **22**, 355
DOUGLAS, T. A., JENNINGS, S., LONGSTREETH, J. and WEAVER, A. D. (1964). *Vet. Rec.* **76**, 615
EPSTEIN, R. M., RACKOW, H., SALANITRE, E. and WOLF, G. L. (1964). *Anesthesiology*, **25**, 364
FABRY, A. (1963). *Vet. Rec.* **75**, 1049
FISHER, E. W. and JENNINGS, S. (1961). *Am. J. vet. Res.* **22**, 279
FORD, E. J. H. (1951). *Vet. Rec.* **63**, 636
FOWLER, N. G. and STEVENSON, D. E. (1961). *Vet. Rec.* **73**, 917
——— ——— (1964). *Small Animal Anaesthesia.* Oxford: Pergamon Press
FRITSCH, R. (1959). *Berl. Münch. tierärztl. Wsch.* **72**, 423
GRAHAM, J. D. P. (1958). *Br. med. Bull.* **14**, 15
GREGORY, R. A. (1947). *Vet. Rec.* **59**, 377
HALL, L. W. (1957). *Vet. Rec.* **69**, 615
——— (1964). *Vet. Rec.* **76**, 650
HARRIS, T. A. B. (1951). *Mode of Action of Anaesthetics.* Edinburgh: Livingstone
HIME, J. M. (1963). *Vet. Rec.* **75**, 426
HUDSON, F., JACQUES, A. and BOIVIN, P. A. (1958). *Can. Anaesth. Soc. J.* **5**, 384
IMRAY, J. McG., KENNEDY, B. R. and KILPATRICK, S. J. (1964). *Anaesthesia*, **19**, 33
JONES, E. W., JOHNSON, L. and HEINZE, C. D. (19660). *J. Am. vet. med. Ass.* **137**, 119
——— VASKO, K. A., HAMM, D. and GRIFFITH, R. W. (1962). *J. Am. vet. med. Ass.* **140**, 148
——— STOCKTON, F. and TIGERT, C. (1962). *J. Am. vet. med. Ass.* **141**, 1043
JONES, R. E., DEUTSCH, S. and TURNDORF, H. (1961). *Anesthesiology*, **22**, 67
JUMES, M. G. and SIEBECKER, K. L. (1960). *Postgrad. Assembly Anesth. New York*
LAUBACH, G. D., P'AN, S. Y. and RUDEL, H. W. (1955). *Science, N.Y.* **122**, 78
LURIE, A. A., JONES, R. E., LINDE, H. W., PRICE, M. L., DRIPPS, R. D. and PRICE, H. L. (1958). *Anesthesiology*, **24**, 346
LEVY, A. G. (1912). *Heart*, **4**, 319
LONGLEY, E. O. (1950). *Vet. Rec.* **62**, 17
MARKEE, G., WANE, H. H. and WANE, S. C. (1963). *Anesthesiology*, **27**, 742
MARRETT, H. R. (1959). *Anaesthesia*, **14**, 28
MERKEL, G. and EGO, E. I. II (1963). *Anesthesiology*, **24**, 346
MONAHAN, C. M. (1964). *Vet. Rec.* **76**, 1333
NEWMAN, H. C. (1958), *Br. J. Anaesth.* **30**, 555
NORMAN, N. and LOFSTRÖM, B. (1955). *J. Pharmac.* **114**, 231
NORTH, W. C., KNOX, P. R., VARTANIAN, V. and STEPHEN, C. T. (1961). *Anesthesiology*, **22**, 138
O'MULLANE, E. T. (1957). *Br. J. Anaesth.* **29**, 71
PRICE, H. L., COOK, W. A. and DEUTSCH, S. (1963). *Anesthesiology*, **24**, 1
——— LINDE, H. W. and MORSE, H. T. (1963). *Anesthesiology*, **24**, 770
——— PRICE, M. L. and MORSE, H. T. (1965). *Anesthesiology*, **26**, 55
——— WARDEN, J. C. and COOPERMAN, L. H. (1969). *Anesthesiology*, **30**, 426
PURCHASE, I. F. H. (1964). Ph.D. Thesis, University of Cambridge
RAVENTÓS, J. (1956). *Br. J. Pharmac.* **11**, 394
REICHART, H., WIQUIST, N. and YLLNER, S. (1960). *Acta obst. gyn. scand.* **39**, 661
REUTNER, T. F. and GRULZIT, O. M. (1948). *J. Am. vet. med. Ass.* **113**, 357

ROBERTSON, J. D., SWANN, A. A. B. and WHITTERIDGE, D. (1956). *J. Physiol.* **131**, 463
ROBERTSHAW, D. (1964). *Vet. Rec.* **76**, 357
SHEPPARD, M. and SHEPPARD, D. H. (1937). *Vet. Rec.* **49**, 424
STEVENSON, D. E. (1959) Ph.D. Thesis, University of Cambridge
STOELTING, R. K. and EGER, E. I. II (1969). *Anesthesiology*, **30**, 273
TAVERNOR, W. D. (1962). *Vet. Rec.* **74**, 595
TYAGI, R. P. S., ARNOLD, J. P., USENIK, E. A. and FLETCHER, T. F. (1964). *Cornell Vet.* **54**, 584
VASKO, K. A. (1962). *Am. J. vet. Res.* **23**, 248
VICKERS, M. D. and DINNICK, O. P. (1964). *Anaesthesia*, **19**, 124
WADDINGTON, F. G. (1950). *Vet. Rec.* **62**, 100
WARREN, A. G. (1960). Thesis, D. Vet. Med. Zurich
WATERS, R. M. (Ed.) (1951). *Chloroform—A Study after 100 Years.* University of Wisconsin Press
WRIGHT, J. G. (1937). *Vet. Rec.* **49**, 27
ZIMA, O., WERDER, F. VON and HOTOVY, R. (1954). *Anaesthestist*, **3**, 224

13

The Administration of Anaesthetic Agents

The Administration of Intravenous Agents

For agents which are intended to reach the central nervous system and produce narcosis or anaesthesia the intravenous route is obviously more direct than the one through the respiratory tract. But it must always be borne in mind that unlike the respiratory pathway the intravenous one does not provide an exit as well as an entrance. Gases and volatile drugs have the advantage of being eliminated through the pulmonary epithelium according to the physical laws governing the diffusion of gases through membranes, there being very little actual breakdown of the agent by the tissues of the body; thus ether passes as a vapour from the alveoli into the blood and nearly all returns to the alveoli unchanged when the administration ceases. With the commonly used intravenous agents (chloral hydrate and the barbiturates), on the other hand, the speed of elimination depends on such factors as the speed of injection and the rate of distribution and detoxication of the drug in the tissues. The rates of distribution and detoxication are subject to a number of variable factors such as the age and metabolic rate of the patient and the chemical structure of the substance injected.

Nevertheless, very considerable control can be exercised over the action of the intravenous agents. By careful assessment of the condition of the animal, whereby allowance is made for such factors as renal and hepatic disease, lowered metabolic rate and increased circulation time, the dose and rate of administration of the drug can be judged so as to ensure that overdosage does not occur. The variation in the circulation time is a most important factor for whenever the circulation is sluggish (e.g. in shocked or elderly animals) there will be an increase in the delay between the commencement of the intravenous injection and the onset of narcosis.

Intravenous Technique

Although any superficial vein may be used, in veterinary practice injection is usually made into the external jugular vein, the cephalic vein or the recurrent tarsal vein. The choice of the vein used and the technique of venepuncture are largely governed by the kind of animal in which the injection is to be made.

Venepuncture in the Horse

In horses intravenous injections are usually made into the jugular vein about half-way down the neck.

The horse should be handled quietly and the use of a twitch is to be avoided for its application often tends to provoke rather than prevent head movement. Many horses will tense their neck muscles and obscure the jugular furrow whenever a twitch is applied. With the usual aseptic precautions 1 or 2 ml of procaine or lignocaine hydrochloride are injected through a short fine needle into the dermis and subcutaneous tissue to produce an insensitive area over the jugular furrow. The importance of this cannot be overemphasized for the insertion of a stout intravenous needle through skin which has not been desensitized may be associated with such pain that young or nervous animals will become uncontrollable.

When local analgesia has developed, the intravenous needle (about 6 to 7 cm long and 2 to 2·5 mm bore)* is thrust through the skin over the vein with its point directed towards the head. Often the needle cuts out a plug of skin which occludes its lumen and it is advisable to pass a stilette through the needle before attempting to introduce it into the blood vessel. Next the vein is distended by the application of pressure. This pressure is best applied by pressing the thumb into the jugular furrow just below the site of puncture for this tenses the skin (Fig. 75). The distended vein is easily palpable and the point of the needle is directed towards the vein, thrust into it and advanced up its lumen for about 2 to 3 cm. It is important that a good length of the needle shall be introduced into the vein otherwise there is a risk that as the vein subsides, on release of pressure, it will be drawn off the needle because the position of the needle is fixed by the skin. Moreover, if this provision is not made the slightest movement is likely to cause the needle to leave the vessel. A free flow of blood through the needle indicates that it is well placed in the lumen of the vein. If only a few drops of blood fall from the hub of the needle it may be concluded that either (*a*) the needle is in a perivascular haematoma or (*b*) the needle is in the vein but the lumen of the needle is

---

* The relationship of the British Wire Gauge to Metric measurement is shown in Appendix i.

partially blocked. Once it is certain that the needle is correctly placed in the vein the thumb pressure is relaxed, the syringe or infusion apparatus attached and the injection made. The needle should be held and pressed gently and continuously against the animal's neck during the injection so that should the animal move its neck the hand (and needle) will move with it and thus overcome any tendency for the needle to be pulled out of the vein.

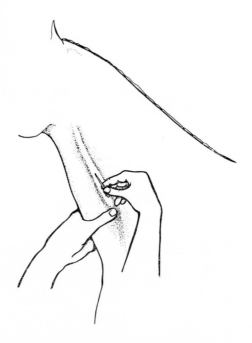

FIG. 75.—Raising the jugular vein in the horse.

There is no advantage to be gained from introducing the needle into the vein in a downwards direction away from the head. Indeed, technical errors are much more likely to arise if attempts are made to perform venepuncture in this manner. The operation is more awkward; it is more difficult to assess the depth to which the needle is being inserted and if the animal moves its neck the direction of movement will be against the point of the needle thus tending to transfix the vein.

When irritant substances (such as chloral hydrate) are being given by slow administration, and injection occupies several minutes, restive animals frequently move so that the needle is pulled out of the vein during the course of the injection. In such animals the risk of perivascular deposition of the irritant solution is high. Greater certainty of correct intravenous injection is obtained when plastic catheters are used instead of needles. There are today numerous types of disposable polythene and nylon intravenous catheters which may be bought sterile, in packets, ready for immediate use. The 'Portex' nylon intravenous cannulae, 12 in long, Luer fitting, gamma-ray sterilized (Portland Plastics Limited, Hythe, Kent) and the 'Bardic Intracath' (Murray Hill, New Jersey—obtainable in Great Britain from Chas.Thackray Ltd., Leeds) are excellent examples of such catheters. Up to 10 in (25 cm) of catheter may be introduced into the lumen of the vein and the risk of complete dislodgement during the course of injection is slight.

Venepuncture in Cattle

The technique of venepuncture in cattle is very similar to that described for the horse. Injection is made through a needle (about 6 to 7 cm long and 2 to 2·5 mm bore) inserted through a desensitized area into the external jugular vein about half-way down the neck.

As in the horse the vein should be distended by pressing the thumb into the jugular furrow below the site of puncture. 'Neck-ropes' or 'bleeding-ropes' should not be used for they cause puckering of the skin and make accurate palpation of the vein more difficult. The skin is tensed and identification of the vein is easier if an assistant bends the animal's head and neck away from the side on which the injection is to be made.

Disposable plastic intravenous catheters may also be used in cattle and are most convenient when chloral hydrate is to be given by slow injection.

Venepuncture in Pigs

Intravenous injections are best made into one of the auricular veins on the external aspect of the ear-flap. Small pigs are restrained on their side on the table. One assistant leans on the neck and trunk, at the same time gripping the legs, while a second assistant holds the uppermost ear at the base of the conchal cartilage and applies pressure to the vein as near to the base of the ear-flap as possible. If a second assistant is not available a rubber band is applied around the base of the ear. In large pigs, a noose is applied around the upper jaw behind the tusks, drawn tight and secured to a post or other suitable object. As in small pigs the ear veins are distended by the application of pressure.

Venepuncture is carried out as shown in Fig. 76 using a needle about 2·5 cm long and, depending on the calibre of the vein, 0·6 to 1·0 mm bore with a 'short bevel' point. The veins become more obvious if the ear-flap is made hyperaemic by gentle slapping and brisk rubbing with an alcohol-soaked piece of gauze. In large pigs blood can be aspirated into the syringe once the needle has been inserted into the vein but in small pigs the amount of blood in the vein between the points of pressure and insertion of the needle may be so small that it is impossible to withdraw any into the syringe. In such cases injection must be attempted and if the needle is not in the lumen of the vein a subcutaneous bleb will develop. When it is certain that the needle is in the vein the pressure is released (if a rubber band has been applied to the base of the ear the band must be cut with scissors) and the injection made. It will be

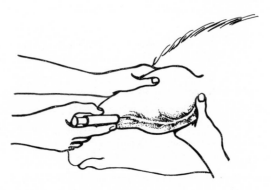

FIG. 76.—Intravenous injection in the pig using the marginal ear vein.

noticed that the solution injected washes the blood out of the vein and this affords further evidence that the needle is correctly placed in the lumen of the vessel.

Venepuncture in Dogs and Cats

In dogs and cats intravenous injections are best made into the cephalic vein.

The animal should be handled quietly and forcible restraint should not be used unless the animal is vicious or unusually restive. Cats should not be handled by gripping the skin at the back of the neck for even the most placid pet cats resent being handled in this manner. Tape muzzles should only be applied to dogs which show an inclination to bite.

The animal is placed in a sitting position on a table of convenient height. If the vein on the right fore-leg is to be punctured an assistant stands on the left side of the animal, passes his or her left arm around the animal's neck and raises its head (Figs 77, 78). The assistant's right hand grips the animal's right fore-leg so that the middle, third and fourth fingers are immediately behind the olecranon and the thumb is round the front side of the limb. The limb is extended by pushing on the olecranon and the vein is raised by applying pressure with the thumb. Venepuncture must, of course, be carried out with the usual aseptic precautions so the hair over the vein is clipped and the skin is disinfected.

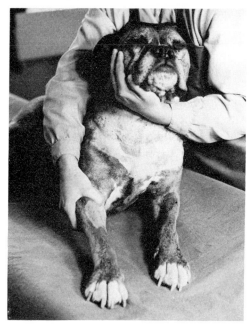

FIG. 77.—Restraint for injection into the cephalic vein in a dog.

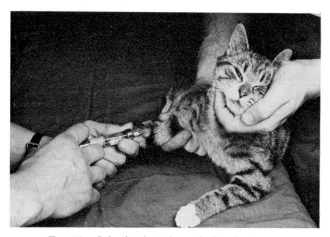

FIG. 78.—Injection into the cephalic vein in a cat.

It is an advantage to use a syringe which has an eccentrically placed nozzle for this allows the syringe to rest securely on the fore-arm with the needle more or less flush with the vein. In this way the angle of entrance, that is, the angle between the needle and the vein, is small and consequently there is much less risk of the needle being pushed right through the vein. For dogs a needle 2·5 cm long and 0·6 mm bore should be used while a needle 1·5 cm long with a bore of 0·4 mm is suitable for cats. The points of the needle should not be cut too acutely, the so-called 'short bevel' or 'dental cut' is to be preferred.

The skin over the vein is kept taut by the thumb and fore-finger of the anaesthetist's left hand which grasps the animal's fore-arm immediately below the site of puncture. In this position it is easy for the anaesthetist to grip the syringe between the left thumb and fore-finger once the vein has been entered (Fig. 79). The skin should be pierced immediately over the vein to avoid the branches of the radial nerve which run on either side of the vein in this region of the limb.

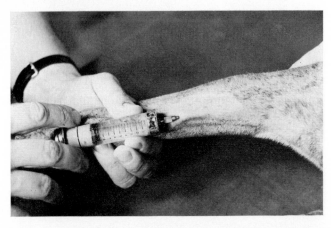

FIG. 79.—Method of holding syringe during injection into cephalic vein.

All air should be expressed from the syringe before venepuncture is attempted and there must be sufficient space left in the syringe to allow slight withdrawal of the piston in order to test whether the needle is within the lumen of the vessel. Blood should enter the syringe when this is done, and no injection must be made if blood does not appear in the syringe. Failure to withdraw blood usually means that either the vein has not been entered, or that the needle has become occluded. Failure to aspirate blood into the syringe is also encountered if the vein is already thrombosed.

In dogs the recurrent tarsal vein may also be used for intravenous injection at the point where it passes upwards and backwards on the lateral aspect of the leg just above the tarsus. Either hind-leg may be used with the animal restrained on its side, but two assistants are always required. One places an arm under the animal's neck and grips both fore-legs, and with the other arm exerts pressure on the neck and head. The other assistant holds the limb to be used for the injection in a state of full extension and raises the vein as shown in Fig. 80. The recurrent tarsal vein is usually more prominent than the cephalic vein but it is more mobile and therefore more difficult to puncture. When the needle has been introduced well into the vein the syringe is fixed to the leg by pressing on the needle hub with the thumb while the fingers encircle the limb (Fig. 81).

The femoral vein in the middle part of the medial aspect of the thigh may also be used. It is rendered obvious by pressure applied to the inguinal region and is usually more prominent in the proximal part of the thigh. Care should be taken to ensure that injections are not made into the femoral artery which lies directly beneath the vein. Puncture of the femoral vein is not difficult in

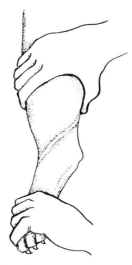

FIG. 80.—Method of extending the limb and raising the vein when using the recurrent tarsal vein.

cats, but fairly heavy sedation is usually necessary before the cat can be restrained in a position in which the vein is accessible. Intravenous injections may also be given into one of the sublingual veins in anaesthetized dogs and cats. Injection into the jugular vein has already been described (page 19).

Venepuncture in Sheep and Goats

In sheep and goats intravenous injections are best given into the cephalic vein or the recurrent tarsal vein as in dogs. However, injections can also be made into the external jugular vein. For this, an assistant sits on a chair and holds the animal between his knees so that it is actually sitting on its rump. His left hand grasps the animal's front legs while his right hand holds the animal's head back so as to stretch the neck. In large heavy animals injections may be made into the external vein with the animal standing.

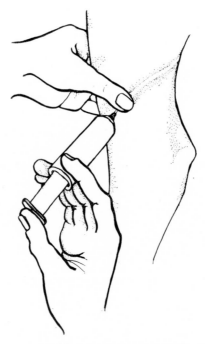

FIG. 81.—Method of holding the syringe and needle during injection when using the recurrent tarsal vein.

Apparatus

Syringes and Needles

The largest syringe which can be conveniently handled is one of 50 ml capacity and it is most desirable that all syringes of more than 2 ml capacity which are used for intravenous injections should have eccentrically placed nozzles.

Needles must be sharp and their points should be of the 'short bevel' or 'dental cut' variety to reduce the risk of transfixing the vein. However, in horses and cattle needles with more tapering points or special 'Analgic' needles (Arnold and Sons) (Fig. 82) may be used for they are more easily

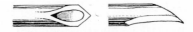

FIG. 82.—'Analgic' needle (Arnold & Sons).

introduced through the skin. The 'Analgic' needle is so designed that penetration of the skin is easier and puncture of the vein wall is more precise— distinct advantages in cattle in which penetration of the skin with a large needle of the standard pattern may be difficult and in which the skin tends to hold the needle so firmly that accurate puncture of the vein is not easy.

When anaesthesia has been induced with any intravenous agent it may be maintained in the required plant by intermittent small doses of the drug. In the larger farm animals the jugular vein may be punctured frequently and without much difficulty, so that it is not necessary to keep the needle in the vein between each dose. In pigs, dogs and cats, however, attention must be concentrated on keeping the needle in the vein and free from blood clot. In dogs and cats the syringe may be secured to the fore-arm, and in pigs to the ear-flap, with adhesive plaster; the needle may then be kept patent by making frequent very small injections to clear it of blood. Nevertheless, in all animals other than horses and cattle it is more convenient to inject the intermittent

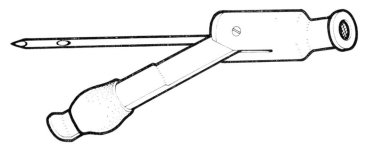

FIG. 83.—Mitchell needle.

doses through an indwelling intravenous needle, such as the Mitchell needle, or into the tubing of a slow-running intravenous infusion because it is not then necessary to secure the heavy syringe to the patient.

The needle designed by Dr. Mitchell (Messrs. Vann Bros. Ltd.) has proved to be a very satisfactory and reliable indwelling intravenous needle in veterinary anaesthesia. The design is simple, allowing the needle to be left in place ready for repeated injections, but with the syringe detached. The orifice of the needle is in the side of the shaft about 1 cm from the point and the needle is solid between the orifice and the point so that repeated sharpening is possible. A metal spring with a rubber pad is pivoted in the hub so that it can be swung laterally (Fig. 83). Venepuncture is carried out with the spring swung to one side and when the needle is in the vein blood can be aspirated into the syringe. The spring is then swung across to be above the line of the needle and the rubber pad on the spring presses the skin, subcutaneous tissues and vein wall against the needle orifice, effectively preventing back flow of blood into the lumen of the needle. The injection of a small volume of the intravenous agent from the syringe clears the needle of blood and as long as the spring is in position above the needle blood never flows back into the lumen. The syringe may be detached from the needle as soon as the needle has been cleared of blood. Three sizes of the needle are manufactured: 1·25, 0·9, and 0·55 mm bore.

Another very useful type of needle is the Guest cannula (Fig. 84). It consists of a stainless steel narrow-bore cannula fitted with a fine hollow needle as a trocar. When the two are assembled, the extremity of the needle projects just beyond that of the cannula. The proximal ends are both Record or Luer fitting. The cannula is inserted into the distended vein, with the trocar needle in position and the needle is withdrawn when blood flows from its proximal end. The blunt-ended cannula is then pushed well home up the distended vein and secured in position with adhesive plaster. Because it has blunt end,

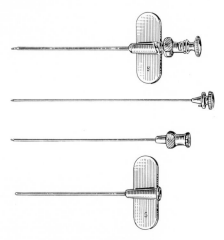

FIG. 84—Guest cannula.

transfixion of the vein does not occur and the cannula is less apt to be displaced from the vein than is an ordinary needle. It is particularly useful for the administration of intravenous infusions.

Disposable cannulae are also obtainable (e.g. The 'Bardic Deseret Angiocath', supplied by Chas. Thackray Ltd., Leeds). These are similar in pattern, and in use, to the Guest cannula, but the cannula part is of polythene or nylon, and the whole unit is supplied sterile, in a sterile packet, ready for immediate use. However, if an attempt is made to introduce one of these plastic units through the intact skin of an animal it usually results in the end of the plastic portion opening out into a bell mouth which is almost impossible to advance into the vein. To avoid this, these cannulae should be introduced through a very small incision in the skin or through a hole made in the skin by a large-bore needle.

The number of proprietary needles, cannulae and catheters for use when giving intravenous infusions is now bewilderingly large and choice is difficult.

Because the wrong choice is made intravenous infusions which appear to run smoothly when originally set up with saline or glucose solutions may prove infuriatingly slow when blood has to be given. Such a disadvantage may cost an animal's life. Consideration of some of the factors influencing fluid flow makes the choice of needle, cannula or catheter more rational and less dependent on the information given on the packet by the manufacturers of any particular appliance.

The flow through a tube is proportional to the driving pressure, which is equal to the pressure difference between the two ends of the tube, multiplied by a constant, $\pi/8$. Flow is also inversely proportional to the viscosity of the fluid, since the more viscous the fluid the harder it will be to force it through the tube. The final factor governing the flow is the size of the tube, flow being directly proportional to the fourth power of the radius, and inversely proportional to the length of the bore. Thus, for maximum flow of any given fluid at any given pressure, the tube should be as short and of the maximum diameter possible. It must be noted that a small change in diameter has a large effect on flow.

At very high flows it may be found that the resistance is disproportionately high. There is a critical flow velocity at which the flow changes from stream line to turbulent. During turbulence the driving pressure is largely used up in creating the kinetic energy of the turbulent eddies. The flow no longer depends on the viscosity of the fluid but on its density. However, the critical velocity at which turbulence occurs depends mainly on its viscosity, its density and the radius of the bore of the tube through which it is flowing. In an intravenous infusion system the critical velocity is likely to be exceeded at very high flow rates and also at local points in the apparatus at which, because of a sudden change in internal configuration, the velocity of flow momentarily rises. Thus, at points at which the internal diameter changes suddenly, turbulence will occur.

The viscosity of blood is considerably greater than that of water, mainly because of the presence of erythrocytes. The viscosity of blood increases with the haematocrit and above about 60% haematocrit blood hardly behaves as a fluid. Viscosity is also increased by a drop in temperature, and the viscosity of blood at 0°C is about $2\frac{1}{2}$ times as great as at 37°C. Blood warming coils are, therefore, justified on grounds of increasing the speed of transfusion as well as of preventing the development of hypothermia in the recipient.

There is a large variety of plastic cannulae with internal needles, and more than 25 different cannulae are commercially available in the United Kingdom alone. They are designed for general intravenous work and they have the advantages of the Guest cannula of being easy to insert, while at the same time not cutting out of the vein. There is some variation in their general shape but most have small handles to aid insertion. Most have plastic needle hubs which allow the operator to see the blood which runs back when the needle punctures the vein. Three important factors govern the choice of cannula. First, it should be no longer than strictly necessary. The length of most cannulae (up to 7 cm) is always adequate and there is no need for the larger diameters to be longer. The second important feature is the wall thickness. It is the external diameter which largely determines the size chosen in any given situation and cannulae with thinner walls obviously permit more rapid infusions. The third factor is that the external shape should be as smooth as possible, for cannulae with smooth contours are the easiest to insert. In animals, all cannulae may become damaged at the tip during insertion unless the skin is nicked with a sharp knife where the cannula is to be introduced.

There are at least nine types of venous needles currently available. All are attached to lengths of plastic tubing and some have winged handles to aid insertion and subsequent fixation to the patient. The flow performance of most of the 'small vein sets' (often called 'infant scalp-vein sets') is surprisingly poor, and it is usually best to choose one with the shortest length of tubing attached.

Longer catheters are available for special purposes such as central venous or arterial pressure measurement (see Chapter 1). Most are not provided with introducing needles, although the type of needle described by McGregor can be used for them. They are usually introduced by cutting down on to the vein, for which purpose they are mostly far too long. They should, therefore, be cut in half whenever possible.

A slightly different design, which is particularly easy to introduce, is the E–Z Cath (Macarthy Ltd.). A needle lies inside the tip of the catheter to assist introduction; it is attached to a wire which passes throughout the length of the catheter. A split inserting handle attached to a protective sleeve surrounds the catheter, and the catheter can be worked up the vein by advancing it with the inserter, using one hand, and holding it inside its protective sleeve with the other.

The danger that catheters which pass through needles may become severed by forcible and ill-advised attempts to withdraw them is well known and the needle and catheter should always be withdrawn together. The use of an internal needle attached to a guide-wire, as in the E–Z Cath, does away with this danger.

Infusion Apparatus

In the larger farm animals intravenous infusions are usually given from one of the types of apparatus shown in Fig. 85. The 'Simplex' or 'flutter' valve is most useful for the administration of sterile solutions prepared by the various manufacturers for it fits on to the narrow-necked bottles in which these solutions are supplied. Solutions prepared immediately before injection (e.g. chloral hydrate) are usually sterilized by boiling in a flask and are administered either directly from the flask in which they have been prepared or from a gravity cylinder. The solution flows under the influence of gravity from the apparatus into the vein and when running from a flask or cylinder the speed of infusion depends more on the bore of the needle than on the pressure (i.e. the height above the needle at which the container is held). It has been shown

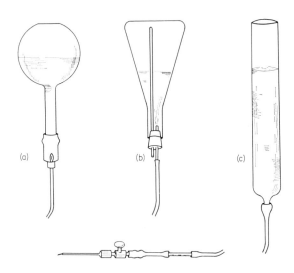

FIG. 85. Gravity apparatus for intravenous injection.
(*a*) 'Flutter valve'; (*b*) Flask with inlet and outlet tubes; (*c*) Gravity cylinder.

that doubling the diameter of the needle gives a 16-fold increase in the rate of flow, whereas a 4-fold increase in the pressure is required to double the rate. In the case of the 'flutter valve' apparatus, however, the vertical distance between the needle and the air inlet opening determines the rate at which air enters the system; increasing this distance increases the rate of air entry and hence the speed of infusion.

In the smaller animals intravenous infusions must be given more slowly and a fairly accurate control of the flow rate is essential. A most convenient apparatus is the standard 'giving set' introduced by the Medical Research Council which fits all standard size transfusion bottles. Essentially, the M.R.C. giving set consists of a rubber bung through which passes a glass air inlet, a filter covered outlet tube, rubber tubing, a glass drip chamber and a screw clip (Fig. 86). The flow rate is controlled by means of the screw clip and can be estimated by counting the number of drops which pass through the drip chamber in 1 minute. For example, 40 drops/minute means the administration of approximately 500 ml in 4 hours.

The use of the safety drip chambers designed by Macintosh and Pask

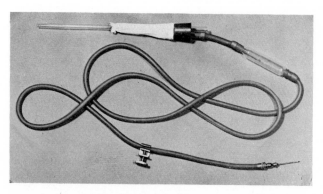

FIG. 86.—Standard M.R.C. giving set for transfusions.

This apparatus is of rubber and glass and is now being superseded by plastic disposable sets such as that shown in Fig. 88.

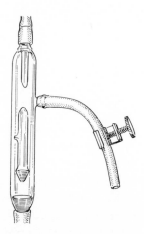

FIG. 87.—Macintosh and Pask's safety drip chamber with float to prevent air embolism.

(Fig. 87) in place of the ordinary drip chamber allows the infusion to be left running unattended for air embolism cannot occur; the cone stopper only floats whilst there is sufficient solution in the drip chamber and should the bottle empty while the infusion is unattended the float will sink into its seating at the bottom of the drip chamber and prevent the entry of air into the rubber tubing to the needle.

The use of rubber tubing and non-disposable apparatus must always expose the recipient of a transfusion or infusion to the risk of a reaction to foreign protein or other antigenic material. No cleaning process which is compatible with a reasonably useful length of life of the apparatus, in particular of rubber tubing, can be relied upon to remove completely all traces of such materials. However, the use of one of the many types of disposable, plastic apparatus, such as the giving set shown in Fig. 88, removes this risk. These plastic sets are cheap enough to be thrown away after use and there is no doubt that in veterinary practice there is much to commend them. This

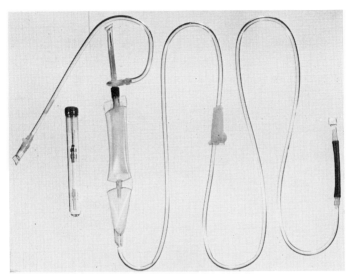

Fig. 88.—Disposable plastic giving set.
(Capon Heaton & Co., Ltd., Birmingham.) Note the air inlet tube above the filter chamber.

practice of using disposable, plastic sets can be extended still further for many pharmaceutical firms now supply infusion fluids not in bottles, but in plastic, collapsible, disposable bags, each bag being complete with a giving set (Fig. 89). Because the plastic bags are collapsible, no air inlet is necessary and the type of giving set incorporated is simpler than the one shown in Fig. 88 which, because it is intended for the administration of fluids from a rigid, glass bottle, has a device for filtering all the air which enters the bottle through the air inlet tube. When a plastic bag container is empty it collapses and air embolism cannot occur, so that the infusion can be left running unattended. All plastic giving sets should have a short length of rubber tubing included near the needle mount so that injections can be made through it into the infusion fluid while the administration proceeds.

An intravenous drip, set up primarily for fluid replacement therapy before operation, is a most useful vehicle for the introduction of an anaesthetic drug into the bloodstream. Injection is made through a fine-bore needle into the lumen of the rubber tubing as close as possible to the intravenous needle or cannula. While the anaesthetic drug is being injected into the drip in this manner the tubing between the point of injection and the drip chamber should be compressed by pinching with the finger and thumb, otherwise the pressure created will dam back fluid in the drip chamber and may stop the flow.

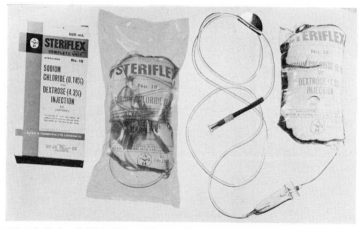

FIG. 89.—Infusion fluid in disposable plastic bag complete with giving set. (Allen & Hanbury's Ltd.)

The Administration of Inhalation Agents

At normal atmospheric pressure and temperature some of the inhalation anaesthetic agents are liquid (e.g. chloroform and ether), whilst others such as nitrous oxide and cyclopropane are in the gaseous state. The methods by which the vapours of the volatile liquids and the gaseous anaesthetic agents are delivered to the animal can be classified in various ways and as yet there is no universally agreed terminology to describe the variety of systems employed. The system of classification in common use in Great Britain is as follows:

1. The open method.
2. The semi-open method.
3. The closed method with carbon dioxide absorption.
4. The semi-closed method.

1. The Open Method

This is used to volatilize agents such as chloroform and ether. They are dropped on to the surface of gauze or lint which is held over the animal's nostrils. The gauze or lint may be stretched over a wire frame such as that illustrated in Fig. 90 to make a mask. The method is often referred to as 'rag and bottle anaesthesia' and is one which has survived through over a hundred years of anaesthetic history. When Sir James Simpson first administered chloroform in 1847 he used a pocket handkerchief placed over the mouth and nostrils, but today chloroform is volatilized, perhaps less elegantly, on common gauze or lint.

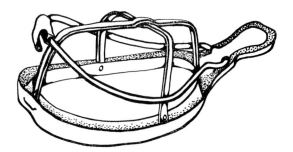

FIG. 90.—Schimmelbusch mask.

The term 'open' is only truly applicable when a mask such as the Schimmelbusch is used. The mask must not fit the contour of the animal's face for an essential feature of the method is that there shall be a free flow of air between the mask and the face. The dropper bottle may be one designed by Bellamy Gardner (Fig. 91) which allows a good control over the rate of

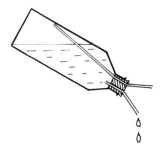

FIG. 91.—Bellamy Gardner dropper bottle.

dropping, but a very satisfactory bottle may be improvised by cutting a groove in the cork of an ordinary medicine bottle and using a little ribbon of gauze to act as a wick (Fig. 92).

2. The Semi-open Method

In the semi-open or 'perhalation' method all the inspired air is made to pass through the mask on which the vaporization of the agent occurs.

When using a mask such as the Schimmelbusch for semi-open administration two thick layers of Gamgee are employed to ensure that all the respired air passes through the mask. The first layer has a small hole in its centre so that when it is in position the nose and mouth are the only exposed parts of the face (Fig. 93). The nose and mouth are then covered by the mask and the

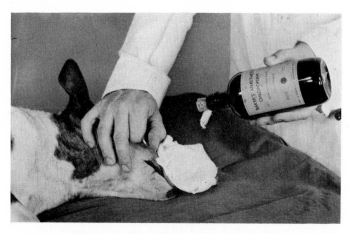

FIG. 92.—Open administration of chloroform.

second layer of Gamgee, which has a larger hole in its centre, applied over the mask as shown in Fig. 94.

In horse and cattle special masks (Fig. 95) are often used for the semi-open administration of chloroform. These masks are cylinders of leather and canvas and they are applied over either the upper or both jaws. Chloroform is applied to a sponge which is inserted in the open end of the cylinder. In the cruder types of mask the sponge is actually in contact with the nostrils, but in more refined patterns a wire mesh partition prevents this direct contact.

Today, the open and semi-open methods of administration are seldom used from choice because with them it is difficult to maintain a stable anaesthetic state. The anaesthetic agents are diluted, to an unknown extent, by air and this dilution is greatest when the minute volume of breathing is large and the inspiratory gas flow rate high. The greater the ventilation (and hence, the dilution of the anaesthetic inhaled), the closer the alveolar concentration of the anaesthetic will approach zero, and the plane of anaesthesia will thus lighten as ventilation increases. Depression of breathing, on the other hand, decreases the air dilution and thereby increases the concentration of anaesthetic inspired. Under these circumstances, unless there is an increase in the uptake of the anaesthetic by the body, the alveolar concentration of the anaesthetic must rise. A rise in the alveolar concentration produces deeper anaes-

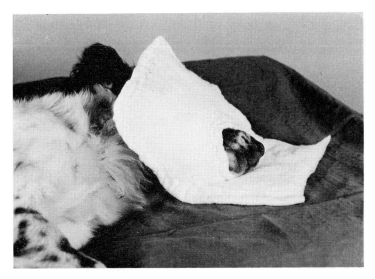

Fig. 93.—Semi-open method. Application of first piece of Gamgee tissue.

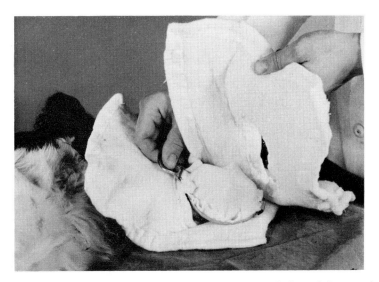

Fig. 94.—Semi-open method. Application of mask and second piece of Gamgee tissue.

thesia and further respiratory depression. In addition, deepening anaesthesia reduces the cardiac output and hence the uptake of anaesthetic by the body, thus adding still further to the rise in the alveolar concentration. If this process is allowed to proceed unchecked, anaesthesia deepens until the ventilation becomes inadequate. In other words, with the open and semi-open methods of administration, animals which become more lightly anaesthetized tend to continue awakening and animals which become more deeply anaesthetized tend to continue becoming more depressed and nearer to death.

The open and semi-open systems have other disadvantages. The anaesthetist lacks control of ventilation and if respiration fails there is no way of applying intermittent positive pressure ventilation; artificial respiration must be carried out by compression of the thoracic cage and this is not very effective in large animal patients. Moreover, there is now evidence to suggest that air

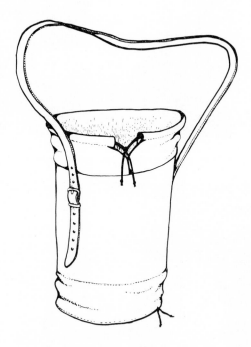

FIG. 95.—Face mask for horses and cattle.

does not supply adequate oxygen when there is respiratory depression so that oxygen enrichment should always be given during general anaesthesia. When the open and semi-open methods are employed this means that a stream of oxygen from a cylinder must be run in under the mask. Both systems are very wasteful and because large quantities of anaesthetic agent have to be volatilized the atmosphere around becomes charged with the agent. This concentration of the agent in the surrounding air is not only unpleasant for the surgical team—when agents such as ether are used there is also considerable risk of fire or explosion.

Although the limitations and dangers inherent in the use of the simple apparatus for the open and semi-open administration of volatile anaesthetic agents must be recognized, the virtues of simplicity and portability will always guarantee them a sphere of utility in remote places or when skilled assistance is not available.

3. The Closed Method with Carbon Dioxide Absorption

Anaesthetic gases and vapours are physiologically 'indifferent', in that they are exhaled from the body unchanged, but when exhaled they are mixed with carbon dioxide. The exhaled mixture can be directed into a closed bag and if the carbon dioxide is removed, and sufficient oxygen to satisfy the metabolic requirements of the animal is added, the same gas or vapour can be rebreathed continuously from the bag. This is the principle of closed circuit anaesthetic administration.

In anaesthesia, the carbon dioxide is usually removed by directing the exhaled mixture over the surface of soda lime. This is a mixture of 90% calcium hydroxide and 5% sodium hydroxide together with 5% of silicate and water to prevent powdering. It is used in a granular form, the granules being 4 to 8 mesh in size, and is packed into a canister so that, ideally, the space between the granules is at least equal to the tidal volume of the animal. Some brands of soda lime contain an indicator dye which changes colour when their carbon dioxide absorbing capacity is exhausted.

Theoretically, once anaesthesia has been induced and a state of equilibrium established, all that the animal requires from the apparatus is a continuous stream of oxygen and efficient absorption of carbon dioxide. In practice, however, most periods of anaesthesia are too short to allow a state of equilibrium to be reached and the body continues to take up the anaesthetic agent throughout the administration, so that the agent has to be given all the time in order to maintain the alveolar concentration.

The closed method of administration is simple, and much less anaesthetic is used than in open and semi-open methods because there is no wastage to the atmosphere. The chief disadvantage of closed circuit anaesthesia is the resistance to respiration due to the packed soda lime. This resistance is sufficiently great to render the method unsuitable for cats, puppies and very small adult dogs. Another disadvantage is that the conservation of heat and water vapour afforded by the method may give rise to heat-stroke in dogs and sheep.

There are two systems in use for closed-circuit carbon dioxide absorption techniques of anaesthesia:

(i) The 'to-and-fro' system.
(ii) The 'circle' system.

The 'To-and-fro' System

A canister full of soda lime is interposed between the animal and the rebreathing bag, fresh gases being fed into the system as close to the animal as possible to effect changes in the mixture rapidly (Fig. 96). This system is simple and efficient but has several drawbacks. It is difficult to maintain the heavy, awkward apparatus in a gas-tight condition and the inspired gases become undesirably hot due to the chemical action between the soda lime and the carbon dioxide. Furthermore, irritating dust may be inhaled from the soda lime and give rise to a bronchitis. Nevertheless the system is the one most commonly used in veterinary anaesthesia for the necessary apparatus is relatively inexpensive and indeed may be improvised.

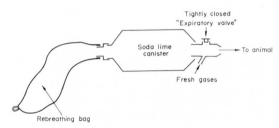

FIG. 96.—To-and-fro absorption system.

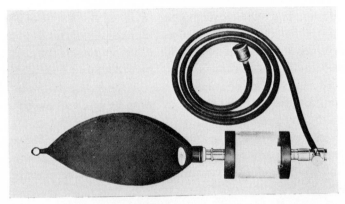

FIG. 97.—Waters's carbon dioxide absorber with transparent canister.

For small animal anaesthesia (dogs, sheep and goats, young calves, young foals and small pigs) the standard soda lime canisters used in man, which are known as Waters's canisters (Fig. 97) after their designer, are quite satisfactory. They are available in various sizes and one canister to contain 1 lb (approx. 0·5 kg) and a second one to contain 10 oz (approx. 0·3 kg) of soda lime are adequate for most veterinary purposes. For cats and small dogs, in order to keep resistance to breathing and apparatus dead-space volume to a minimum, special absorbers as designed for small infants (Fig. 98) should be used. All these canisters are used horizontally and unless the soda lime is tightly packed when the canister is filled it tends to settle, leaving a channel along the top of the canister through which gases pass without being subjected to the action of the soda lime. Robson and Pask (1954) suggested that in the larger canisters a domestic nylon pot-scrub may be used to pack the soda lime. The canister is filled and shaken down as well as possible and the nylon scrub inserted so as to leave about half of it to be compressed by the wire gauze in the lid of the canister when the cap is screwed on.

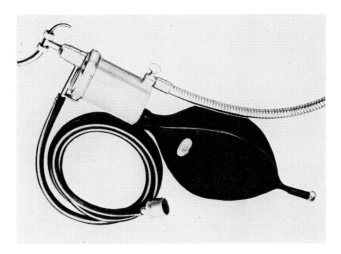

FIG. 98. Infant size absorber (Sandford's).

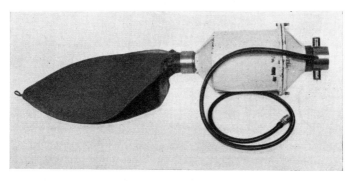

FIG. 99. To-and-fro absorber for horses and cattle.

Adult horses and cattle and large pigs need much larger soda lime canisters. They are designed on the principle that for efficient absorption of carbon dioxide the whole of the animal's tidal volume should be accommodated in the spaces between the soda lime granules. The canister shown in Fig. 99 which has been in use in the Cambridge School for over 15 years has been found to be reasonably efficient yet not too awkward or cumbersome. It measures approximately 20 cm long and 81 cm in diameter (internal measurements) and contains about 10 lb (approx. 4·5 kg) of soda lime. The connections to the rebreathing bag and to the expiratory mount are 5 cm internal diameter. Because of the difficulty experienced in packing this canister sufficiently tightly with soda lime, a special to-and-fro canister has been designed and developed for large animals (Fig. 100). The vertical position of this soda lime canister means that tight packing is not necessary, and the cross-sectional area is large to ensure that the respired gases move through the absorbent slowly.

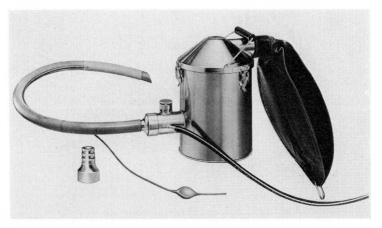

FIG. 100.—To-and-fro absorber with vertical canister (British Oxygen Co. Ltd.)

Single-ended rubber rebreathing bags of 2 to 4 litres are used in conjunction with the Waters apparatus, while a bag from a B.L.B. (Boothby, Lovelace and Bulbulian) oxygen inhalation apparatus is most suitable for use with the infant size absorbers. For adult horses and cattle a rebreathing bag having a capacity of about 15 litres is used.

The to-and-fro systems can never be really efficient absorbers of carbon dioxide. As pointed out by Pas, Brown and Elam (1958), the exhaled gases all come into contact with the soda lime at the end of the canister nearest to the patient and the absorbent in this region is quickly exhausted. Thus, as this occurs, the gases have to travel further and further into the canister before carbon dioxide is absorbed or, in other words, the apparatus dead-space steadily increases during anaesthesia.

The performance of soda lime canisters used in man has been studied by Walls (1950). Purchase (1965) investigated the performance of the two large to-and-fro absorbers described above with regard to resistance to breathing and carbon dioxide absorption, using a mechanical analogue of a horse's lung.

Both absorbers were found to offer a resistance to breathing of approximately 1·2 cm of water per 100 litres/minute at a flow of 600 litres/minute (a flow rate of the order encountered during the respiratory cycle in horses), and both provided a similar mean inspired carbon dioxide concentration. Their dead-space increased steadily as the proximal soda lime became exhausted, but starting with a fresh charge of absorbent, the mean inspired carbon dioxide concentration should not, in practice, exceed 3% for over 4 hours.

The 'Circle' System

The circle system for carbon dioxide absorption incorporates an inspiratory and an expiratory tube with unidirectional valves to ensure a one-way flow of

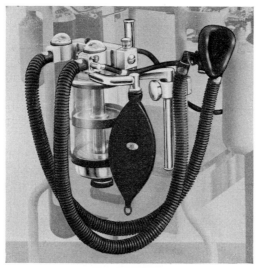

Fig. 101.—Boyle circle absorber Mark 3 fitted to Boyle anaesthetic apparatus.

gases; the rebreathing bag and soda lime canister are placed between these tubes. The valves and tubing offer an appreciable resistance to breathing and unless the apparatus is carefully designed with regard to the diameter of airways in relation to flow rates, breathing through the apparatus can impose a considerable strain on the animal. Circle type absorber units are not, as a general rule, suitable for cats and small dogs of less than about 15 kg body weight because of the resistance offered by even the best designed units and because of the inevitable degree of rebreathing which occurs at the T-piece connection to the patient. This rebreathing can be prevented by placing the unidirectional valves at the face-piece or connection to the endotracheal tube, but it is difficult to design robust, competent valves for use in this situation. In the majority of modern circle type units the unidirectional valves are of the turret type (Fig. 101); some however, employ rubber flaps. The turret

9

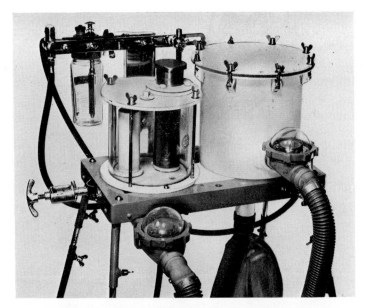

FIG. 102.—Fisher and Jennings circle absorber unit.

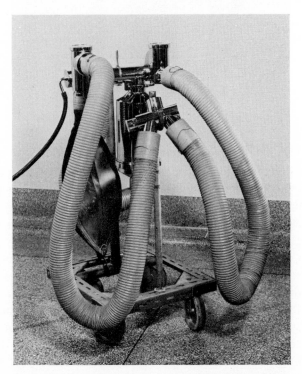

FIG. 103.—The Weaver circle absorber unit.

type is robust and competent but it has the disadvantage that it must be kept upright and of necessity, therefore, has to be mounted on the apparatus at some distance away from the animal.

Circle absorber units are more efficient absorbers of carbon dioxide than are to-and-fro units because their dead-space is constant since all the charge of soda lime is available to the respired gases. Exhaustion of the soda lime is noticed more suddenly than in to-and-fro absorbers and once it occurs the inspired carbon dioxide concentration may soon become excessive.

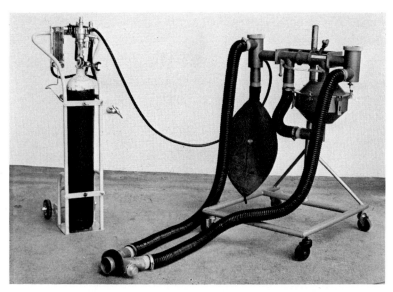

FIG. 104.—The modified Weaver circle absorber unit used at the Cambridge School. The canister is shorter and wider than in the original apparatus.

Standard circle absorbers designed for man, such as that illustrated in Fig. 101, are satisfactory for young foals, young calves, sheep, goats, large pigs and dogs over 15 kg body weight. Circle absorbers for large animal patients have been described by Fisher and Jennings (1957), Hansson and Johannisson (1958), Weaver (1960), Jones (1961) and Fowler, Parker, McLaughlin and Tyler (1963). Purchase (1965) studied the resistance to breathing offered by the Fisher-Jennings apparatus (Fig. 102) and the modified Weaver circle absorber (Fig. 104), and compared their efficiency as carbon dioxide absorbers, using a mechanical analogue of a horse's lung. The modified Weaver circle absorber had a resistance about equal to that of the two to-and-fro absorbers described on page 255, i.e. approximately 1·2 cm of water/100 litres per minute gas flow of 600 litres/minute. The Fisher-Jennings apparatus offered more resistance to gas flow (3·3 cm of water/100 litres/minute at a flow of

600 litres/minute). It is interesting to note that the figures obtained by Purchase for the modified Weaver circle absorber showed that this apparatus apparently afforded less resistance to breathing than does the to-and-fro absorber of Westhues and Fritsch (1961). A fresh charge of soda lime was found to keep the mean inspired carbon dioxide concentration to below 3% in the Fisher-Jennings apparatus for 2 hours, and for 5 hours in the modified Weaver apparatus (which has a larger soda lime canister).

All available information suggests that, although the ideal circuit for large animal patients has yet to be designed, the Weaver circle absorber or the modified version of this apparatus as used at the Cambridge School provides the best available combination of efficient carbon dioxide absorption with low resistance to breathing. However, all circle absorption systems are relatively

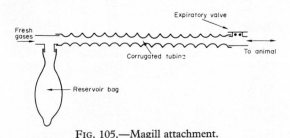

FIG. 105.—Magill attachment.

cumbersome and expensive and are only likely to find favour for hospital use. For field use less cumbersome and less expensive apparatus is desirable. The Weaver circle absorber is the only available apparatus designed for use under both sets of conditions—it has a soda lime canister which may be used in the field as a to-and-fro absorber. For general practice the vertical to-and-fro canister by virtue of its low resistance, relatively good carbon dioxide absorption characteristics, and portability, appears to be the most satisfactory. One other point which must be considered when apparatus is to be selected is that under hospital conditions animals are anaesthetized on raised operating tables and it becomes difficult to support the heavy soda lime canister near the head. Consequently, the circle system is more convenient for hospital use, but in the field where animals are anaesthetized lying on the ground this difficulty does not arise.

4. The Semi-closed Method

The general principle of the semi-closed method is that gases and vapours flow from the anaesthetic apparatus into a reservoir bag from which the animal inhales, while part of all of the exhaled mixture passes out through an expiratory valve into the atmosphere.

The Magill attachment, which incorporates a reservoir bag, wide-bore corrugated tubing and a spring-loaded expiratory valve (Fig. 105), is probably the most generally useful of all the semi-closed systems. With this system rebreathing is prevented by maintaining the total gas flow rate from the cylinders slightly in excess of the patient's respiratory minute volume. The animal inhales from the bag and wide-bore tubing; the exhaled mixture passes back up the tubing displacing the gas in it back into the bag until this is full.

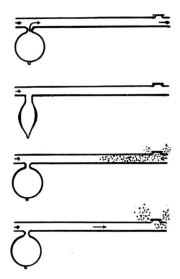

FIG. 106.—Magill attachment.
Exhaled gases indicated by shading.

The exhaled gases never reach the bag because the capacity of the tube is too great and once the bag is distended the build-up of pressure inside the system causes the expiratory valve to open so that the terminal part of the expiration passes out of the valve into the atmosphere. During the pause which follows expiration and before the next inspiration fresh gas from the anaesthetic apparatus sweep the remainder, or first part of the exhaled gases, from the corrugated tube out through the expiratory valve (Fig. 106).

Another commonly used system is shown in Fig. 107. It is obviously more difficult to prevent rebreathing with this system since the inflowing gases from the anaesthetic apparatus will not wash expired gases out through the expiratory valve. This difficulty is usually overcome by interposing a soda lime canister between the animal and the bag, as in the Waters's apparatus. This arrangement is then referred to as a 'semi-closed system with absorption'. A similar system can also be arranged with a circle-type absorber unit by opening the expiratory valve near the face-mask or endotracheal tube. By the use of soda lime canisters with semi-closed systems it is possible to effect a very great economy in the consumption of gases, but the use of these methods requires considerable practice because the expiratory valve setting and the gas flow rates require almost continuous adjustments throughout the anaesthesia.

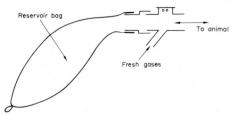

Reservoir bag

To animal

Fresh gases

FIG. 107. Semi-closed system without absorption.

For small dogs and for cats none of the above systems is suitable and for these animals the T-piece system (Fig. 108) is used. The open tube acts as a reservoir and there are no valves. The exhaled gases are swept out of the open end of the reservoir tube by fresh gases flowing in from the anaesthetic apparatus during the expiratory pause. Unless the capacity of the reservoir tube is at least equal to the tidal volume of the animal the inspired gases will be diluted with air.

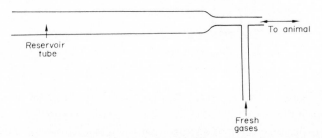

Reservoir tube

To animal

Fresh gases

FIG. 108.—T-piece system.

The modifications of the T-piece system can be divided into three types. In the first there is no expiratory limb, in the second the capacity of the expiratory limb is greater than the tidal volume, and in the third the capacity of the expiratory limb is less than the tidal volume. On the basis of previous mathematical and laboratory investigations by other authors, Harrison (1964) discussed these three types with reference to resistance to respiration and the minimum fresh gas flow required to prevent rebreathing and air dilution during both spontaneous and controlled ventilation. The resistance and fresh gas requirements are obviously related to the expiratory flow rates and respiratory flow patterns which occur in patients of any particular size. Harrison concluded that the most convenient system is one in which the expiratory limb volume is greater than the tidal volume and which has an open-ended bag attached to the distal end of the expiratory limb. With such an arrangement fresh gas flows of up to $2\frac{1}{2}$ to 3 times the minute volume of respiration are required to eliminate rebreathing.

Recently various non-return valves (Ryan's valve, Ruben's valve, Emerson's valve, Hewer's valve and, in veterinary anaesthesia, Weaver's valve) have been incorporated in semi-closed systems in place of the simple spring-loaded expiratory valves. All these valves prevent any rebreathing of the exhaled gases other than those contained in the 'dead-space' of the valve itself and its connections. When these valves are used the gas flow rates from the apparatus require frequent adjustment for any alteration in the rate or depth of the patient's breathing affects the degree of distension of the reservoir bag. If the gas flow rate is constant, deep or rapid breathing empties the bag quickly, while slow or shallow breathing allows the bag to become over-distended. These non-return valves can, therefore, be used to measure the minute volume of respiration, for if gas flow rates are adjusted to maintain the bag at a constant average size at the end of expiration the total gas flow rate as read at the flowmeters will equal the respiratory minute volume. In practice, to avoid the necessity for repeat adjustments of the total gas flow rate, an excessive flow is employed and a relief, or spill, valve is incorporated in the circuit between the reservoir bag and the non-return valve.

Definition of Anaesthetic Circuits

There have been many multiple and inconsistent definitions in British and American literature and as yet there is no universal nomenclature. The following summary may serve to illustrate some of the differences between British and American usage of terms:

(a) American nomenclature

	Reservoir bag	Rebreathing	Examples
Open	No	No	Open drop Insufflation T-piece
Semi-open . .	Yes	No	T-piece with bag Magill Non-rebreathing valves
Semi-closed . .	Yes	Partial }	Carbon dioxide absorbers
Closed . . .	Yes	Complete }	

(b) British nomenclature

	Reservoir bag	Rebreathing	Examples
Open . . .	No	No	Open drop Draw over systems with non-rebreathing valves
Semi-open . . .	No	Partial	Open drop + occlusive packing
Semi-closed (i) without absorption	Yes	Partial	Magill. T-piece T-piece with bag
(ii) with absorption .	Yes	Partial	Carbon dioxide absorbers
Closed . . .	Yes	Complete	Carbon dioxide absorbers

From this summary it is apparent that the present systems of terminology consist of 'closed' and 'open' themes with variations, but that this terminology is now of very little value. Moreover, these systems attempt to use rebreathing as the distinguishing factor. No one would deny that rebreathing is an extremely important variable, yet it is impossible to describe accurately variations which occur in the degree of rebreathing by the use of such terms as semi-closed, semi-closed absorption, partial rebreathing, etc. For example, it appears to be agreed upon by most workers that semi-closed refers to partial rebreathing techniques. Thus, a system which has nearly complete rebreathing of the expired gases might have the same label as a system which has almost no rebreathing.

As pointed out by Hamilton (1964), when considering the effect of rebreathing and variation in degrees thereof upon the constitution of the inspired gases, it is unwise to use terms which give incomplete and inaccurate information concerning this important variable. Gas, inspired by an animal being anaesthetized, is a mixture of fresh and previously expired gas. When previously expired gas is excluded, a non-rebreathing system results. With such a system, inspired gas tensions may be held constant, and reasonably accurately defined, by calibrated vaporizers and flowmeters. Changes of flow or vaporizer setting produce rapid changes in inspired concentrations. On the other hand, maximal rebreathing occurs when oxygen is added to a system in amount just to satisfy the animal's metabolic requirements, and anaesthetic agent in amount just sufficient to satisfy its uptake by the animal. In this system changes in inspired tensions are very gradual. The inspired tension is seldom, if ever, constant. All degrees of variation may occur between these two extremes of rebreathing. For example, a semi-closed system with absorption (see page 261) might be used with fresh gas added only just in excess of absolute minimal requirements, or it might be used with very high fresh gas flow rates. In the first instance the inspired gases would consist mainly of previously expired gases; in the second the inspired volume would consist mainly of fresh gas. Some gas would have to escape in each case, and although there would be rebreathing in both instances it would be complete in neither. It is variations such as this which are incompletely described by the use of current nomenclature.

Variations in the degree of rebreathing are particularly important when it is intended to follow some particular method described in the literature, for unless the degree of rebreathing is known it may be impossible, at first, to repeat the results obtained by the author of the article. Various degrees of rebreathing will affect the rate of nitrogen elimination and rise in inspired oxygen tension in an inhalation system connected to an animal which was previously breathing room air. Moreover, these rates will also be affected by the rate of fresh gas flow into the system.

The introduction of agents such as halothane into anaesthetic practice has further emphasized this need for more accurate nomenclature. Vaporizers have been constructed which deliver an accurately known concentration of halothane and other agents. However, since such wide variations in the degree of rebreathing are possible, the inspired tension of the agent will be constantly changing even with a known amount of agent being added to the system. In addition, the inspired concentration will be influenced by the volume of fresh gas being added to the circuit. Clearly, the present systems of nomenclature may allow erroneous concepts concerning the actual inspired concentration or tension of any inhalation anaesthetic.

In order to clarify matters so that any reader of an article can obtain an exact picture of what has actually been performed on any occasion, regardless of variations of teaching, practice and geographical location, it is only necessary for an author to give two simple pieces of information. First, the actual equipment used needs to be described, e.g. circle absorber, to-and-fro absorber, T-piece, etc., and second, the fresh gas flow rate should be stated. These two basic items of information need only be supplemented to provide complete data under certain, special circumstances. For example, in certain communications it might be necessary to give such details as exact apparatus dead-space volume, types of valves, type and location of vaporizer (in or out of breathing circuit) etc. For the majority of communications this might well be unnecessary and simply stating the apparatus used and the flow rate of gases would be quite adequate. It is to be hoped that authors will adopt this simple expedient so that the easy exchange of accurate information so vital to patients' welfare, teaching and research, will become a possibility in veterinary anaesthesia.

Anaesthetic Apparatus

Basically, an anaesthetic apparatus for inhalation anaesthesia consists of a vaporizing bottle for the volatile anaesthetic liquids linked to an oxygen cylinder through a reducing valve and flowmeter (Fig. 109). Although such a simple apparatus is not as versatile as the more complicated pieces of equipment commonly used today, it is quite adequate for all veterinary purposes. In such simple apparatus the vaporizer is invariably outside the breathing circuit and the implications of this will be considered later (page 275).

Reducing Valve

The reducing valve is necessary for three reasons:

(i) Once the flow has been set for any particular level, frequent readjustment of the flowmeter control, which would be necessary as the pressure in

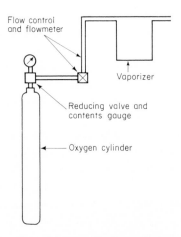

FIG. 109.—Essential parts of an anaesthetic apparatus.

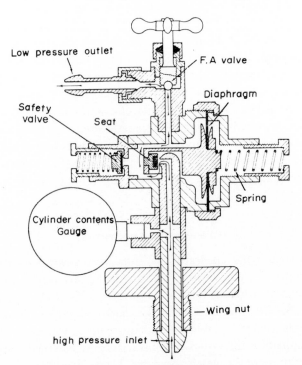

FIG. 110.—Endurance regulator.

the cylinder fell off, is obviated. In early days of gas cylinders the anaesthetist had to readjust the flow control every few minutes in order to keep the flow steady since there were no reducing valves, and a demand arose for an automatic regulator which would render this continuous adjustment unnecessary.

Because the reducing valve exerts this automatic control it is often referred to as a 'regulator'.

(ii) By supplying a low gas pressure to the control valve spindle small variations in the gas flow can be made easily. When a high pressure cylinder is controlled directly by a simple needle type valve large changes in flow rate result from very small movements of the control valve spindle.

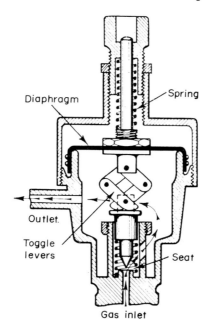

FIG. 111.—Adam's pressure reducing valve.

(iii) The reducing valve limits the pressure within the connecting tubing to a low level and the likelihood of bursting the connecting tubes when the flow is shut off by the flowmeter control is very much reduced.

The reducing valves in use in anaesthesia are known as 'endurance regulators' and 'Adam's pressure reducing valves' (Figs. 110 and 111). The setting of the endurance regulator can be adjusted by the anaesthetist, but the Adam's valve is pre-set to a given reduced pressure to 6 to 10 lb/sq in. Further details of the working of these regulators can be obtained from such sources as Macintosh, Mushin and Epstein (1958), and will not be considered here.

Flowmeters

Today, most of the flowmeters used in anaesthesia are known as 'rotameters' (Fig. 112). They make use of the interdependence of flow rate, size of orifice and pressure difference on either side of an orifice. The rotameter consists of a glass tube inside which a rotating bobbin is free to move. The bore of the tube gradually increases from below upwards. The bobbin floats up and down the tube, allowing gas to flow around it. The higher the bobbin in the tube the wider the annular space between the tube and bobbin (orifice) and the greater the flow rate through it. The bobbin, usually made of aluminium, has an upper rim which is of a diameter slightly greater than that of the body, and in which specially shaped channels are cut. As the gas enters the rotameter tube it impinges on the bobbin and causes it to rise. As the gas passes between the rim of the bobbin and the wall of the tube the bobbin is

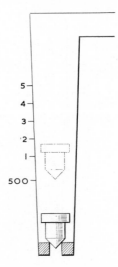

FIG. 112.—Rotameter.

made to spin because the rim with its set of channels acts like a set of vanes. The result is that the bobbin rides on a cushion of gas, and this eliminates errors due to friction between the tube and bobbin. If the tube is mounted in a truly upright position these meters are capable of readings of an accuracy of $\pm 2\%$.

The anaesthetist may wish to measure with a rotameter a gas other than the one for which the meter is calibrated. Unfortunately this is not a simple matter. The characteristics of a gas which influence its rate of flow through a given constriction are its density and its viscosity. If the constriction through which the gas flows is an orifice, the density of the gas plays a much more important part than does the viscosity in determining the rate of flow through the orifice. On the other hand, if the constriction is in the form of a tube, viscosity plays the dominant role in controlling the rate of the gas and the effect of density becomes negligible.

The clearance between the rotameter bobbin and tube is annular but may be considered as equivalent to a circular channel of the same cross section area. At low flows the bobbin is nearer the lower end of the tube and the diameter of the equivalent channel is smaller than its length or, in other words, the constriction is tubular in nature. As the bobbin rises the diameter of the equivalent channel increases, but the length remains that of the rim of the bobbin, and thus the constriction becomes more like a simple orifice. Therefore, when the float spins at the lower part of the tube the viscosity of the gas plays a more important part than does its density in determining the rate of

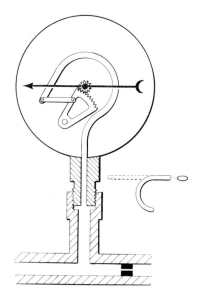

Fig. 113.—Bourdon pressure gauge flowmeter.

flow through the meter, whereas, at high flow rates density plays the more important role in this respect. Because of this there is no single correction factor which can be applied to convert the indicated flow into the actual flow when a foreign gas is passed through a meter which has been calibrated for one particular gas.

A much more crude flowmeter which is also encountered in veterinary anaesthesia utilizes a Bourdon pressure gauge (Fig. 113). The gas flowing from the cylinder issues from the reducing valve and is made to pass through a small orifice. A pressure builds up proximal to the constriction and this pressure is transmitted to the flexible metal Bourdon tube of oval cross section. This tube tends to straighten out and the degree of straightening depends on the pressure within it which, in turn, depends on the rate of flow of gas through the orifice. The tip of the Bourdon tube is linked by a simple mechanism to an indicator needle which moves over a scale calibrated in terms of rate of gas flow through the constriction. In fact, in this meter the gauge indicates the pressure difference between the proximal side of the orifice and the atmosphere. This is virtually equivalent to measuring the pressure gradient across the orifice, since in anaesthetic practice the pressure on the distal side of the orifice approximates very closely to atmospheric.

The Bourdon type of flowmeter is not satisfactory for measuring small

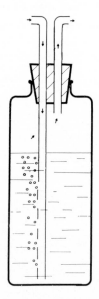

FIG. 114.—Water sight-feed meter.

rates of gas flow. Owing to the pressure necessary to cause the Bourdon tube to straighten out, a very small orifice must be used to provide the resistance to gas flow. If this orifice becomes partially blocked by dirt, the meter reading increases, whereas the actual flow of gas is decreased; if the orifice becomes completely blocked the meter reading suggests that the flow is being maintained. On the other hand, if the orifice is enlarged due to wear, the gas flow will be increased while the decreased resistance to gas flow will lead to a low meter reading.

A meter which can be improvised is the water sight-feed meter (Fig. 114). In this meter the gas flows through a tube which dips into water contained in a bottle. The part of the tube below the surface of the water is perforated with a number of holes placed one below the other. As the gas flows it escapes through the holes, bubbles through the water and is led away from the top of the bottle. The greater the flow of gas the greater the number of holes through which the gas will emerge into the water. A rough measure of the rate of flow of the gas is therefore provided by noting the number of holes from which the gas is bubbling. Owing to the disturbance of the water which would result this method is not suited to the measurement of large flows of gases. Although grossly inaccurate this is the only meter in which the volume of gas passing to the patient is actually seen. The only other positive evidence that gas is actually flowing through a meter is the spinning of the rotameter bobbin.

Vaporizers

In Britain the Boyle pattern vaporizer (Fig. 115) is probably the one most frequently encountered. These vaporizers are so designed as to allow for a fairly fine control of the strength of the anaesthetic vapour delivered. The

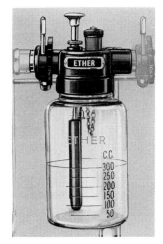

FIG. 115.—Boyle pattern vaporizer.

method of varying the concentration of anaesthetic vapour utilizes a permanent partition to prevent the direct passage of gases from the flowmeters to the patient. When the control lever is in the OFF position all the gases are diverted around the partition but away from the bottle. With the tap in the ON position all the gases pass through the bottle containing the liquid anaesthetic agent. The control tap can be placed in any intermediate position and this determines how much of the total gas flow passes through the bottle. A further means of controlling the vapour concentration is also provided. The gases are made to pass through a J-shaped tube before emerging into the space above the liquid anaesthetic in the bottle. The open end of the J-tube is covered by a metal hood which can be positioned as required by moving the rod attached to it up or down. As the hood is pushed downwards, the gas is deflected nearer and nearer to the surface of the liquid and finally, when the open end of the hood is pushed below the surface of the liquid the gases are made to bubble through the liquid anaesthetic. With the tap in the ON position and the hood, or cowl, fully depressed, the whole of the gas flow is made to bubble through the liquid and a maximum concentration of the anaesthetic vapour is picked up. The actual concentration of anaesthetic vapour delivered from any particular bottle depends on the diameter of the airways and the diameter of the bottle but some idea of the concentrations obtained from a typical bottle can be seen in Fig. 116.

When air or other gas flows over the surface of a liquid, the vapour of the liquid is carried away, and is replaced by fresh vapour. This continuous

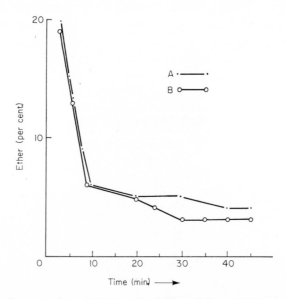

Fig. 116.—Concentration of ether and trichloroethylene delivered from Boyle vaporizer bottle with gas flowing at 8 litres/minute. Vapour concentration measured by gas chromatography.

Above: 200 ml of ether in bottle. Room temperature 16°C.
    A. Control tap 'Full on', plunger fully depressed, gases bubbling through ether.
    B. Control tap 'Full on', plunger 5 mm above surface of liquid ether.

Below: 50 ml of trichloroethylene in bottle. Room temperature 16° C. Control tap '¾ on', plunger fully withdrawn.

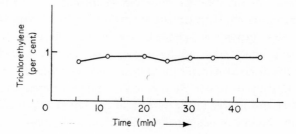

process of vaporization is accompanied by a corresponding loss of heat, the magnitude of which is determined by the rate at which the vapour is removed and by the latent heat of vaporization of the liquid. The loss of heat results in a fall in the temperature of the liquid unless heat is conducted to the liquid from some outside source. With the fall in the temperature of the liquid there is a corresponding decrease in the speed of vaporization and, as can be seen in Fig. 116, if the gas flow remains constant, the concentration of anaesthetic vapour in the gas stream from a Boyle pattern vaporizer decreases with time until the heat loss due to vaporization is balanced by the conduction of heat through the glass of the bottle from the surrounding atmosphere to the liquid anaesthetic.

There are today many precision vaporizers on the market, all designed to deliver an accurately known concentration of volatile anaesthetic agents over a wide range of gas flow rates. Among the best known of these are the Copper Kettle (Foregger Co. Inc.), the various ''tecs' (e.g. Fluotec, Pentec, etc., Cyprane Ltd.) and the Vapor (Drägerwerk). All these consist of a vaporizing chamber and a bypass. The fresh gas stream flowing into the vaporizer is divided into two portions, the larger of which passes straight through the bypass. The smaller portion is ducted through the vaporizing chamber, where it becomes saturated with the vapour, and this ensures that (a) there is no sudden burst of high vapour concentration when the vaporizer is first switched on, and (b) the output of the vaporizer is unaffected by shaking.

As already pointed out, the vaporization of the liquid anaesthetic results in the removal of heat from the liquid with a resultant fall in its temperature. If this fall is not checked the rate of vaporization will fall and the output concentration of the vaporizer decreases with time. In the various ''tecs' (e.g. Fluotec for halothane) temperature compensation is achieved by means of a bimetallic strip valve. This valve is arranged to act as a control of the volume of gas passing through the vaporizing chamber. As the temperature of the liquid falls, the bimetallic strip opens the valve further, allowing more gas to pass through the chamber. In the Copper Kettle and the Vapor, the vaporizer is constructed from a large mass of copper. The high thermal conductivity of copper allows heat to pass into the liquid from the room and this, together with the high thermal capacity of the copper mass, supplies the necessary heat for vaporization, holding the liquid temperature constant. In the ''tec' vaporizers, temperature compensation is automatic and there is only one control to set the output concentration. In the Copper Kettle the output concentration must be calculated from the liquid temperature as read from a thermometer, and the values of the vaporizing chamber and bypass gas flows read on flow-meters. The Vapor combines these principles.

A major problem in vaporizing design lies in the design of the splitting valves. The flow division ratio of this valve should remain constant over a wide range of flow rates but it is impossible to achieve this uniformity with the thermostatic valve; hence the ''tec' vaporizers are provided with auxiliary graphs for use with gas flows below 4 litres/minute.

It is known that the pressure fluctuations produced by intermittent positive pressure ventilation may have a considerable effect on the output concentration of vaporizers (Hill and Lowe, 1962). This 'pumping effect' can result in doubling the output concentration at low fresh gas flow rates, and the anaesthetist must allow for this or serious overdosage may occur.

When circle systems are used for the administration of inhalation anaesthetics the vaporizer may be placed either inside the breathing circuit or outside the breathing circuit. In the to-and-fro breathing circuits the vaporizer is almost invariably outside the breathing circuit, in the fresh gas supply line, so that the circuit receives a steady supply of anaesthetic. With the vaporizer in the breathing circuit the patient's inspirations and/or expirations pass through the vaporizer. The influence of the location of the vaporizer on the inspired tension of the anaesthetic agent has been considered in some detail by workers in the Welsh National School of Medicine, Cardiff (Galloon, 1960; Mapleson, 1960; Mushin and Galloon, 1960). These workers concluded that each system has its own advantages and disadvantages, but that in the hands of an experienced anaesthetist either arrangement is equally safe (or unsafe). The inexperienced anaesthetist is advised, especially with potent anaesthetics such as halothane, to use a calibrated and preferably thermostatically controlled vaporizer placed outside the breathing circuit. All anaesthetists using vaporizers with rebreathing systems must understand clearly the way in which the alveolar concentration, and hence the depth of anaesthesia, is dependent on the factors of ventilation, fresh gas flow and vaporizer characteristics.

In general, *when the vaporizer is in the breathing circuit:*

1. If anaesthesia is too light surgical stimulation will lead to an increase in ventilation and a deepening of anaesthesia.

2. If the vaporizer setting is too high, deepening anaesthesia depresses the ventilation and reduces vaporization. This acts to some extent as a built in safety factor.

3. If the animal stops breathing no fresh vapour enters the circuit.

4. The smaller the fresh gas flow the greater the economy in the use of the volatile agent.

5. A simple, low efficiency vaporizer is all that is required (e.g. The Goldman vaporizer for halothane shown in Fig. 117 which limits the concentration delivered to less than 3% by volume whatever the gas flow through it).

6. A sudden increase in ventilation and, therefore, of inspired concentration may be dangerous.

7. The fact that respired gases pass through the vaporizer introduces problems of resistance to breathing.

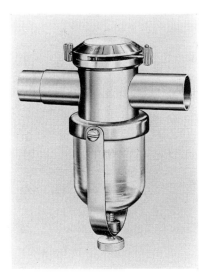

FIG. 117.—Goldman vaporizer for halothane.

When the vaporizer is outside the breathing circuit:

1. Ventilation has no effect on vaporization. Assisted or controlled respiration by intermittent positive pressure ventilation of the lungs has little effect on the depth of anaesthesia and is therefore much safer than is the case when the vaporizer is in the breathing circuit.

2. In most instances for any particular setting of the vaporizer control the smaller the fresh gas flow, the lower is the inspired concentration. (This is not always so in the ''tec' vaporizers.)

3. Too deep anaesthesia with respiratory depression does not have the built in safety factor found when the vaporizer is in the breathing circuit and the animal is breathing spontaneously.

Delivery of Inhalation Anaesthetics to the Patient from Closed and Semi-closed Systems

Anaesthetics given by the closed and semi-closed circuit methods must be delivered to the animal through a well fitting face-mask or endotracheal tube otherwise the anaesthetic agent will be diluted and inhaled with an unknown quantity of air.

Anaesthetic Face-masks

In domestic animals there are wide variations in the configuration and size of the face, so that it is difficult to obtain an accurate air-tight fit between the face and mask. However, this difficulty can be overcome by the use of malleable latex rubber masks (Fig. 118) which can be moulded around the face and

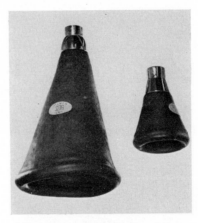

FIG. 118.—Malleable face-masks.

held in position with a simple headstrap (Fig. 119). The lower jaw must be pushed forward into the mask for if it is displaced backwards the airway may become obstructed by the base of the tongue coming into contact with the posterior wall of the pharynx.

After use these masks should be thoroughly washed with soap and hot water and then disinfected.

Endotracheal Intubation

The history of endotracheal intubation in animals is older than that of anaesthesia. In 1542 Vesalius passed a tube into the trachea of an animal and inflated the lungs by means of a bellows to keep the animal alive while the anatomy of its thoracic cavity was demonstrated. Similar demonstrations were given before the Fellows of the Royal Society by Robert Hook in 1667.

There are two methods by which inhalation anaesthetics can be administered through an endotracheal tube, and the first to be used was that of 'insufflation' in which the anaesthetic agents are blown through a narrow-bore tube, the distal end of which lies in the trachea near to the carina. Respiration and the return flow of gases and vapours takes place around the tube. The insufflation technique is said to render respiratory movements unnecessary but has the great disadvantage of causing a considerable loss of heat and water vapour from the body. It has fallen into disuse and has given place to the second method, that of inhalation, in which to-and-fro respiration takes place through one large-bore tube.

The standard endotracheal tubes used in man in the United Kingdom were designed by Magill and two kinds ('oral' and 'nasal') are available. The 'oral' tubes have comparatively thick walls and are intended for intubation through the mouth, while the 'nasal' tubes, designed for passage through the nostril into the trachea, have comparatively thin walls. The tubes

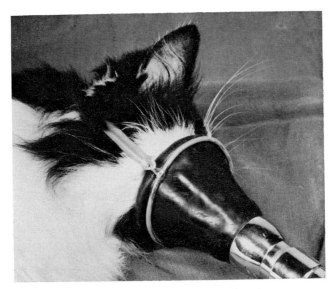

FIG. 119.—Harness for fixing face-mask.

are obtainable in 'Portex' plastic or red rubber. The red rubber 'oral' tubes may be either plain or fitted with a cuff which can be inflated with air from a syringe after the tube has been passed into the trachea (Fig. 120). The inflated cuff provides an airtight seal between the wall of the trachea and the tube so that all the respired gases must pass through the lumen of the tube.

Through the offices of the British Standards Institution the range of tubes for use in man are designated by reference to the internal diameter expressed in millimetres and tubes for veterinary use are, in future, to be designated in the same way.

Although not strictly essential, a laryngoscope greatly facilitates the process of intubation in many animals and is a piece of equipment which is most desirable if endotracheal intubation is to be widely practised. A suitable laryngoscope is one which holds a dry electric battery in the handle and has a detachable blade in order that blades of different sizes can be fitted to the instrument. The blades should be designed so as to enable the passage of a large-bore endotracheal tube to be made as easily as possible. For veterinary purposes one standard human adult and one child size 'Magill pattern' blades and one special blade are the minimum requirements. The special blade should be of the Macintosh pattern, ¾ in (1·9 cm) wide, and between 9 and 12 in (23 to 30 cm) long. The blades should be separate from the lamp and its electrical connections so that they can be sterilized by boiling without risk of damage to the electrical system. Various types are available and one

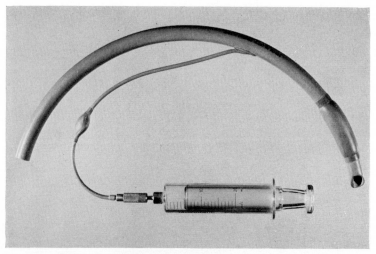

FIG. 120.—Cuffed endotracheal tube, non-return valve and inflating syringe.

suitable instrument is shown in Fig. 121. Recently, the Rowson laryngoscope (Fig. 122) has been introduced for use in large pigs and adult cattle (Rowson, 1965). This instrument is employed in a special manner (see page 280) and it makes the intubation of adult cattle and pigs a simple matter.

Wide-bore tubes may be introduced into the trachea by various methods. The method adopted in any particular case will be decided by the experience and skill of the anaesthetist and by the kind of animal in which the tube is to be passed. The following descriptions are of techniques which students and anaesthetists in training have found to be relatively simple to acquire.

Endotracheal Intubation in Horses

In horses the passage of an endotracheal tube presents no great problem. With the anaesthetized horse in lateral recumbency the head is moderately extended on the neck, the mouth opened and the tongue pulled forward. The tube, lubricated on its outside with a suitable lubricant (K-Y Jelly, Johnson and Johnson), is introduced into the mouth with the concave side of its curve directed towards the hard palate and advanced, keeping to the mid-

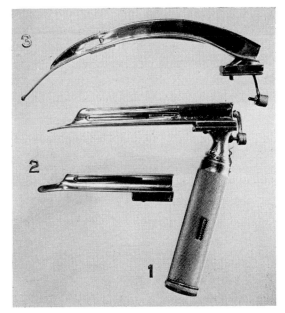

FIG. 121.—Laryngoscope with child, adult and special blade.

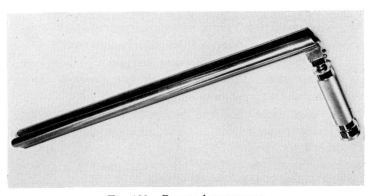

FIG. 122.—Rowson laryngoscope.

line, until its tip is in the pharynx. It is then rotated so that the concavity of its curve is towards the tongue (Fig. 123) and at the next inspiration it is pushed rapidly on into the trachea. The rotation of the tube when its tip is in the pharynx ensures that it does not become impacted on the epiglottis. Failure of the tube to enter the trachea indicates that the alignment of the head and neck is incorrect.

Intubation through the mouth permits the use of the largest tube which will comfortably fit the trachea. A 16·0 mm tube is suitable for ponies up to about 150 kg (330 lb) body weight, while a 30 mm tube is adequate for small thoroughbreds. Heavy hunters often take surprisingly large tubes. Endo-tracheal tubes can be passed through the inferior nasal meatus but this limits the size of the tube to that which can be accommodated by the nostril. Such tubes are often too small to allow free unobstructed respiration and their introduction and removal entails the risk of damaging the turbinate bones

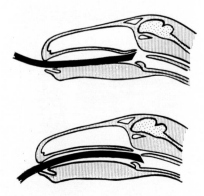

FIG. 123.—Passage of an endotracheal tube in a horse.

Endotracheal Intubation in Adult Cattle

In adult cattle the larynx cannot be seen without the use of the Rowson laryngoscope and 'blind' intubation through the mouth is successful only on rare occasions. However, when a Rowson laryngoscope is not available, a tube may be introduced into the trachea with certainty if the procedure known as 'intubation by palpation' is adopted.

For this, a wedge-shaped gag is insinuated between the molar teeth of the anaesthetized animal and a hand is passed through the mouth to identify the epiglottis and arytenoid cartileges (Fig. 124). The finger-tips are placed on the arytenoid cartileges and the lubricated tube is passed between the dorsum of the tongue and the arm. The tube is directed through the glottis by the exploring hand which is then withdrawn from the mouth as the tube is pushed on into the trachea.

A 25·0 mm tube is suitable for cattle of about 450 kg (1000 lb) body weight.

The use of the Rowson laryngoscope (Longworth Scientific Instrument Co. Ltd) makes intubation a relatively simple matter. The head and neck of the anaesthetized animal are positioned so that the head is in full extension and a wedged-shaped mouth gag is introduced between the molar teeth. The blade of the laryngoscope is inserted into the pharynx with the open side of the C-section blade against the hard palate, until contact is made with the epiglottis. The handle is then moved to the left or right so as to rotate the blade, when one of the two distal tips will lift the epiglottis, exposing to view the vocal cords and the interior of the larynx. No attempt is made to lift the jaw of the animal during this procedure. A large endotracheal tube cannot be passed down the blade of the instrument so a rubber-covered, fairly stout wire guide is introduced down the blade and into the trachea. The laryngoscope is withdrawn as soon as the guide is in position and the endotracheal tube is passed around the guide wire. The guide must be about three times as long as the endotracheal tube to avoid the possibility of its being lost into the trachea during this manoeuvre, and it is, of course, withdrawn from the lumen of the tube once this has been introduced.

The lubricant applied to any endotracheal tube used in ruminant animals

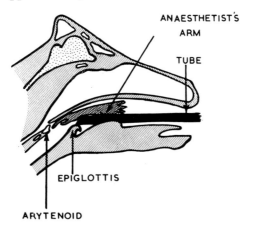

FIG. 124.—Intubation by palpation.

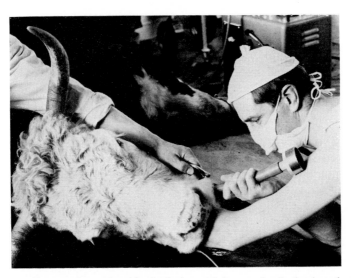

FIG. 125.—Passage of an endotracheal tube in an adult cow—intubation by palpation.

should never contain a local analgesic drug for if it does the mucous membrane of the trachea and larynx may remain desensitized for some time after the tube is withdrawn. The protective cough reflex will then be absent and foreign material may be inhaled into the bronchial tree.

Endotracheal Intubation in Calves, Sheep and Goats

In calves, sheep and goats endotracheal intubation is best performed with the aid of a laryngoscope. The anaesthetized animal is placed on its back with its head and neck in full extension. An assistant draws the tongue well

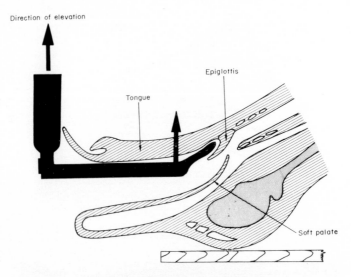

FIG. 126.—Use of the laryngoscope.

out of the mouth and fixes the upper jaw by pulling on the ends of a tape placed just behind the dental pad. The laryngoscope is then introduced so that the tip of the blade is behind the base of the tongue and in front of the epiglottis. The laryngoscope blade is lifted as shown in Fig. 126 to expose the larynx and vocal cords and the tube passed into the trachea under direct vision. It is important to note that the larynx is brought into view by a lifting movement and not by employing the laryngoscope blade as a lever using the incisor teeth as a fulcrum.

Endotracheal tubes may also be passed through the mouth and 'threaded' through the larynx which is gripped between the anaesthetist's finger and thumb (Fig. 127). When using this method it is sometimes necessary to stiffen the tube by passing down a piece of straight brass rod of suitable length which is withdrawn as soon as the tube is in the trachea. It is difficult to pass tubes of adequate size by this method but the method is useful if a laryngoscope is not available.

A 16 mm tube is suitable for large sheep (such as Dorset Horn) and for calves, while 11 and 12 mm tubes are adequate for most adult goats.

Endotracheal Intubation in Pigs

In pigs intubation of the trachea is not easy. The anaesthetized pig is placed on its back with its head and neck fully extended. An assistant pulls on the tongue and fixes the upper jaw while the laryngoscope is introduced and the

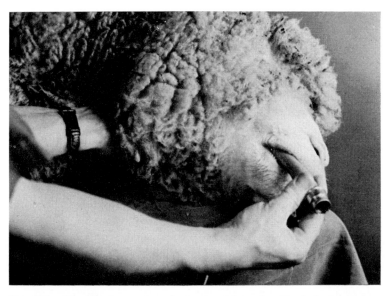

FIG. 127.—Passage of an endotracheal tube without the aid of a laryngoscope.

larynx brought into view. Under direct vision the tube is passed between the vocal cords and kept dorsal to the middle ventricle of the larynx. Its progress is usually arrested at the cricoid ring for in pigs the larynx is set at an angle to the trachea and before the tube can be advanced the head must be slightly flexed on the neck. Laryngeal spasm is easily provoked and endotracheal intubation is greatly facilitated by the use of relaxant drugs.

The Rowson laryngoscope was designed for use in large pigs where the larynx cannot be seen with the aid of a conventional instrument. It is used in pigs in a similar manner to that used in cattle (page 280) but because the endotracheal tubes are much smaller the use of a guide is usually not necessary. The endotracheal tube can be passed down the blade of the laryngoscope. Intubation is sometimes facilitated by the use of a gum elastic bougie as a stiffener inside the endotracheal tube.

A 9·5 mm oral tube is required for pigs weighing about 50 kg and for large sows and boars 15 to 20 mm tubes should be employed.

Endotracheal Intubation in Dogs

The anaesthetized dog is placed in lateral recumbency, its mouth open and its tongue pulled well forward. The lubricated tube is introduced into the mouth and the epiglottis exposed by reflecting the soft palate upwards and backwards with the end of the tube. The tube is then used to depress the epiglottis anteriorly on to the base of the tongue and to keep it there as the tube itself is advanced on into the trachea (Fig. 128). Should any difficulty be

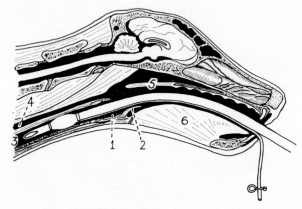

FIG. 128.—Endotracheal intubation in the dog.
(1) Vocal cords.   (2) Epiglottis.   (3) Trachea.   (4) Oesophagus.
(5) Soft palate.   (6) Tongue.

experienced a laryngoscope may be used and the tube introduced under direct vision or, alternatively, a finger may be inserted into the pharynx and employed to direct the tube into the glottis.

Care should always be taken to avoid injury to the larynx and forceps should never be applied to the epiglottis, or to the fold of mucous membrane between the epiglottis and the tongue, in order to expose the laryngeal opening. Trauma to the larynx or to the tissues around it may give rise to local oedema which can, when the tube is removed, cause complete obstruction of the airway and necessitate the performance of an emergency tracheostomy.

The diameter of the largest tube which can be introduced into the trachea of a dog is related both to the dog's size and to its breed. For example, a 16 mm tube can usually be passed into the trachea of an adult Alsatian dog while in an Airedale dog of similar size and age a 12 mm tube may be the largest tube which will pass between the vocal cords.

Endotracheal Intubation in Cats

In cats laryngeal spasm is easily provoked and atraumatic intubation is only possible after adopting one of the following methods:

(i) deep anaesthesia has been induced, or
(ii) the laryngeal mucous membrane of the lightly anaesthetized animal has been desensitized by spraying the region with a solution of a local analgesic drug such as cocaine or lignocaine hydrochloride, or
(iii) the anaesthetized animal has been paralysed by the administration of a relaxant drug.

Whichever course is adopted the lubricated tube is passed under direct vision using either a laryngoscope or a wooden tongue spatula to expose the larynx.

To avoid hypoxic episodes when a relaxant drug is employed the animal must be allowed to inhale oxygen or an oxygen-rich mixture through a face mask for 30 to 60 seconds before the relaxant is injected. After intubation artificial respiration must be performed until normal spontaneous breathing is resumed.

For most adult cats either a 5·0 or 5·5 mm Magill tube will be required and because no tube smaller than size 5·5 mm is fitted with a cuff it may sometimes be necessary to pack ribbon gauze into the pharynx around the tube to enable positive pressure respiration to be carried out through the tube.

Apparatus for Endotracheal Intubation

Length of endotracheal tubes. An endotracheal tube which is too long may be inadvertently introduced into one or other of the main bronchi and the lung on the non-intubated side will then act as a venous-arterial shunt. This may give rise to persistent cyanosis and endobronchial intubation should always be suspected if an animal shows cyanosis when breathing an oxygen-rich mixture through an endotracheal tube.

All new Magill tubes must be cut to the correct length both to ensure that endobronchial intubation is impossible and to minimize the respiratory dead space. They should be cut so that when their bevelled tip lies in the trachea about midway between the larynx and carina their cut end is immediately below the nostrils. Also, the connecting piece between the tube and any closed or semi-closed anaesthetic apparatus should be as short as possible.

Reinforced endotracheal tubes. Frequent use, with the associated cleaning and sterilizing processes, makes red rubber endotracheal tubes soft, and plastic tubes may soften when warmed to body temperature. Soft tubes flatten out when bent, and are easily compressed by pressure. Obliteration of the lumen from either of these causes may give rise to serious obstruction of the airway. Patency of the airway, when the animal has to be placed in any position which may cause flattening or kinking of the tube, can be assured by the use of an armoured, or reinforced, endotracheal tube. These special tubes are made of latex rubber and incorporate a wire spiral in their walls. They are more expensive than the standard tubes, and because there are not many occasions when their use is desirable, most veterinary anaesthetists consider their purchase to be unjustified. On the occasions when compression or kinking of the endotracheal tube is likely to be encountered, the use of a new red rubber tube is usually quite satisfactory.

REFERENCES

FISHER, E. W. and JENNINGS, S. (1957). *Vet. Rec.* **69**, 769
FOWLER, M. E., PARKER, E. E., McLAUGHLIN, E. F. and TYLER, W. S. (1963). *J. Am. vet. med. Ass.* **143**, 272
GALLOON, S. (1960). *Br. J. Anaesth.* **32**, 310
HAMILTON, W. K. (1964). *Anesthesiology*, **25**, 3
HANSSON, C. H. and JOHANNISSON, D. (1958). *Nord. Vet. Med.* **10**, 469
HARRISON, G. A. (1964). *Br. J. Anaesth.* **36**, 115
HILL, D. W. and LOWE, H. J. (1962). *Anesthesiology*, **23**, 291
JONES, E. W. (1961). *J. Am. vet. med. Ass.* **139**, 785
MACINTOSH, R., MUSHIN, W. W. and EPSTEIN, H. G. (1968). *Physics for the Anaesthetist.* Oxford: Blackwell
MAPLESON, W. W. (1960). *Br. J. Anaesth.* **32**, 298
MUSHIN, W. W. and GALLOON, S. (1960). *Br. J. Anaesth.* **32**, 324
PAS, TEN, R. H., BROWN, E. S. and ELAM, J. O. (1958). *Anesthesiology*, **19**, 231
PURCHASE, I. F. H. (1965). *Vet. Rec.* **77**, 913
ROBSON, J. G. and PASK, E. A. (1954). *Br. J. Anaesth.* **26**, 333
ROWSON, L. E. A. (1965). *Vet. Rec.* **77**, 1465
WALLS, N. S. (1950). *Anaesthesia*, **5**, 171
WEAVER, B. M. Q. (1959). *Vet. Rec.* **71**, 11
——— (1960). *Vet. Rec.* **72**, 1121
WESTHUES, M. and FRITSCH, R. (1961). *Die Narkose der Tiere.* Berlin: Paul Parey (Eng. ed. 1964. Edinburgh: Oliver and Boyd)

14

Intravenous Anaesthesia in Horses and Farm Animals

The Horse

Chloral Hydrate

Among the pioneers of chloral hydrate anaesthesia in equine surgery was Degive, a prominent Belgian professor. Writing in 1908, he stated: 'Chloral hydrate injected into the jugular vein of the horse in a dose of 10 g/100 kg, in a 20% solution, produces in 1 to 2 minutes complete general anaesthesia without causing preliminary excitement in the animal. The method is most valuable when practised with full aseptic precautions but it has been followed by several accidents which have put its value in doubt.' Even today, it is the opinion of many that it is still a valuable method of inducing general anaesthesia in the horse. It is probable that the accidents referred to by the professor were related not so much to a lack of surgical cleanliness as to technical errors during injection. Solutions of chloral hydrate are particularly irritant and it is essential that none shall be introduced into the perivenous tissues or into the wall of the vein itself, for otherwise a serious obliterating and perhaps septic thrombophlebitis may result.

During the First World War officers of the Royal Army Veterinary Corps (Gillett, Crawford, Malone and others) recorded their experiences with the drug administered in the standing position and expressed the most favourable conclusions while acknowledging technical failure with serious consequences in a small proportion of cases. Such complications are less likely to have disagreeable repercussions when dealing with Army horses than when one is engaged in civil practice and thus it is understandable that in general practice chloroform continued to be the equine anaesthetic of choice. The work of Marcenac in France in the thirties again brought chloral hydrate into prominence and since that time it is probably true to say that it has been the most widely used anaesthetic for horses, certainly among veterinary surgeons on the Continent of Europe, in South Africa, Australia and the United States of America, but still to a considerably less extent in the British Isles. The practice of combining chloral hydrate with magnesium sulphate and/or the barbiturates has been introduced but it is unlikely that these combinations have advantages over the single drug while their inclusion in the injection may have disadvantages.

J. G. Wright used chloral hydrate almost solely for the induction of deep narcosis or general anaesthesia in horses for 25 years and during that time treated some 600 animals. They comprised horses of all ages and sizes. Two deaths occurred, both during the course of anaesthesia, and there were 4 cases of jugular thrombosis.

The advantage of the method are:

1. The regularity of response to a unit dosage by body weight.
2. The absence of excitement during either induction or recovery.
3. The wide safety factor in reasonably healthy subjects.
4. The absence of any post-anaesthetic nausea or malaise.

Against these must be set the following disadvantages:

1. Satisfactory results are dependent upon perfect technique in relation to the injection, and the introduction of the chloral solution either into the wall of the vein or into the perivascular tissues will provoke serious consequences.
2. The duration of recumbency $1\frac{1}{2}$ hours or so after the induction of marginal anaesthesia and over 2 hours after full anaesthesia is a significant inconvenience.

Chloral hydrate is used as an induction anaesthetic. In the case of rapidly performed interferences such as castration, it is likely that the induction dose will suffice, or that in the case of longer but relatively simple interferences local anaesthesia will be used in addition. In cases in which more prolonged general anaesthesia is required, such as operation for fistulous withers or intra-abdominal interferences such as cryptorchid castration or ovariectomy, it is not advised that additional chloral hydrate be used for the continuation of anaesthesia, for it must be borne in mind that being a halogen derivative the drug has a toxic effect on parenchymatous cells similar to that of chloroform, and thus a switch should be made to a relatively non-toxic inhalation anaesthetic or an ultra-short or short-acting barbiturate.

It has been found that a dosage of 6·5 g/50 kg in horses in the weight range 450 to 650 kg (9 to 13 cwt) which have not been fasted, will provoke a state just over or just under the borderline of consciousness. In heavier animals a slightly reduced dose will have the same effect, while in lighter ones rather more will be required, in fact for yearling horses a dose of 7 g/50 kg is given. A point to be considered is the concentration in which the drug shall be used. The higher the concentration the greater will be the degree of local inflammation should technical error occur. Conversely the lower the concentration the greater will be the volume of solution to be injected, and when using the gravity method of injection (the one recommended) the time occupied in its administration will be inconveniently long. Ten% is considered to be the optimum; when dealing with a horse of 550 kg (11 cwt), this represents about $\frac{3}{4}$ litre. The optimum time in which to induce anaesthesia is from 4 to 5 minutes and care should be taken when a horse struggles vigorously after casting that injection is made very slowly during this period. Administration is both easier and safer in the cast and restrained position than in the standing one, for in the former accurate penetration of the vein throughout injection is much more certain, the speed of injection can be more effectively controlled, while in the later stages the degree of narcosis can, with reasonable accuracy, be assessed and the total amount given thereby modified.

Quite apart, however, from the dangers of technical error in the standing position, the floundering which may be associated with the animal's fall is a grave inconvenience. It has long been recognized that casting, particularly by the hobble method, is attended by a risk of fracture, particularly of the lumbar vertebral column. The accident occurs almost immediately after the animal falls and is due to the powerful contraction of the longissimus mass with the limbs fixed. It is prevented by keeping the head and neck well extended during casting and until the horse is anaesthetized. Experienced assistance is essential. In this connection, premedication is a valuable aid. By its use, the application of tackle is facilitated and the degree of struggling on casting reduced. The use of the sedative does not reduce the amount of chloral hydrate required to induce full anaesthesia but it does tend to increase the total recumbency time.

The assessment of depths of anaesthesia is, perhaps, particularly difficult in the horse. One of the first indications that the animal is passing into a state of profound narcosis is that the eyeballs commence to rotate laterally. At first this movement is slow but as the stage of anaesthesia is reached it becomes faster. The condition persists with progressively deepening anaesthesia almost to the point of death. Thus it is important to observe its onset for it is likely that from that point an additional one-eighth to one-tenth of the dose already given will bring the animal to a state of medium depth anaesthesia. At the stage of deep narcosis also it is noted that if the tongue is withdrawn through the interdental space the animal is unable to draw it back and also that there is no response to vigorous pinching. (In many superficial operations in which local analgesia will also be used, narcosis will not be deepened beyond this point for unless there is some severe pain stimulus there will be

10

no movement.) In the horse the tail reflex is a lowly one which serves as a useful guide. If the tail is suddenly but gently raised there will be a definite response when deep narcosis only has been attained but this response will be lost with the onset of anaesthesia. In the male and the gelding it will be noticed, just as anaesthesia is developing, that the penis is relaxing and slowly protruding from the prepuce. In the mare the vulval lips relax and urine often seeps away. The anus relaxes with the onset of anaesthesia although the sphincter reflex remains brisk. The corneal reflex although sluggish in anaesthesia can be provoked almost to the point of death. In light anaesthesia there is slight pupillary construction but this may be impossible to determine because of the varying light intensities. In deep anaesthesia there is marked constriction. In anaesthesia the pulse rate is accelerated to from 60 to 80 beats/minute. (*It should be noted that when phenothiazine derivatives are used for premedication, many of the muscle-relaxation guides to depth are lost for among the actions of such drugs as promazine are relaxation of the tail, penis and tongue together with drooping of the eyelids. In horses so treated, movement of the eyeballs and the pulse rate are the most reliable guides.*)

There is no doubt that the margin between the anaesthetic and the paralytic doses is wide in the healthy animal.

Dumas (1935) states that harmful effects are not seen until 18·5 g/50 kg have been given. J. G. Wright has given a dosage of 10 g/50 kg to an animal in poor condition by slow intravenous injection in a period of 20 minutes without appreciable toxic effect on the respiratory centre or the heart.

Chloral Hydrate–Magnesium Sulphate

Vladutiu recorded the use of a mixture of chloral hydrate and magnesium sulphate administered by intravenous injection as a general anaesthetic for the horse. He employed a dose of 5 g of each/50 kg body weight in 10% solution and claimed that the inclusion of the magnesium sulphate hastened the onset of anaesthesia, increased its depth and reduced the toxicity of the chloral. Since that time a number of American records of the use of the mixture have been published. Danks (1943) recommends a mixture of 2 parts of chloral hydrate to 1 of magnesium sulphate. He claims that solutions are less irritant than those of chloral hydrate alone and that the mixture eliminates the reflex irritability seen in some horses when using chloral hydrate alone. Coffee (1949) prefers the proportions 3 of chloral hydrate to 1 of magnesium, given by slow intravenous injection until the desired degree of anaesthesia is attained.

In the United Kingdom these mixtures have received very little attention, the general practice being to give chloral hydrate alone either in full anaesthetic doses or in doses provoking deep narcosis only and augmented by inhalation, a barbiturate or local infiltration. Moreover, experience in this country is that chloral hydrate given alone in adequate quantities does not cause excitability.

Chloral Hydrate–Magnesium Sulphate–Pentobarbitone (Equithesin)

Millenbruck and Wallinga in America speak highly of this mixture as a general anaesthetic for the horse when administered by intravenous injection. Millenbruck records a total experience of 250 cases in which no death occurred and of 90 cases under conditions of general veterinary practice in which results were consistently satisfactory. Advantages claimed for the method are: the mixture is of low toxicity, there being approximately a 100% margin over the quantity required for anaesthesia, excitement during induction is negligible or completely absent, there is no floundering during the recovery period and surgical anaesthesia is complete.

The solution used comprises:

Chloral hydrate	28 g (1 oz)
Magnesium sulphate	14 g ($\frac{1}{2}$ oz)
Pentobarbitone sodium . . .	6·5 g (100 grains)
Distilled water	1000 ml (1$\frac{3}{4}$ pints)

The solution must be prepared within an hour before administration so as to prevent precipitation which occurs as the result of a reaction between the chloral hydrate and the barbiturate.

Administration. Administration is by slow infusion into the jugular vein, using one of the common forms of gravity apparatus. In a 450 kg (1000 lb) horse about 325 ml are allowed to gravitate into the vein in a period of 3 minutes by holding the flask at about shoulder height. When the horse commences to lose muscular coordination the flask is raised as high as possible to increase the rate of flow before the horse collapses. Efforts should be made to keep the animal on its feet as long as possible. This is best done by a man on each side applying support in the region of the hips. When the horse has fallen its head should be restrained for a short time in case there are efforts to rise. If narcosis is not complete in a few minutes, the needle should be reintroduced into the vein and a little more of the solution slowly run in until the desired degree is obtained. When oscillatory movement of the eyeball almost ceases and the horse takes a deep sigh, the stage of surgical anaesthesia has been reached. The average quantity taken by horses of 450 kg was 670 ml of the solution. This represents: chloral hydrate, 20 g ($\frac{2}{3}$ oz); magnesium sulphate, 10 g ($\frac{1}{3}$ oz); pentobarbitone sodium, 4·3 g (67 grains).

Course. With minimum doses required to get only a slight corneal reflex, the surgical stage persists for 15 to 30 minutes, whereas an addition of 15% will maintain the stage for from 40 to 60 minutes. Muscular relaxation is good. Recovery is rapid, the animal regaining consciousness at about the same rate as muscular coordination is restored. The total recumbency period is usually about 1 hour.

Toxicity is claimed to be negligible; a case is quoted by Millenbruck in which a horse was given twice the average dose and still lived in profound narcosis with a respiratory rate of 2/minute.

Pentobarbitone Sodium

Pentobarbitone sodium is considered to be an unsuitable anaesthetic for the adult horse because the recovery period is long, and associated with marked narcotic excitement and struggling.

Fowler (1946) speaks well of pentobarbitone sodium as a general anaesthetic for foals up to a few months old. He reports that the total dose required varied from 0·3 to 1·5 g and that up to 5 g was given to older colts. Somewhat limited experience at the Liverpool School confirms these statements. The secret of success would appear to lie in slow injection with the assessment of depth as injection proceeds, continuing until the tail is completely flaccid and the anal reflex absent. The animal generally remains recumbent for a period of 2½ to 3 hours and the recovery period may be associated with considerable movement of the limbs and head. Usually, these may easily be controlled in a foal without the application of very forcible restraint.

Pentobarbitone sodium has been used in the Liverpool School for the continuation of anaesthesia after induction with chloral hydrate. On the first sign that anaesthesia is lightening (or if only deep basal narcosis has been attained), pentobarbitone sodium is slowly injected into the jugular vein. A quantity of 1 to 1·5 g is injected over about 2 minutes. This is generally sufficient to deepen the anaesthesia to the medium plane. If it is not, injection is slowly continued, making pauses while the depth is assessed. As much as 4 g (60 grains) may be given in this manner during the course of operation. By this method the total period of recumbency is much less than it would have been had pentobarbitone sodium been used alone; in fact it is probable that the horse will be able to regain its feet within 90 minutes of the initial induction. Moreover, the struggling and floundering during the recovery period, which is a feature when the barbiturates are used alone, will be absent.

Thiopentone Sodium

The rapid injection of a solution containing 1 g of thiopentone sodium for every 90 kg (200 lb) of the animal's body weight into the jugular vein of the unrestrained horse will induce anaesthesia. The majority of horses sink quietly to the ground within 20 to 30 seconds of the injection being made and a brief period of unconsciousness is produced. Surgical anaesthesia is present for 3 to 4 minutes and then signs of recovery become apparent. Injection of the drug causes apnoea but this seldom lasts for longer than 15 to 20 seconds and artificial respiration is not required. A slight fall in blood pressure is also produced and there may be a small increase in the pulse rate. Recovery is complete within 35 to 45 minutes *and is usually violent in nature*. Most horses make galloping movements as soon as narcosis begins to lighten and attempt to stand long before they are even capable of maintaining the dog-sitting position. As might be expected, the violent struggling which occurs during the recovery period not infrequently causes injury to the animal.

It is obvious that while this method of using thiopentone is attractive, in that anaesthesia can be induced in the unrestrained horse so that casting is unnecessary and only minimal assistance is required, the violent recovery period renders it a dangerous method. Moreover, although most animals sink quietly to the ground some rear up immediately after injection of the drug and then fall to the ground so heavily that they sustain injuries which may be as severe as those associated with forcible casting by ropes or hobbles. The need for very rapid injection may also constitute a hazard for it necessitates the use of concentrated solutions of the drug. These concentrated solutions are very irritant to the tissues so that necrosis, sloughing and even aneurism formation may follow accidental perivascular injection (Neal, 1963).

Until quite recently these disadvantages prevented the widespread use of the drug in horses. There was no way of preventing some horses from falling heavily to the ground and the only certain way of preventing injury during recovery was to apply hobbles to the unconscious animal and to maintain restraint until full consciousness was regained. Now, however, thanks to the introduction of relaxants and phenothiazine ataractic drugs, the anaesthetist has means of overcoming both these major disadvantages and thiopentone has become popular in equine anaesthesia. It is being used together with these other drugs either to provide full surgical anaesthesia for operations of short duration or to induce anaesthesia which is then maintained by inhalation agents such as chloroform, halothane, or cyclopropane.

If the intravenous injection of thiopentone is immediately followed by the intravenous injection of the relaxant suxamethonium chloride (0·15 mg/kg), it becomes easier for the man at the head of the animal to ensure that it sinks quietly to the ground. When, as advocated by Messervy (1967), additional protection in the form of a foam-rubber padded horse-rug and head gear is used, there is then no risk of injury even in heavy subjects. The use of suxamethonium does not in any way do away with the necessity of having 'a good man on the head' but it makes it very much easier for him to control the animal as it goes down. When given in this way the use of suxamethonium is not attended by undesirable side-effects since the action of the thiopentone prevents the rise in blood pressure and serum potassium, and minimizes the release of adrenaline from the adrenal glands caused by this relaxant drug (see page 409).

When the phenothiazine ataractic drugs are used for premedication (see Chapter 9) a quiet recovery, with a most noticeable absence of struggling and excitement, can be expected. Moreover, their use facilitates the intravenous injection of thiopentone and makes it easier to avoid extravenous injection of this drug. Given in appropriate doses by intramuscular or intravenous injection, all the various phenothiazine derivatives appear to be effective but acetylpromazine possesses certain properties which probably make it the one of choice.

The use of the phenothiazine ataractics for premedication does not reduce the dose of thiopentone necessary for the induction of anaesthesia, nor does it render the very rapid injection of the barbiturate unnecessary. The injection must be complete within 10 to 15 seconds for the dose of thiopentone used is only sufficient to produce unconsciousness when given in this manner. Such a rapid injection secures a very high concentration of the drug in the blood flowing through the vein and although this blood is diluted with blood from other regions of the body as it enters the right side of the heart and passes through the pulmonary circulation, a substantial portion of the drug injected is delivered from the left side of the heart direct to the cerebral vessels. Thus the brain is exposed, for a short space of time, to blood which contains a high concentration of thiopentone and unconsciousness is produced. The remainder of the drug diffuses rapidly from the blood into the body tissues, so that after receiving the initial dose, the brain is perfused by blood which contains very little thiopentone and the concentration in the brain falls as the drug passes back into the blood to be redistributed to the non-fatty tissues of the body. This results in a rapid return of consciousness unless more thiopentone is given or some other agent is administered.

Although it is recognized that the need for such rapid injection is associated with a risk of perivascular deposition of the drug, in practice it has been found that the rapid injection actually makes for safety because it reduces to a minimum the length of time for which the needle has to be maintained in the lumen of the vein. *Provided that the needle is inserted through the skin and into the vein within an area which has been infiltrated with local analgesic solution, there are very few premedicated animals which cannot be restrained long enough for the injection of the thiopentone to be made with precision.*

In horses, the sequence of premedication with a phenothiazine derivative, induction of anaesthesia by the rapid intravenous injection of thiopentone followed by suxamethonium and maintenance, where necessary, with an inhalation anaesthetic agent such as halothane, provides a very useful technique of anaesthesia. It is a technique which can be carried out anywhere with the minimum of assistance and apparatus, avoids the risks associated with forcible casting, and is followed by a quiet, reasonably quick, recovery. The main disadvantage of the technique is that on occasion the horse may not 'go down' after injection of thiopentone. This may be due to one of three reasons:

1. *The injection may have been perivascular. If so, the region around the site of injection should be infiltrated with 0·5 to 1·0 litre of saline to which the enzyme hyaluronidase has been added. When dilution with saline is carried out without undue delay surprisingly little tissue reaction follows the subcutaneous injection of even very concentrated solutions of thiopentone. Poultices should not be applied to the site for they provoke excessive reaction and sloughing of tissue.* Although a second injection of thiopentone may then be made into the jugular vein on the other side of the neck it is probably better to postpone any further attempt at inducing anaesthesia for 3 to 4 days.

2. Under field conditions it is not always possible to weigh animals before anaesthesia and their weight has to be guessed so that underdosage may occur. If this is believed to be the reason for the failure to induce anaesthesia, then another, slightly larger dose should be injected without delay. Because the total quantity of thiopentone used will be larger than 1 g/90 kg recovery from anaesthesia will be delayed to some extent but no other harmful effects need be anticipated.

3. The injection may not have been made quickly enough. In this case a second dose may be injected without delay and apart from a slight prolongation of the recovery period no harm will result. When a dose of thiopentone fails to induce anaesthesia the horse does not become excited and the injection of a further dose (or even of two more doses) presents no greater difficulty than the injection of the first. No matter what dose of thiopentone is to be employed it should never be dissolved in more than 50 ml of water for very rapid injection cannot be made from syringes of more than 50 ml capacity.

The technique is safe since the margin of error is wide. Serious overdosage of thiopentone is impossible unless there is a very gross mistake in the estimation of the weight of the horse. A gross mistake of this nature will not be made when the weight of the horse is estimated from the formula given on page 176. Nevertheless, the technique is not to be recommended for use in horses suffering from shock or non-compensated cardiovascular disease for in such animals all intravenous injections must be made very slowly.

In foals up to 4 or 5 weeks of age the use of thiopentone, even in very small doses, is probably unwise, for in these young animals recovery may be very prolonged.

Methohexitone Sodium

Methohexitone sodium may be better than thiopentone sodium for the induction of anaesthesia in horses (Monahan, 1964) although it is very much more expensive. At the Cambridge School it has been used to induce anaesthesia in horses premedicated with Acetylpromazine (0·04 mg/kg), and the results obtained compared to those in similar cases where thiopentone was used. Methohexitone sodium is approximately twice as potent as thiopentone sodium, so that the dose for induction was fixed at 1 g/180 kg body weight (i.e. approximately 1 g/400 lb, or 5·5 mg/kg). This dose was dissolved in not more than 50 ml of water and injected rapidly into the jugular vein. Because at the Cambridge School it is customary to administer suxamethonium chloride (0·1 mg/kg) intravenously immediately after the dose of barbiturate, this practice was followed when methohexitone sodium was employed. In all cases the induction of anaesthesia was smooth and rapid. The use of methohexitone rather than thiopentone produced no obvious major differences in the nature of the subsequent anaesthesia although it is possible that respiration was more depressed after methohexitone than after thiopentone. Recoveries were uneventful. Horses given methohexitone appeared to recover completely more quickly than those which received thiopentone. Because of this apparently more rapid recovery it is believed that the use of methohexitone sodium in equine anaesthesia is well worth while when its expense can be justified (Grono, 1966).

The Ox

Chloral Hydrate

Chloral hydrate has been used extensively for inducing deep narcosis and light general anaesthesia in cows for such operations as extirpation of an eyeball, amputation of a digit and Caesarean section, and in young adults for umbilical hernia. (At the Liverpool School Field Station, the drug has been used in more than 150 cases of Caesarean section without a death ascribable to the anaesthetic occurring.) Administration is by slow intravenous injection into the external jugular vein, occupying from 4 to 6 minutes in induction. Injection is sometimes made with the animal in the standing position, slowly continuing until it sinks to the ground, when a state bordering between deep narcosis and light anaesthesia is attained, generally after a dose of from 6 to 7 g/cwt (6 to 7 g/50 kg) has been given. It is preferable, however, that it shall be injected after the animal has been cast and restrained when a computed dose of 6 to 7 g/cwt (6 to 7 g/50 kg or 0·12 to 0·14 g/kg) is given to healthy animals. (The higher dosage is used for animals in the 6 to 8 cwt range and the lower for those weighing 8 to 11 cwt.) It cannot too often be reiterated that the intravenous use of chloral hydrate requires great technical precision, precision which cannot be ensured when the animal is standing up and is free to move. When administration is in the cast position assessment of depth should be made in the later stages and slowing of the lateral nystagmus, limpness of the tail, flaccidity of the anus and absence of the anal reflex taken as indications of the onset of anaesthesia. The method of preparation of the solution of chloral hydrate and the technique of injection are the same as described for the horse.

In cases in which the anaesthesia produced is insufficiently deep it may be augmented by subcutaneous or perineural infiltration of local analgesic, or by inhalation anaesthesia. For prolonged operations in which full anaesthesia throughout is necessary, the practice in the Liverpool School is to augment with pentobarbitone sodium when evidence of lightening is noted. Full anaesthesia is usually attained once again by the injection of 1 to 1·5 g of pentobarbitone sodium. A further injection of a similar quantity may be necessary some 10 minutes or so later. This method can easily be followed if an indwelling Mitchell needle is left in place during the operation.

The operation of Caesarean section requires special consideration. Having particular regard for the welfare of the foetuses, minimal doses of anaesthetic should be employed, especially during the period before the foetus is removed from the uterus. Thus, when performing Caesarean section in the cow, the total dose for healthy animals should be kept within the range 40 to 60 g according to size. This will cause the animal to lie completely still, but it is often an advantage to infiltrate the line of incision with local analgesic in addition, particularly for the ultimate suturing of the abdominal wound. Moreover, a barbiturate should be at hand in case it is necessary to deepen anaesthesia during the later stages of operation.

Calves require a higher unit dose and quantities as great as 140 mg/kg body weight (7 g/112 lb) have been given, but again care must be taken. In these animals the most convenient vein is the saphena on the inner aspect of the thigh. The animal is restrained on its side and the under hind-leg held firmly during injection.

During anaesthesia, both respirations and pulse rate are accelerated; the former to about 36 and the latter between 100 and 120/minute. Anaesthesia persists for about 20 minutes and is followed by a progressively lightening narcosis. The animal is able to raise itself on to the brisket in about an hour and regains the standing position in from 2 to 3 hours. The periods of induction and recovery are quiet and there is no post-anaesthetic malaise.

Bulls

Young bulls and relatively small adults present no special difficulty provided their temperament is such that they can be effectively restrained for the precise intravenous injection of anaesthetic agents. Very heavy bulls, however, comprise a very difficult problem for the mere restraining of such an animal in lateral recumbency may cause great respiratory difficulty due to compression of the undermost lung and restriction of the diaphragm by pressure of the abdominal viscera, in fact breathing may cease unless the animal is quickly returned to the breast position. The precise intravenous injection of drugs in the standing position may not only be uncertain on account of difficulties in satisfactorily introducing the needle into the vein but sometimes impossible on account of movement by the animal. In many instances the temperament of the animal to be dealt with is such that large doses of chloral hydrate have to be given by the mouth in order to obtain sufficient sedation to allow of the application of casting tackle. The further administration of the drug by intravenous injection after casting gives rise to a danger of fatal overdosage consequent on continued absorption from the stomach. When chloral hydrate is given to the bull by intravenous injection at the usual rate, the dose required to bring the animal to the borderline of general anaesthesia is the same as for the big cow, about 6 g/50 kg body weight. For a 800 kg bull (16 cwt approx.) this represents a dose of about 100 g, yet to induce a degree of sedation whereby the animal may be safely handled an oral dose of 150 to 200 g (or even more) may be required, and even after such a quantity (i.e. 5 to 7 oz) the animal is still able to stand.

Pentobarbitone Sodium

Satisfactory anaesthesia can be induced in small bovine animals by the slow intravenous injection of pentobarbitone sodium. The injection should occupy at least 4 minutes. Induction is quiet and the dose taken to induce light anaesthesia varies from 1 to 1·45 g/50 kg body weight ($\frac{1}{7}$ to $\frac{1}{5}$ grain/lb). Surgical anaesthesia persists for about 30 minutes and is followed by a lightening narcosis. The animal will not be able to regain its feet in less than 3 hours. For the very young calf—animals up to 1 month old—pentobarbitone is unsuitable. Narcosis is prolonged for 2 days or even longer, and there is a grave danger that during this period the animal will succumb from oedema of the lungs, or that it may subsequently develop pneumonia.

Thiopentone Sodium

In recent years thiopentone sodium has come to be used in adult cattle either alone to provide full anaesthesia for operations of short duration or to induce anaesthesia which is then maintained by inhalation agents. It enables anaesthesia to be induced in the standing animal so that casting tackle is unnecessary and only one assistant is required to hold the animal while the injection is being made.

Premedication is seldom indicated but if essential it must be remembered that its use will delay recovery from anaesthesia. Thiopentone sodium is injected rapidly into the jugular vein in a dose of 1 g/90 kg (200 lb) estimated body weight. (The 5 g pack of the drug is particularly convenient.) The dose should be dissolved in a maximum of 50 ml of water for larger volumes cannot be injected rapidly enough to produce unconsciousness when this minimal dose is employed. The animal sinks quietly to the ground within 20 to 30 seconds of injection and there is a brief period of apnoea. Apnoea seldom lasts for more than 15 to 20 seconds and artificial respiration is not required. Surgical anaesthesia of about 3 to 4 minutes' duration is followed by recovery which is usually complete within 45 minutes. Recovery is invariably quiet and free from excitement. The animal can be propped up, and will maintain a position of sternal recumbency, about 12 to 15 minutes after the injection of the drug. The period of surgical anaesthesia, although brief, is adequate for operations of very short duration or the performance of endotracheal intubation, and can be prolonged by the administration of inhalation agents such as halothane or cyclopropane.

Apart from the usual risks of general anaesthesia in ruminant animals the method is safe. The margin of safety is wide and serious overdosage is impossible unless there is a gross error in the estimation of body weight. Underdosage, on the other hand, is not infrequent and when subanaesthetic doses are given the animal remains standing. Subanaesthetic doses do not cause excitement. Another reason for failure to induce anaesthesia is slow injection of the drug; it is essential that the injection should be completed within 8 seconds. When subanaesthetic doses are given, or the injection is made too slowly, a second injection of the drug may be made without delay and apart from some delay in recovery no harmful effects occur. Perivascular injection will also account for failure to induce anaesthesia and should this mishap occur the site of injection must be infiltrated with 0·5 to 1·0 litres of saline to which the enzyme hyaluronidase has been added. Severe tissue reaction will not occur if the irritant thiopentone is promptly diluted with saline in this manner, but it is unwise to persist with attempts to induce anaesthesia by further injections of thiopentone once a perivascular injection has been made.

Thiopentone should not be administered by this rapid injection technique to shocked animals or to animals suffering from non-compensated cardiovascular disease. Young calves up to 14 days old are not good subjects for thiopentone anaesthesia as in these animals recovery may be very prolonged and the use of even very small doses for induction of anaesthesia is probably unwise.

Methohexitone Sodium

Because recovery after methohexitone sodium is so much more rapid than it is after thiopentone sodium, it might appear to be the better of the two compounds for use in ruminants. However, preliminary trials at the Cambridge

School have shown that, in cattle, the action of methohexitone sodium is rather unpredictable. The reason for this is unknown and, at the moment, the rapid intravenous injection of a computed dose cannot be recommended. Given to cows by slow intravenous injection, assessing the effects produced as injection proceeds, the compound has so far proved to be quite satisfactory. Slow injection is usually associated with the occurrence of muscle tremors during induction but these seem to be of no importance. Methohexitone sodium appears to produce better conditions for endotracheal intubation than are produced by thiopentone sodium. The jaw is more relaxed and the laryngeal closure and cough mechanisms appear to be less active. Adult cows have been given up to 2·5 g of methohexitone sodium by slow intravenous injection for induction, anaesthesia has been uneventful, and recovery has been smooth and extremely rapid.

Tavernor (1964) has suggested the use of methohexitone in young calves and comments that a dose of 1 mg/kg by rapid intravenous injection is sufficient to enable endotracheal intubation to be carried out. Robertshaw (1964) has reported the satisfactory use of methohexitone in castrated Ayrshire calves whose ages ranged from $1\frac{1}{4}$ to 10 months.

Sheep and Goats

In veterinary clinical practice the call for surgical interference in sheep and goats is very limited. What little surgery has to be performed under general anaesthesia is best carried out under inhalation anaesthesia, but the intravenous drugs have a place as induction agents. Intravenous anaesthesia alone may have a limited place in the laboratory for non-survival experiments and interferences of short duration.

Chloral Hydrate

Although in the past chloral hydrate has been used as an anaesthetic in sheep and goats, much better agents are available today. Further information on the use of chloral hydrate in these animals may be obtained from the articles by De Koch and Quinlan (1926), Bessalaar and Quin (1935) and Dukes and Sampson (1937).

Pentobarbitone Sodium

Phillipson and Barnett (1939) reported on the use of pentobarbitone sodium in sheep. They found that in lambs up to 2 months old a dose of 29 mg/kg by slow intravenous injection gave anaesthesia of sufficient depth and duration for abdominal surgery. With adult sheep they found great variation in response to the drug. In all cases the duration of anaesthesia was shorter than in lambs— about 15 minutes only. In adult sheep they found that the dose for induction varied from 28 to 33 mg/kg. Two very exceptional cases were encountered. The first, a yearling ewe, took a dose of 51 mg/kg, and the second, a 3-year-old castrated animal, only 17·3 mg/kg. (American workers have also observed the greater susceptibility of castrated animals to pentobarbitone sodium.)

Phillipson and Barnett assessed the depth of anaesthesia as injection proceeded (see pentobarbitone sodium anaesthesia in the dog, page 313), and continued the injection until the interdigital reflex was just lost. This reflex was elicited by pressing the finger- and thumb-nails into the skin between the digits. They found that the corneal reflex was also a useful guide, and injection was continued until only a weak corneal reflex could be demonstrated. The form of restraint used by these workers was to sit the animal up on its hind-quarters and to hold the head back to stretch the neck. Injection was made into the jugular vein. In very large animals the injection was given with the animal standing, the needle being withdrawn from the vein as soon as relaxation sets in. The animal was then laid on the floor and the injection completed.

Their conclusion was that pentobarbitone sodium is a satisfactory anaesthetic for minor operations of short duration in sheep but that, as detoxication is rapid, the duration of anaesthesia from a single injection is short and thus it is not satisfactory for prolonged intra-abdominal surgery.

Today, most workers prefer to use pentobarbitone simply as an induction agent and to maintain anaesthesia with an inhalation anaesthetic administered through an endotracheal tube.

Hill, Turner, Uren and Gomez (1935) and Lukens (1937) were probably the first to report the use of pentobarbitone sodium in goats. More recently Linzell (1964) has recorded his experiences. According to Linzell the full anaesthetic dose for a goat is about 30 mg/kg for an adult animal and the animal is on its feet in 20 to 60 min from the time of injection. To maintain anaesthesia further doses of 6 to 36 mg/kg per hour (according to the depth of anaesthesia required) must be administered. Usually, he prefers to induce with pentobarbitone sodium and then to maintain with an inhalation anaesthetic after intubation. He reports that the dose required to induce and intubate varies from 10 to 42 mg/kg, depending upon the rate of injection.

It is important to note that commercially available solutions of pentobarbitone sodium often contain propylene glycol and this causes haemolysis and haematuria in both goats and sheep (Potter, 1958; Linzel, 1964). Pentobarbitone sodium solutions for use in these animals should be made up from powder, using 10% ethyl alcohol in saline as the solvent.

Thiobarbiturates

Titchen, Steel and Hamilton (1949) have reported on the use of thiopentone sodium and thialbarbitone sodium for experimental surgical procedures in sheep. Both drugs were given by injection into the jugular vein, and the depth of anaesthesia was assessed as injection proceeded. With both drugs induction was smooth, rapid and unassociated with excitement. Thiopentone was used as a 5% aqueous solution and thialbarbitone as a 10% solution. Injection was at first rapid and then slow, occupying a period of 30 to 60 seconds, and continued until apnoea, lasting about 15 seconds, resulted. Apnoea generally ended with 1 or 2 sighing respirations which were followed by rapid, shallow breathing. The progressive onset of muscular relaxation, loss of corneal reflex, quickening and decrease in depth of respirations and the disappearance of the interdigital reflex were the signs used in judging the degree of response prior to the onset of apnoea. The first signs of lightening anaesthesia were a deepening of respirations, the onset of incoordinated limb movements and sometimes swallowing movements. Defaecation always occurred during the course of anaesthesia, and in some instances, more often with thiopentone, ruminal regurgitation occurred.

Induction and Maintenance Doses

These workers stress the point that injection was continued until the desired effect was obtained and that this was the final criterion of dosage. Individual susceptibility varied. Six lambs of 15 to 17 kg received induction doses of thiopentone sodium varying from 0·15 to 0·25 g and anaesthesia was maintained for periods varying from 12 to 22 minutes. Recovery was complete within 45 minutes of induction. In sheep weighing 20 to 30 kg the induction dose of thiopentone averaged 0·56 g with a range of 1·0 to 2·0 g. The average time after induction at which a maintenance dose was given was 20 minutes in the case of thiopentone and 13 minutes with thialbarbitone. With thiopentone the average maintenance dose was 0·2 g, and with thialbarbitone, 0·37 g, with an interval between the doses of thiopentone of 26 minutes, and between the doses of thialbarbitone of 14 minutes (average).

Although Titchen *et al.* encountered several deaths due to respiratory failure or the aspiration of ingesta, they concluded that both drugs were satisfactory anaesthetics for sheep. They preferred thialbarbitone sodium because of its shorter action and because it appeared to produce less respiratory depression.

Today, thiopentone sodium is extensively used to induce anaesthesia which is to be maintained by endotracheal inhalation methods.

Precautions to be observed during Anaesthesia

Phillipson and Barnett have instructive comments to make on precautions to be observed when subjecting sheep to prolonged anaesthetization especially when endotracheal intubation is not practised.

Ruminants secrete large quantities of saliva at all times, and if this is allowed to collect in the pharynx it may be inhaled and so cause temporary respiratory failure. It is therefore necessary to keep the animal's head inclined downwards throughout, so that saliva escapes from the mouth. The previous administration of atropine sulphate (13 mg ($\frac{1}{5}$ grain), to adult sheep by subcutaneous injection) greatly reduces, but does not completely stop, this flow of saliva. Spontaneous regurgitation of the rumen ingesta is an alarming accident. It is best prevented by tilting the operating table, so that the hind-part of the body is about 6 inches lower than the fore-part. Even so the head must be inclined downwards, so that ingesta may escape from the mouth if necessary. In case of respiratory failure, artificial respiration must not be applied by pressure on the abdomen, for this will cause ingesta to be forced up into the mouth. It should be applied only to the thorax and in a gentle manner until endotracheal intubation can be performed and intermittent positive pressure ventilation of the lungs commenced. Tympany of the rumen may become a nuisance to the operator within an hour and unless steps are taken to relieve it causes danger to the animal.

It is most likely to occur in animals brought in from grass; it is reduced or prevented if the animal is kept on a hay diet for 24 hours or so prior to operation. When it occurs the animal should, if possible, be lifted into the sitting position. The gas may then escape, otherwise the rumen should be punctured with a trocar and cannula.

Methohexitone Sodium

In both sheep and goats the intravenous injection of 4 mg/kg of a 2·5% solution of methohexitone sodium produces anaesthesia of 5 to 7 minutes' duration. Recovery to the standing position is complete within 10 to 14 minutes of the injection but the recovery may be associated with violent jerking or convulsive movements if the animal is disturbed by noise during this period. Anaesthesia may be prolonged by the injection of 50 to 75 mg of the drug/minute (Robertshaw, 1966).

The Pig

The subject of general anaesthesia in pigs is one which has received considerable attention during recent years. Although there has been a tendency towards the use of inhalation methods, the intravenous agents still have an important place.

Chloral Hydrate

The intravenous administration of chloral hydrate to pigs is not easy. Klarenbeek and Harthog (1938) described the infusion of a 20% solution into one of the ear veins, in doses of 7·5 to 8·5 g/50 kg body weight. They found that anaesthesia developed while the injection was being made and that recovery was complete in about 3 hours. It is claimed that the method is safe and satisfactory, but it is pointed out that it is unsuitable for the operation of Caesarean section as the foetuses die soon after delivery. Slatter (1948) records similar results. He used a 33% solution injected by gravity into an ear vein through an 18 or 19 s.w.g. needle until the desired degree of anaesthesia was attained. Slatter claims that should a little of the chloral hydrate solution accidently infiltrate the perivenous tissues it is unlikely that sloughing will result.

All anaesthetics given by intravenous injection should always be injected slowly, the depth of narcosis being assessed, as far as possible, as injection proceeds. The object of computing a dose is to ensure that a sufficient quantity is available.

In the pig the technique of intravenous injection employing comparatively large quantities of fluid is not easy and in adults, particularly, inability to prevent movement often causes failure. In such cases it is often necessary to resort to inhalation methods.

Because of the difficulty of injecting large volumes of solution into an ear vein some workers prefer to give chloral hydrate to pigs by stomach tube or by injection into the peritoneal cavity. Although these methods are now mainly of historical interest, they are included here for the sake of completeness.

Into the Stomach

Bemis and his colleagues (1924), after an extensive experience of the method, speak highly of its value. The drug is administered directly into the stomach by stomach tube, using Juhl's technique. They found that by using 3 drachms of chloral hydrate/50 lb body weight (approx. 13 g/50 kg) satisfactory general anaesthesia was obtained in $\frac{4}{5}$ of the subjects after a lapse of 20 to 30 minutes. Their maximum dose was $2\frac{1}{2}$ oz dissolved in a quart of warm water. In those cases in which surgical anaesthesia was not present after a wait of 30 minutes, a little chloroform by inhalation was given.

Intraperitoneal Injection

The intraperitoneal method is employed in young pigs. A dose of 0·3 g/kg

(2·3 grains/lb) in 5% solution is injected after fasting the animal for 24 hours. The site for injection is midway between the umbilicus and the pubic brim. Anaesthesia attains its maximum depth in 20 to 30 minutes and persists for 1 to $1\frac{1}{2}$ hours, followed by a period of progressive recovery up to 4 hours. During the recovery period the animal should be kept warm. The solution may cause some slight peritoneal inflammation but this is not of practical significance.

Pentobarbitone Sodium

The most satisfactory method of administration of pentobarbitone sodium to pigs is slow intravenous injection into the ear vein, continuing until the desired depression of the central nervous system is obtained. However, intraperitoneal injection using a computed dose or intra-testicular injection may be adopted.

Intravenous Injection

For healthy male and female pigs up to 50 kg (approx. 1 cwt) live weight, the average dose necessary to induce medium depth anaesthesia is about 30 mg/kg ($\frac{1}{5}$ grain/lb). In small pigs there is a considerable margin of safety, but in larger ones great variations in susceptibility may occur. Castrated animals appear to be slightly more susceptible than entires. Provided that the injection is made slowly and the onset of muscle relaxation is observed, the method is safe. Induction is not associated with narcotic excitement; in fact, in the case of a squealing animal, the progressive reduction, and finally cessation of squealing, is a good guide to the progress of narcosis. Depths of anaesthesia may be difficult to assess in pigs. The presence of complete relaxation of the abdominal muscles and the absence of response to pricking of the skin is evidence that anaesthesia has been attained. Its duration will be sufficient for the performance of rapid operations such as castration. For very large subjects the dosage per kg must be reduced and marked variations in suscepti-bility will be encountered.

Kernkamp (1939) records that while the average anaesthetic dose for pigs of all sizes was $\frac{1}{7}$ grain/lb, in 2 exceptional cases—sows of 127 kg (280 lb)—anaesthesia was provoked with a dosage of $\frac{1}{16}$ and $\frac{1}{18}$ grain/lb. Ritchie (1961) records even wider variations. In a series of pigs weighing up to 200 kg, he found that the dose required to induce deep anaesthesia varied from 9 to 56 mg/kg ($\frac{1}{18}$ to $\frac{1}{3}$ gr/lb). The duration of the surgical plane will depend upon the initial depth of anaesthesia induced. As a rule it is shorter than in the dog. With light anaesthesia—a brisk corneal reflex and a reflex response to skin pricking—it is of 10 to 15 minutes only; when medium depth is attained—a sluggish corneal reflex and loss of reflex response to pricking—20 to 25 minutes. When deep anaesthesia up to the point of respiratory failure is induced, its duration is 30 to 45 minutes. Anaesthesia is followed by a period of progressively lightening narcosis which persists for 3 to 8 hours. The period of recovery is not accompanied by narcotic excitement and the animal usually passes into a state of sleep.

When dealing with fat pigs, cessation of breathing is a common complication of deep anaesthesia. A striking feature of this apparent respiratory failure is that it is different from that seen in other species, for expulsion of the air from the lungs by pressure on the abdomen is immediately followed by a spontaneous deep inspiration of the type seen when there is some mechanical obstruction to respiration during anaesthesia. It is possible that in the fat pig mere extension of the head is enough to cause pressure on the larynx sufficient to arrest breathing. The animal's head should be placed at the natural angle and artificial respiration applied. This is performed by applying pressure to the abdomen about every 4 seconds and unless spontaneous breathing returns within 1 to 2 minutes, endotracheal intubation to facilitate intermittent positive pressure ventilation of the lungs should be considered. Intermittent positive pressure ventilation may also be carried out through a closely applied face-mask without endotracheal intubation, but if it is, care must be taken to avoid inflation of the stomach.

Intraperitoneal Injection

In small subjects in which intravenous injection may be found to be difficult, the intraperitoneal route may be adopted, although in general, it is not to be recommended. It becomes necessary to compute an anaesthetic dose. For animals up to 20 kg (45 lb) this is put at 30 mg/kg ($\frac{1}{5}$ grain/lb); for those between 20 and 30 kg (45 to 65 lb), at 24 mg/kg ($\frac{1}{6}$ grain/lb). Variations in response are inevitable with such a method. In some cases narcosis only will be obtained and it will be necessary to augment it by inhalation or local injection, while in others anaesthesia may become alarmingly deep and even fatal. Provided a careful watch is kept on respirations and artificial respiration applied should they cease, fatalities will be of rare occurrence. In fat subjects there is a possibility that, despite the length of the needle employed, the injection will be made into retroperitoneal fat. In this case absorption will be so slow it is improbable that even light narcosis will develop. When employing this route of administration, the action of the drug will attain its maximum depth in a period of 20 to 30 minutes after injection. The duration of the periods of anaesthesia and of narcosis tends to be rather longer than with the intravenous method. The technique of intraperitoneal injection is similar to that described for the dog (page 314).

Intra-testicular Injection

A strong solution of pentobarbitone sodium, such as one commercially available for the euthanasia of small animals (300 mg/ml) may be administered by intra-testicular injection prior to castration (Henry, 1968). A dose rate of about 45 mg/kg is employed, a very large boar being given 20 ml of solution into each testicle, and adequate anaesthesia for castration develops within 10 minutes of injection. Removal of the testicle removes any excess drug and recovery follows in the normal manner.

Thiopentone Sodium

Muhrer (1950) has recorded an extensive experience of thiopentone sodium as an intravenous anaesthetic in pigs. He used a 5% solution (1 g in 20 ml) injected into the ear vein, half the computed dose being injected rapidly and the remainder more slowly over the next 2 to 3 minutes. He found that the dose required to produce his desired degree of anaesthesia varied considerably, for quite apart from weight factors pigs showed marked differences in their susceptibility to the drug. In his experience, induction doses generally gave 5 to 10 minutes' anaesthesia with a total recovery period of 30 to 60 minutes.

Experience at the Cambridge School has been that the quantity of thiopentone taken to induce medium surgical anaesthesia and the duration of the anaesthetic period are chiefly governed by the speed at which the injection is made. When rapid injection techniques are practised in healthy pigs, the quantity used will be surprisingly small, and the recovery period short. Surgical anaesthesia can be induced in sows weighing about 100 kg by the injection of no more than 500 mg of the drug. Moreover, it has been observed that the use of a 2·5% solution decreases the total dose required for any operation. Induction of anaesthesia with thiopentone sodium is greatly facilitated by the use of azaperone premedication (see page 169). Provided the pig is left undisturbed for 20 minutes after the injection of the azaperone, controlled injection into an ear vein is easy and complete anaesthesia can be obtained with surprisingly small quantities of a 2·5% solution of thiopentone. It seems that the butyrophenone antagonizes the respiratory effect of the thiopentone, but this clinical impression still awaits controlled investigation.

As with pentobarbitone sodium, respiration may fail with the onset of anaesthesia. When rapid injection techniques are used this period of apnoea is short and should not necessitate the use of artificial respiration. Apnoea of more than a few seconds' duration must, of course, be treated by artificial respiration and, provided this is applied efficiently, spontaneous breathing soon returns. Recovery after a very great overdose of thiopentone may be expected if efficient artificial ventilation of the lungs is performed until the concentration of thiopentone in the brain has diminished.

Methohexitone Sodium

It would seem that provided the anaesthetist is aware of the basic principles underlying the use of intravenous anaesthetic agents, and has some knowledge of the special characteristics of methohexitone (such as its tendency to produce muscle tremors during induction), it can be used quite safely in pigs (Emberton, 1966). At the moment, however, its cost probably prohibits its use in this species of animal. Anaesthesia can be produced by the intravenous injection of 11 to 12 mg/kg as a 2·5% solution and recovery is complete 10 to 15 minutes after the injection of a single induction dose (Noakes, 1966).

REFERENCES

BEMIS, H. E., GUARD, W. F. and COVAULT, C. H. (1924). *J. Am. vet. med. Ass.* **64**, 413
BESSALAAR, H. J. and QUIN, J. I. (1935). *Onderstepoort J. vet. Sci.* **5**, 501
COFFEE, W. F. (1949). *J. Am. vet. med. Ass.* **114**, 291
DANKS, A. G. (1943–44). *Rep. N.Y. State vet. Coll.* p. 180
DEGIVE, A. (1908). *Précis de Médécin Operatoire Veterinaire*. Brussels and Paris
DE KOCH, G. and QUINLAN, J. (1926). *Dept. Agric. Union of S. Africa*, 11th and 12th reports, part *i*, p. 361.
DUKES, H. H. and SAMPSON, J. (1937). *Cornell Vet.* **27**, 139
DUMAS, A. (1935). *Bull. Acad. vét. France*, **8**, 275
EMBERTON, G. A. (1966). *Vet. Rec.* **78**, 541
FOWLER, G. R. (1946). *J. Am. vet. med. Ass.* **96**, 210
GILLET, E. S. and CRAWFORD, A. (1917). Cited by Malone, P. J.
GRONO, L. R. (1966). *Aust. vet. J.* **42**, 398
HENRY, D. P. (1968). *Aust. vet. J.* **44**, 418
HILL, R. T., TURNER, C. W., UREN, A. E. and GOMEZ, E. T. (1935). *Res. Bull. Mo Agr. Exp. Sta.*, No. 230
JUHL, C. E. (1923). *J. Am. vet. med. Ass.* **63**, 60
KERNKAMP, H. C. (1939). *J. Am. vet. med. Ass.* **94**, 207
KLARENBEEK, A. and HARTOG, J. H. (1938). *Proc. XIIIth Int. vet. Congr. Zurich*
LINZELL, J. L. (1964). *Small Animal Anaesthesia*. Oxford: Pergamon Press
LUKENS, F. D. W. (1937). *Am. J. Physiol.* **122**, 729
MALONE, P. J. (1917). *Vet. Rec.* **29**, 531
MARCENAC and LEMETAYER (1930). *Bull. Acad. vét. France*, **3**, 141
MESSERVY, A. (1967). Private communication
MILLENBRUCK, E. W. and WALLINGA, M. H. (1946). *J. Am. vet. med. Ass.* **108**, 148
MONAHAN, C. M. (1964). *Vet. Rec.* **76**, 1333
MUHRER, M. E. (1950). *J. Am. vet. med. Ass.* **117**, 293
NEAL, P. A. (1963). *Vet. Rec.* **75**, 289
NOAKES, D. E. (1966). *Vet. Rec.* **78**, 669
PHILLIPSON, A. T. and BARNETT, S. F. (1939). *Vet. Rec.* **51**, 869
POTTER, G. B. (1958). *Br. J. Pharmac.* **13**, 385
RITCHIE, H. E. (1961). Private communication
ROBERTSHAW, D. (1964). *Vet. Rec.* **76**, 357
———— (1966). *Vet. Rec.* **78**, 433
SLATTER, E. E. (1948). *N. Am. Vet.* **29**, 157
TAVERNOR, W. D. (1962). *Vet. Rec.* **74**, 595
TITCHEN, D., STEEL, J. D. and HAMILTON, F. J. (1949). *Aust. Vet. J.* **25**, 257
VLADUTIU, O. (1938). *Revista Veterinara Militara*, Nos. 2 & 3: *Abst. Rec. Med. vet.* (1939). **115**, 236

15

Intravenous Anaesthesia in Dogs and Cats

The introduction of the barbiturates some 30 years ago brought about a revolution in the subject of general anaesthesia in the dog and cat. Of recent years there has been a swing away from the use of a barbiturate as the sole anaesthetic agent to a combination of an ultra-short-acting barbiturate with an inhalation anaesthetic, but there is no doubt that under conditions of general practice and in laboratories with poor facilities and without skilled assistance, the longer-acting barbiturates which can be relied on to give full anaesthesia for the whole duration of an operation will continue to be used.

The barbiturates may be regarded as derivatives of malonic acid with urea. They all possess powerful narcotic actions and the chief differences between the various members of the series are related to duration of action and toxicity. These factors would appear to be controlled by the rate and degree of completeness with which they are destroyed in the body or otherwise eliminated from it.

Among the first members of the series of compounds to be introduced were barbitone (diethyl barbituric acid) and phenobarbitone (phenyl-ethyl barbituric acid), which prior to their inclusion in the Pharmacopoeia were known by the trade names of Veronal and Luminal. They are still extensively employed in human medicine as sedatives and soporifics and occasionally in animals as sedatives. They are, however, too toxic for use as general anaesthetics. Later, amylobarbitone (Amytal), butobarbitone (Soneryl, Neonal), cyclobarbitone (Phanodorm, Pernocton) and others were introduced, and sometimes used as anaesthetics, but their action was undesirably long and the safety margin narrow.

Pentobarbitone sodium and thiopentone sodium, selection between them depending chiefly on the duration of anaesthesia required, have for a number of years been the standard barbiturates used in animals, and while other thiobarbiturates have been recently introduced there are no substantially significant differences between their actions and that of thiopentone sodium, and thus comparisons become matters of slight degree.

Pentobarbitone Sodium

Pentobarbitone was first used as a general anaesthetic in veterinary surgery in America in 1931, and Kreutzer, Haigler and Sweeb were amongst the first to record its use. At the outset the drug was administered orally or by intraperitoneal injection, and despite variations in results it became quite evident that it represented a marked advance in the subject of anaesthesia in dog and cat. These methods necessitated the computation of an anaesthetic dose and this was originally put at 29 mg/kg for healthy animals. Results were more regular by the intraperitoneal than the oral method, for in the latter the presence of food in the stomach caused great variation. At the same time this dosage by the intraperitoneal route did not give entirely consistent results. Cases were met in which narcosis only (often accompanied by excitation) was obtained, while in others anaesthesia became alarmingly deep, and in a very occasional case fatal. It soon became evident that while for healthy animals of from 11 to 16 kg (25 to 35 lb) this dosage gave satisfactory results, in animals below these weights the quantity must be slightly increased and in those above them reduced. In 1934 Wright recommended the following dosage:

Body weight (kg)					Dose (g)
4·5	.	.	.	.	0·16
7·0	.	.	.	.	0·22
9·0	.	.	.	.	0·28
11·0	.	.	.	.	0·33
13·5	.	.	.	.	0·37
16·0	.	.	.	.	0·40
18·0	.	.	.	.	0·44
22·5	.	.	.	.	0·52
27·2	.	.	.	.	0·56

In a series of 300 cases, results were, on the whole, consistent, although there was variation in the depth of anaesthesia obtained. In two cases the drug proved fatal. At the same time, from the standpoint of toxicity, the agent compared more than favourably with the then accepted inhalation methods. It was soon realized that computation of a dose was not the proper method of administering non-volatile anaesthetic agents, for, apart from body weight, there are other factors which influence their action even in healthy subjects. Amongst these are individual idiosyncrasy, the degree of fasting and the nature of the diet before operation. When dealing with diseased animals, variations were more marked. Toxaemia greatly increases susceptibility, and as there are no accurate clinical methods of assessing its degree, fatalities were inevitable. It was quickly learned that in cases of liver dysfunction the dose should be reduced to two-thirds the normal. It was thus decided to adopt the method of intravenous injection, but instead of injecting an estimated dose, to make the injection slowly and assess the degree of narcosis present as one proceeded, stopping when the required depth was obtained. Auchterlonie had already adopted this method, using hexobarbitone sodium. By this means varying depths of anaesthesia could be induced at will, overdosage avoided, and the safety factor greatly increased. By the end of 1938 the method had been used by Wright and his colleagues in the Beaumont Hospital of the Royal Veterinary College, London, in more than 2000 operation cases, and in over 800 consecutive ones without a death attributable to the anaesthetic. Since that time pentobarbitone sodium has become one of the standard methods of inducing anaesthesia of medium duration in the dog.

The agent in solution is non-irritating and no undesirable local effects result from its use or misuse. When given by intravenous injection, induction is generally quiet, although an occasional subject will be encountered in which excitement and struggling occur as the animal passes through the phase of narcosis. Not infrequently it is the animal which is normally lethargic and quiet, not the nervous one, which behaves thus. It has been noticed that the greyhound and Dalmatian breeds are particularly susceptible to excitement during induction. The aim always should be to produce anaesthesia, its depth depending on the interference to be performed. If narcosis only ensues, the animal tends to become hyperaesthetic and interference may cause uncontrollable movement and/or barking. This is in contrast to man, in which pentobarbitone is used as a hypnotic or basal narcotic. In anaesthesia of medium depth respirations remain good, regular, and numbering 30 to 40/minute. The pulse is full and its rate accelerated—in the dog to 150 to 170, and in the cat to 200 or more. The duration of the surgical plane depends upon the depth of anaesthesia initially induced—when light, it persists for about 15 minutes; when of medium depth, for 30 minutes; and when deep, for an hour or more. The total period of narcosis varies similarly from 3 to 8 hours. The action on the pupil is worthy of notice. In light anaesthesia the reflex response of the iris to light is unaffected, but as anaesthesia deepens the pupil constricts. In dangerously deep anaesthesia the pupil becomes the size of a pinhead in the dog and a mere slit in the cat. In light anaesthesia the eyelids remain open and the corneal reflex is brisk. When medium depth is attained, the lids partially close and the reflex becomes sluggish. In deep anaesthesia it is lost. With toxic overdosage respiratory failure occurs. Respirations become slower and shallower until they are almost imperceptible and finally cease. The heart continues to beat, strongly at first but later becoming weaker, for a period of 4 to 5 minutes after respiratory failure, to cease finally from anoxaemia. As syncope becomes imminent the pupils slowly dilate. When toxic doses have been given by the intravenous route respiratory failure generally occurs in a period of 10 to 15 minutes. Dogs under pentobarbitone anaesthesia develop a metabolic acidosis as well as a respiratory acidosis. Respiratory acidosis occurs first and produces an increase in cardiac output but as the metabolic acidosis develops the cardiac output decreases (Carson, Chorley, Hamilton, Lee and Morris, 1966).

Delayed poisoning does not occur, and as the healthy liver is capable of rapidly and completely breaking down the drug there is no risk of cumulative poisoning. Clinical experience indicates that the drug has no toxic action on the myocardium, for many aged dogs with severe cardiac dysfunction have been safely anaesthetized. Moreover, it has been noticed that chronic nephritis does not increase an animal's susceptibility provided that it is not in a state of acute uraemic intoxication at the time. The dangers associated with general anaesthesia, however produced, in those breeds of dog whose anatomical structure favours respiratory obstruction—a depressed face, fleshy tongue, large soft palate and flaccid pharynx (the bulldog, French bulldog, pug, and Pekingese)—must again be stressed. When pentobarbitone sodium is used in these, light anaesthesia only should be induced. If necessary it may be temporarily deepened with an inhalation agent. Care should be taken to see that the tongue is drawn well out of the mouth until anaesthesia lightens. Of recent years the use of an endotracheal tube to maintain a clear airway has become widely adopted.

Pentobarbitone Sodium in the Dog

Intravenous Injection

The animal is weighed and the approximate dose estimated on a basis of about 30 mg/kg body weight. This dose, together with a little more of the drug, is drawn up into the syringe. This procedure ensures that full anaesthesia can be induced without the syringe needing to be refilled during the injection.

In feeble or toxic animals the injection must be made very slowly from the commencement, for not infrequently in such animals it is found that half the normal dose produces deep anaesthesia. With experience, it becomes possible to assess the degree of debility or toxaemia present, and thus the ultimate prognosis, by the quantity of pentobarbitone sodium taken to anaesthetize the animal. In fit animals, about two-thirds of the computed probable dose is injected rapidly as soon as venepuncture has been performed, in order to ensure that the dog passes quickly through the second (narcotic excitement) stage of anaesthesia. The remainder of the dose is administered over 3 to 4 minutes, pausing after the injection of each increment and assessing its effect.

During the first minute, while the initial part of the dose is being injected, there is no change in the animal and it should be held firmly. At the end of the second minute pressure is removed from the head. The dog generally attempts to raise it; the action, however, is sluggish. It may lick its nose and possibly yawn. A little more of the drug is injected. The first indication of the onset of anaesthesia is muscular relaxation and this is demonstrated by the fact that if the head is lifted it falls limply to the table. During the stage immediately prior to the onset of the anaesthesia the assistant must continue to hold the animal firmly, for stimulation at this point may provoke excitement and movement. When complete relaxation of the head and neck is obtained, the assistant releases the fore-limbs and if a tape muzzle has been used it is removed. Opening the mouth provokes movement of the tongue and jaws varying, according to the depth present, from a complete yawn to a slight curling of the tip of the tongue. A little more of the anaesthetic is injected and after an appropriate wait the jaws are again opened. The aim now is to reach the point at which the jaws are completely relaxed and the tongue, when drawn out, hangs limply. When this is attained, light anaesthesia is present. The corneal reflex is present, the pupil reacts to light and the pedal reflex is brisk. Respirations are regular and deep. This is the degree of anaesthesia to be induced for superficial operations. If an intra-abdominal interference is to be made, it may be decided to deepen from this point during peritoneal manipulations by ether or some other inhalation agent. At any rate, it may be taken that this depth of anaesthesia is perfectly safe. If it is decided to induce deeper anaesthesia with pentobarbitone, the so-called 'pedal reflex' is then used as the index of depth. If the 'web' between the digits is pinched firmly with the finger- and thumb-nails, it will be found that the pedal reflex comprises a definite upward and backward jerking of the limb. Often the response continues for several seconds after the stimulus has ceased. Administration is slowly continued until the reflex is just lost. By this time anaesthesia is deep and beyond this point injection should not proceed. The corneal reflex is generally absent; the pupil is constricted and does not respond. Respirations are slow, shallow, but regular and the pulse is accelerated and forceful. To sum up, assessment of depth is carried out in four stages:

1. The onset of inability to raise the head—deep narcosis.
2. The onset of complete relaxation of the jaws, and inability to move the tongue, but a brisk pedal reflex—light anaesthesia.
3. A sluggish pedal reflex—medium anaesthesia.
4. Loss of the pedal reflex—deep anaesthesia.

The administration of pentobarbitone to a dog causes an immediate large increase in heart rate, decrease in stroke volume and a transient moderate fall in both cardiac output and arterial blood pressure with no change in peripheral resistance. The mean arterial pressure, cardiac output and peripheral resistance are all within normal limits about 5 minutes after the induction of anaesthesia, but the arterial pressure rises steadily for some time after this due to either increased peripheral resistance or cardiac output (Olmsted and Page, 1966).

Death from pentobarbitone overdosage is due primarily to respiratory failure in profound anaesthesia. The pulse is still forceful but the heart ultimately ceases to beat 4 to 5 minutes after respiratory arrest, due to anoxia. Respiratory arrest is most likely to occur during the first 10 to 15 minutes after the drug has been administered intravenously, and if respiration is good 15 minutes after induction by this route it may be taken that there will be little trouble subsequently. It follows, then, that when deep anaesthesia has been induced the animal's breathing should be closely watched during the early part of anaesthesia so that if respiratory arrest occurs artificial respiration may be commenced without delay. As the heart continues to beat vigorously for a time after breathing has ceased, remedial measures should prove successful provided they are applied promptly. For further information in resuscitative measures the reader is referred to page 470. Care must be taken to prevent the onset of hypothermia during pentobarbitone anaesthesia, for this will both prolong recovery and increase fatalities (Dale, Elefson and Niemeyer, 1968).

By Mouth and by Intraperitoneal Injection

As already mentioned, in the past, pentobarbitone sodium has been given by mouth and by intraperitoneal injection, but neither of these routes can be recommended today. Given by mouth on an empty stomach, full depth is generally attained in 15 to 20 minutes, although an occasional case may be encountered in which it is unusually delayed. By intraperitoneal injection it varies from 8 to 20 minutes. In the majority of cases, when adopting the oral or intraperitoneal routes, there is no excitement during the period of induction, provided the animal is allowed to lie quietly, but if disturbed it may become frenzied and noisy.

Before intraperitoneal injection it should be ensured that the case is one suitable for this method, i.e. the peritoneal cavity is not distended due to 'pyometra', pregnancy, the presence of exudate or transudate, or gross enlargement of the liver or spleen. If the animal is grossly fat, it must be borne in mind that there may be difficulty in traversing retroperitoneal fat with the needle. The abdomen should be palpated to ensure that the urinary bladder is empty.

The animal is restrained on its back and an area of skin in the umbilical region clipped, washed, shaved, and disinfected. For the success of the operation it is essential that the needle shall be suitable. Its point should be perfect; it should be sufficiently strong to withstand bending or breaking should the animal suddenly move, and it should be long enough to penetrate the peritoneal cavity with certainty. The needle employed will vary with the size of the animal—21 to 18 gauge, 2 to 6 cm long.

The needle is thrust subcutaneously for a distance of about $\frac{1}{2}$ in and then turned directly downwards into the peritoneal cavity. That the solution is being injected into the peritoneal cavity is indicated by the complete absence of resistance to pressure on the plunger.

The question arises—is there a risk of injury to the abdominal viscera? Provided there is no gross abnormality present, the bladder is empty, and the animal is not heavily pregnant—none. After withdrawal of the needle the animal should be allowed to lie quietly until the onset of anaesthesia.

To ensure that the injection is made accurately and efficiently it is essential that the animal shall be effectively restrained. Apart from the initial prick of the needle the operation is painless. The solution is entirely non-irritating and no abdominal pain or discomfort attends its injection. It is when restraint is ineffective that accidents may occur.

In reasonably healthy animals results will be consistent, but in diseased animals it becomes necessary to make provision for hepatic dysfunction and reduce the dose accordingly. In a number of conditions intraperitoneal injection is contra-indicated. In pyometra and advanced pregnancy there is a risk of puncture of the uterus; in cases of ascites or peritoneal exudate results will be irregular; in grossly fat animals the needle may fail to penetrate the peritoneal cavity and the injection then be made into the retroperitoneal fat.

Today, intraperitoneal injections of pentobarbitone sodium should only be made when inhalation methods cannot be employed on those very rare occasions when venepuncture is quite impossible.

Indications

Pentobarbitone sodium anaesthesia can be used for nearly all extensive surgical operations in dogs and for prolonged diagnostic investigations. There is little doubt that when properly administered it is safe in *reasonably healthy* animals. For simple interferences about the surface of the body and in the mouth, examinations under anaesthesia, the immobilization of fractures, etc., light anaesthesia only is necessary. For intra-abdominal surgery it must be deeper to overcome the tendency to strain provoked by handling the peritoneum. When pentobarbitone sodium *has* to be used in severely toxaemic animals, it is best to adopt light anaesthesia only and to obtain satisfactory operating conditions by the use of other techniques such as regional analgesia, or local infiltration analgesia. It is commonly agreed that pentobarbitone sodium is contra-indicated for Caesarean section when it is desired to obtain living puppies, for if the drug is given in doses which will induce general anaesthesia in the mother, the mortality amongst the puppies will be high.

Premedication

In considering the use of premedication before pentobarbitone sodium anaesthesia, Professor Wright, after a most extensive experience of pentobarbitone anaesthesia, is of the opinion that thought should be given to the purpose of the premedication, especially as the barbiturate alone gives quite satisfactory results in healthy dogs. The reduction in the dose of barbiturate required after premedication has been given is not, in his view, an entirely convincing argument that the combined method is better than the simple administration of pentobarbitone alone, nor is a suggestion that the restraint necessary for the intravenous injection of a barbiturate in a fully conscious animal is distressing to it and that premedication is desirable out of consideration for the dog. In the great majority of cases, provided the restraint is efficiently applied, it and the subsequent intravenous injection cause the dog very little discomfort. The chief indication for a sedative which can be given by the simple method of subcutaneous injection is the dog which it is very difficult effectively to restrain with the assistance available and in which the precision necessary for the intravenous injection is difficult to obtain. This applies to only a small proportion of the dogs.

Other anaesthetists, however, are of the opinion that suitable premedication prevents a household pet becoming apprehensive or frightened by strange surroundings, unfamiliar attendants and the indignities involved in preoperative preparations, and is, therefore, of great value, even before pentobarbitone sodium anaesthesia.

Pentobarbitone Sodium in the Cat

The major part of what has been said about pentobarbitone sodium in dogs is equally applicable to cats.

In the cat the indications for the use of the drug are similar to those in the dog, but there are several factors which make its satisfactory application in this species more difficult. The technique of slow intravenous injection is not easy, and there is a danger that the injection will be made too quickly. As the total dose is a small one as compared with the dog, this may result in toxic overdosage. *It is safer to use a more dilute solution in the cat in order to give greater bulk to the injection and thus a solution of 30 mg/ml is advised.* Nevertheless, provided that these points are borne in mind, full anaesthesia can be induced quite satisfactorily.

Apart from the castration and spaying of kittens, for the performance of which ether anaesthesia may be preferred, the indications for general anaesthesia are probably fewer in the cat than in the dog. The induction of deep narcosis, however, is a great aid for such interferences as clipping and cleansing the skin; operations under local anaesthesia for sepsis and haematoma of the external ear; attention to the teeth; examinations of the pharynx, etc.; and for this purpose the drug may be administered in capsule by the mouth in a dosage of 29 to 24 mg/kg.

Intrathoracic Injection

It would seem that veterinarians sometimes administer pentobarbitone sodium to cats by intrathoracic injection. Scott (1964) states that this practice is much more widely used than the literature would suggest, and claims to have used it extensively in his general veterinary practice without observing any harmful effects. However, as pointed out by Price (1961) in an editorial in the *Journal of the American Veterinary Medical Association*, clinically inapparent lesions (such as scars, ruptured alveoli, torn blood vessels) are likely to result, and the clinical signs of a condition such as pyothorax, pleurisy or pneumonia, may not become apparent until several weeks later, when the clinician is unlikely to relate them to the administration of the anaesthetic agent. Such experimental studies as have been published (Ernold, 1961; Cummings, 1963; Strand, 1964) all indicate that the intrathoracic injection of pentobarbitone may be considered to constitute a serious menace to the future health of the cat. It seems abundantly clear that no further evidence is needed to justify relegation of the procedure to the status of being quite unacceptable (except, possibly, for euthanasia) in modern veterinary practice.

Thiopentone Sodium

Thiopentone sodium closely resembles pentobarbitone sodium chemically, but one atom of oxygen has been replaced by sulphur. Its use in animal surgery was first recorded in America by Sweebe (1936) and it has since been extensively employed throughout the world. In the dog and cat the drug is administered by intravenous injection in a manner similar to that described for pentobarbitone sodium and its anaesthetic potency appears to approximate to that of pentobarbitone in that the dose required to produce full anaesthesia in unpremedicated animals is of the order of 30 mg/kg. As already mentioned, however (pages 202–207), there are several factors which influence the duration and depth of anaesthesia obtained by the intravenous injection of this drug. The most important of these is probably the rate at which the injection is made. When the drug is given rapidly—the total dose being given in a period of 30 to 60 seconds—the onset of anaesthesia is abrupt, the dose required is small, generally in the region of 16 mg/kg, and the duration of surgical anaesthesia short (3 to 5 minutes). When the drug is administered over a period of 3 to 5 minutes the onset of anaesthesia is gradual and its depth is more readily assessed. The dosage required is larger (30 mg/kg), and the duration of anaesthesia is from 10 to 20 minutes.

The type of anaesthesia produced by slow intravenous injection closely resembles that obtained with pentobarbitone sodium. Muscular relaxation is fair, respiration is slow, shallow and regular; the pulse rate increases while the pulse remains strong; the pupils constrict. Induction of anaesthesia is not associated with a period of excitation, although dogs and cats often sneeze during induction. Recovery is also free from excitement, provided that the animal is kept quiet.

The first indication that anaesthesia is passing off is that stiffening of the jaws and curling of the tongue occur when the mouth is interfered with. There may be licking of the nose. From this point recovery is rapid. In five minutes or so the animal will be attempting to raise its head and in a further 10 minutes it will be able to raise itself on to its breast. The dog or cat is obviously quite conscious in a period of 30 to 45 minutes after the induction of anaesthesia. Limb coordination, especially the hind, is delayed, and the animal will stagger in a drunken fashion for an hour or so. Recovery is complete in 2 hours. There is no post-anaesthetic malaise or vomiting, nor has there been any clinical indication of damage to the liver or kidneys. However, Walton, Uhl, Egner and Livingstone (1950) found that small doses of thiopentone were mildly toxic to both the normal and the damaged liver of the dog. This effect was due to hypoxia and could be overcome by adequate ventilation with oxygen. Large doses of thiopentone are probably hepatotoxic, and adequate oxygenation does not reduce their toxic effects (Dundee, 1956).

In the light of its pharmacology (see pages 202–207) attempts to produce prolonged anaesthesia with thiopentone sodium alone, administered by continuous infusion or intermittent injections, are unwise. If sufficient of the drug is given to saturate the body tissues recovery will be very prolonged. Once the body tissues are saturated with the drug, recovery of consciousness depends on detoxication and elimination of the drug from the body and since, in dogs, thiopentone is destroyed more slowly than pentobarbitone, pentobarbitone must remain the drug of choice when long periods of intravenous anaesthesia are required.

Thiopentone Sodium in Dogs

Because of its great practical importance, the use of thiopentone sodium in dogs warrants detailed consideration. As with all anaesthetics, the best results are only obtained by an anaesthetist who is thoroughly familiar with this agent and who is able to exercise a little artistry in its administration. To illustrate this important point it may be noted that anaesthetists beginning their training in the use of thiopentone usually find it necessary to administer far larger doses of this drug than are used in comparable cases by experienced anaesthetists, yet it is often extremely difficult to understand why this should be so. Possibly the manner in which the animal is handled, the difficulty encountered in atraumatic venepuncture, and lack of familiarity with the signs of thiopentone anaesthesia, all contribute to the necessity for a larger dose of thiopentone.

Thiopentone Sodium as the Sole Anaesthetic

It is probable that the largest total quantity of thiopentone which should be administered to even a very large dog on any one occasion is between 1 and 1·25 g. To keep the total dose of thiopentone down to such acceptable limits, careful attention to technique is required. The dog must be handled quietly (soothing words, which have no toxicity, may take the place of premedication), and weighed, or its weight estimated. The appropriate quantity of thiopentone sodium is drawn up in a syringe, the dose being computed at about 30 mg/kg and whenever possible a 2·5% solution of the drug should be employed. When it is likely that more than 500 mg will be required a 5% solution may be used but it must be remembered that the accidental extravascular injection of a 5% solution is a much more serious mishap than a similar accident involving the 2·5% solution. Necrosis and sloughing of the overlying tissues are common when 5% solutions of thiopentone are injected outside the vein, but do not occur when 2·5% solutions are used. In the case of small dogs in which the total dose required is likely to be between 50 and 100 mg, further dilution of the solution to 1·25% is advisable to give the injection bulk, and ensure that the dose is not given too quickly.

In elderly, frail, debilitated or toxaemic animals, injection must be made slowly from the outset. An initial dose of about 5 mg/kg is injected and the animal observed closely. The briskness of the circulation is assessed by noting the time interval between the injection of the drug and the appearance of visible signs of its action. Further small doses are injected, pausing between each and assessing the depth of anaesthesia (making due allowance for any observed abnormality of circulation time), until the desired depth of central nervous depression has been obtained. Anaesthesia may be prolonged by the further injection of small quantities of the drug as required, but care must be taken not to exceed the safe total dose. In this connection it may be noted that small dogs can cope with relatively larger doses of thiopentone than large dogs. Even so, the careful anaesthetist will always use only the smallest quantity of the drug which will allow the operation or examination to be carried out. In order to keep the dose down the surgeon must tolerate slight limb movements or respiratory irregularity during the procedure.

In young or robust, healthy dogs, the initial part of the dose may be injected rapidly. Because rapid injection is permissible it is often possible to carry out brief interferences under very small doses of thiopentone. Usually, a dose of about 7 to 8 mg/kg is injected very rapidly to produce profound anaesthesia. Anaesthesia may again be prolonged by the injection of further small doses as indicated by movement of the animal. Following this rapid injection procedure recovery is fairly rapid if only the initial dose is given, but, even so, dogs will seldom recover completely in less than 1 hour from the time of injection. It must be emphasized that thiopentone should be regarded more as a hypnotic rather than as an anaesthetic agent, and it is better to ignore slight limb movements or respiratory irregularities caused by surgical stimulation than to administer larger quantities of thiopentone in an attempt to abolish them. With experience, the correct dose for the operation or examination procedure may be given in the initial very rapid injection, but if this does not produce satisfactory conditions, further small doses are injected until the desired depression is obtained.

Thiopentone Sodium as an Induction Agent

Thiopentone sodium is widely employed as an induction agent when anaesthesia is to be maintained by inhalation methods. This practice is used:

1. When an ultra-rapid recovery of consciousness is desired. Premedication is usually not given before the injection of the thiopentone, but atropine is sometimes given intravenously as soon as the animal is unconscious.
2. For major surgery or prolonged diagnostic procedures on prepared, premedicated dogs.

In healthy dogs a dose of about 5 mg/kg may be given by very rapid injection before the application of a face-mask. Induction of anaesthesia is then completed with an inhalation agent. No attempt is made to give sufficient thiopentone to allow endotracheal intubation to be performed, and the sole object is to produce just sufficient depression to overcome struggling when the dog is introduced to the inhalation agent. (Too much thiopentone depresses the respiration and interferes with the uptake of the inhalation agent.) This is probably the best way to use thiopentone sodium in outpatients, for if cyclopropane or halothane is employed as the main anaesthetic agent, recovery of consciousness should be complete within very few minutes of the termination of anaesthesia. Because of the rapid recovery, this is a good method to employ in brachycephalic breeds of dogs, although in these the anaesthetist must be prepared to give slightly greater quantities of thiopentone so that endotracheal intubation may be carried out under its influence should respiratory obstruction develop as soon as consciousness is lost. Caution must be exercised in elderly or frail animals (which, in any case, are probably not suitable subjects for outpatient treatment), because the very rapid injection of even very small quantities of thiopentone may prove fatal.

When thiopentone sodium is given to premedicated dogs, endotracheal intubation can usually be performed after the injection of 10 to 20 mg/kg of the drug. The actual dose required depends, of course, largely upon the speed of injection.

Dosage of Thiopentone Sodium

It will be clear from the considerations outlined above that fixed dosage rates cannot be laid down. The dosage of thiopentone for any particular case is just that amount which is required to produce the desired conditions, and neither more nor less should be given. However, because the dose used will depend so much on the anaesthetist's appreciation of the depth of anaesthesia, it must be pointed out that while an anaesthetist will, in learning to give the drug, have to rely upon observation of almost all of the reflex signs in order to assess the depth of anaesthesia, the experienced anaesthetist concentrates attention on only the breathing and the response to surgical or other stimulation. The experienced anaesthetist aims to produce, at all times, the minimum of respiratory depression while only just abolishing, or perhaps on occasion even only modifying, the response to stimulation. This is accomplished by very careful, though sometimes subconscious, attention to detail.

Thiopentone Sodium in Cats

The use of thiopentone sodium in cats presents no major problems other than those which may be associated with venepuncture, and in practice, if assistance is available, it is found that there are very few cats in which venepuncture is impossible. To enable the anaesthetist to control the dose given a 1·25% solution should always be used.

One absolute contra-indication to the use of thiopentone in cats may exist. The harmful effects of barbiturates, especially thiopentone, in porphyria in man have been noted by several writers. Dundee and Riding (1955), reviewing cases reported in two journals between 1948 and 1953, found that in all of 13 patients subjected to anaesthesia who received thiopentone, paralysis followed

11

and proved fatal in 5 instances. According to Dundee (1956), in the light of our present knowledge, porphyria must be considered an absolute contra-indication to the use of barbiturates. Congenital porphyria has been diagnosed in cattle and pigs (Blood and Henderson, 1961) and while it is probably of little importance in these species, the anaesthetist must note that it has also been diagnosed in cats (Tobias, 1964). The aetiology of the condition is unknown; it is a disease of metabolism involving pyrolle pigments which take part in cell respiration. It is characterized by photosensitivity, pigmentation of bones and teeth (which fluoresce under ultra-violet light) and is familial.

Thialbarbitone Sodium

The actions of thialbarbitone sodium in animals were first studied by Carrington and Raventos (1946). When administered by slow intravenous injection the agent has anaesthetic properties very similar to those of thio-pentone sodium, except that about twice the quantity of thialbarbitone sodium is required to induce the same degree of anaesthesia. There is some evidence that of the two drugs thialbarbitone sodium is less depressant to the respiratory centre. In the dog and cat the course of thialbarbitone sodium anaesthesia is very similar to that described for thiopentone sodium, and when the drug is injected slowly, occupying 3 or 4 minutes to induce anaes-thesia, the dose required to attain medium depth varies from 33 to 66 mg/kg. The duration of anaesthesia and of the recovery period are much the same as with thiopentone. The agent is a pale yellow hygroscopic powder freely soluble in water. It is marketed in ampoules containing 1 g and is administered as a 10% solution. Solutions should be freshly prepared.

Thiamylal Sodium

Thiamylal sodium closely resembles thiopentone sodium in chemical structure except that while the latter is the ethyl derivative of the series, the former is the allyl, and thus it would be expected that they had similar actions.

It is claimed that the drug is a more potent and less cumulative anaesthetic than thiopentone and gives rise to fewer signs of excitement during induction and recovery from anaesthesia. The quantity required to induce medium depth anaesthesia when administered by slow intravenous injection to rela-tively healthy dogs of average size lies between 17 and 20 mg/kg. The cus-tomary method of administration is to inject about a third of the estimated anaesthetic dose fairly quickly and then to continue injection very slowly, assessing depth as it proceeds, and occupying about 5 minutes in the total administration. After the induction of medium depth anaesthesia in healthy dogs, commencing return of reflexes occurs in about 10 minutes, and with deep anaesthesia in from 15 to 20 minutes. Animals generally regain their feet some 30 to 40 minutes after injection.

It is also claimed that in the cat laryngeal spasm and also apnoea are less likely to occur with thiamylal than with thiopentone. Thiamylal causes greater salivation than either pentobarbitone or thiopentone and when using it premedication with atropine may be considered.

Borgman (1953) studying its toxicity found that some dogs survived without stimulation after a dosage of 35 mg/kg, and others with the aid of stimulants lived after a dose of 44 mg/kg. He concludes that the margin of safety appears to be less than 1·75 times the anaesthetic dose and that the maximum dose dogs can survive even with stimulation is 2·5 times the anaesthetic dose.

Apart from its depressant action on the central nervous system, which in overdosage causes respiratory failure, the drug is not significantly toxic and administration can be repeated frequently without cumulative effects.

It is generally used as a 4% solution and the greater the concentration used the greater will be the reaction should some of the solution accidently be injected outside the vein.

Methohexitone Sodium

Methohexitone sodium is usually used in both dogs and cats as a 1% solution, injected intravenously at a rate of approximately 1 ml/second, in doses of 4 to 8 mg/kg. If a slow rate of injection is employed, muscle tremors, sometimes violent, can be provoked by auditory stimuli. With the rate of administration as suggested, i.e. approximately 10 mg/second, however, induction is smooth and rapid. The animal is usually sitting up within 5 to 10 minutes of the injection and has completely recovered within 30 minutes. Recovery should be allowed to occur in a quiet place because noise or other stimuli produce muscle tremors or even convulsions during the recovery period (Fowler and Stevenson, 1961). No nausea, vomiting or excessive salivation occurs during the recovery period, and the incoordinated 'drunken' movements often seen after pentobarbitone or thiobarbitone anaesthesia are seldom observed. Because recovery is so rapid and complete, methohexitone anaesthesia is most useful for 'outpatient anaesthesia' in dogs and cats.

REFERENCES

AUCHTERLONIE, L. A. (1934). *Vet. Rec.* **14**, 21
BLOOD, D. C. and HENDERSON, J. A. (1961). *Veterinary Medicine*. London: Baillière, Tindall and Cox
BORGMAN, R. F. (1953). *J. Am. vet. med. Ass.* **122**, 161
CARRINGTON, H. C. and RAVENTOS, J. (1946). *Br. J. Pharmac.* **1**, 215

CARSON, S. A. A., CHORLEY, G. E., HAMILTON, F. N., LEE, D. C. and MORRIS, L. E. (1966). *J. appl. Physiol.* **20**, 948
CUMMINGS, B. C. (1963). *Small Anim. Clin.* **3**, 539
DALE, H. E., ELEFSON, E. E. and NIEMEYER, K. H. (1968). *Am. J. vet. Res.* **29**, 1339
DUNDEE, J. W. (1956). *Thiopentone and Thiobarbiturates.* Edinburgh: Livingstone
────── and RIDING, J. E. (1955). *Anaesthesia,* **10**, 55.
ERNOLD, G. L. (1961). *J. Am. vet. med. Ass.* **140**, 795
FOWLER, N. G. and STEVENSON, D. E. (1961). *Vet. Rec.* **73**, 917
HAIGLER, S. W. (1931). *Vet. Med.* **26**, 424
KREUTZER, B. H. (1931). *Vet. Med.* **26**, 524
OLMSTED, F. and PAGE, I. H. (1966). *Am. J. Physiol.* **210**, 817
PRICE, D. A. (1961). *J. Am. vet. med. Ass.* **139**, 691
SCOTT, W. A. (1964). *J. small Anim. Pract.* **5**, 459
STRANDE, A. (1964). *J. small Anim. Pract.* **5**, 153
SWEEBE, E. E. (1936). *Vet. Med.* **31**, 158
TOBIAS, G. (1964). *J. Am. vet. med. Ass.* **145**, 462
WALTON, C. H., UHL, J. W., EGNER, W. M. and LIVINGSTONE, H. H. (1950). *Archs Surg. Chicago,* **60**, 968
WRIGHT, J. G. (1934). *Vet. Rec.* **14**, 486

16

Introduction to Inhalation Anaesthesia

An inhalation anaesthetic cannot be introduced into the brain without at the same time being distributed through the entire body, and this distribution exerts a controlling influence over the rate of uptake or elimination of the anaesthetic by the brain. All the gaseous and volatile anaesthetic agents, with the exception of trichloroethylene, behave in the body, both physically and chemically, as inert gases. To regulate anaesthesia in a rational manner, therefore, the anaesthetist should have a clear understanding of the processes involved in the exchange of inert gases in the body.

Simplifications

If certain factors are reduced to their simplest possible terms, and certain assumptions are made, it is possible to give approximate predictions relating to inert gas exchange in the body. These predictions are sufficiently realistic for practical purposes and will serve to illustrate the main principles involved. Once these are understood, more elaborate expositions found elsewhere (Mapleson, 1963; Bourne, 1964; Butler, 1964; Eger, 1964; Epstein, 1964) should become reasonably easy to follow. It is possible, once these certain assumptions have been made, to give a mathematical description of uptake under certain conditions and this line of approach has been admirably reviewed by Kety (1951) in an account which includes his own, very large, contributions to this field of knowledge. It is mainly on this review and one other paper (Kety, 1950) that the following outline is based.

For simplicity, the physiological variables such as cardiac output and tidal volume must be assumed to be unaffected by the presence of the gas, and to remain uniform throughout the administration. Allowance cannot be made for alterations in the tidal volume as uptake or elimination proceeds. The blood supply to the grey matter of the brain must be assumed to be uniform and the gas to be evenly distributed throughout the grey matter. Finally, although in practice anaesthetics are seldom administered in this way, the anaesthetic must be assumed to be given at a fixed inspired concentration, and, what is more, it must be assumed that no rebreathing of gases occurs.

Terminology

In the account which follows frequent reference is made to tensions, solubilities and concentrations of gases in solution. These terms may perhaps be best explained by considering specific examples:

The tension of agents dissolved in a liquid. This is the pressure of the agent in the gas with which the liquid would be in equilibrium. (A liquid and a gas, or two liquids, are in equilibrium if, when separated by a permeable membrane, there is no exchange between them.) The statement that 'the tension of nitrous oxide in the blood is 380 mm Hg' means that if a sample of the blood were placed in an ambient atmosphere containing nitrous oxide at a concentration of 50% V/V (and, therefore, according to Dalton's law, exerting a partial pressure of 380 mm Hg) there would be no movement of nitrous oxide into or out of the blood. 'Tension' is a term used by physiologists and anaesthetists, while physicists speak of 'partial pressure'.

Solubility coefficients of gases. At any given temperature the mass of a gas dissolved in a solution, i.e. its concentration in the solution, varies directly with its tension (Henry's law) and is governed by the solubility of the gas in the particular solvent. The solubility of anaesthetics varies widely and, therefore, at any one tension, the quantities of the different anaesthetics in the solvent are not equal. The solubility of anaesthetics in the blood and tissues is best expressed in terms of their partition, or distribution, coefficients. For example, the blood/gas partition coefficient of nitrous oxide is 0·47. This means that when blood and alveolar air containing nitrous oxide at a given tension are in equilibrium, there will be 47 parts of nitrous oxide per unit volume (say per litre) of blood for every 100 parts of nitrous oxide per unit volume (litre) of alveolar air. In general, the partition coefficient of a gas at a stated temperature is the ratio, at equilibrium, of the gas's concentration on the two sides of a diffusing membrane or interface. In the brain and all other tissues (except fat) gases have very nearly the same solubility as they have in blood; their tissue blood partition coefficients are close to unity. Exceptions are substances like halothane which are exceptionally soluble in fat. Halothane is about 60 times as soluble in fat as it is in blood (i.e. its fat/blood coefficient is 60) and because of the lipoid nature of brain tissue the brain/ blood partition coefficient for halothane is 2·6.

Concentration of a gas in solution. The concentration of a gas in solution may be expressed in a variety of ways including (*a*) the volume of gas which can be extracted from a unit volume of solution under standard conditions (V/V); (*b*) the weight of dissolved gas per unit volume of solvent (W/V); or (*c*) the molar concentration, i.e. the number of gram-molecules of gas/litre of solvent. The molar concentration is the most useful—equimolar solutions of gases of different molecular weights contain equal concentrations of molecules. This would not be so if their concentrations in terms of W/V were equal.

Uptake of Anaesthetics

Kety has pointed out that when an inert gas is suddenly introduced at a fixed partial pressure into the inspired air of a non-rebreathing system, the tissues of the body do not immediately acquire the gas at this tension. The tensions of the gas in the alveolar blood and tissues all tend to move towards inspired tension but a number of processes, each of which proceeds at its own rate, intervene to delay the eventual saturation of the tissues. In other words, the tension of the gas in the brain follows, with a slight delay, its tension in the alveolar air. Since both the rate of induction and recovery from inhalation anaesthesia are governed by the rate of change of the tension of the anaesthetic in the brain, and this in turn is governed by the rate of change of its tension in the alveoli, the factors which determine the tension of the anaesthetic in the alveoli are obviously of very great importance to the anaesthetist.

The rate at which the tension of an anaesthetic in the alveoli air approaches its tension in the inspired air depends on the pulmonary ventilation, the uptake of the anaesthetic by the blood and tissues and the inspired concentration. First, by means of pulmonary ventilation the gas is inhaled, diluted with functional residual air, and distributed to the alveolar membrane. This is where diffusion occurs and normally the alveolar gas equilibrates almost immediately with the pulmonary blood which is then distributed throughout the body. A second diffusion process occurs across the capillary membranes of the tissues into the interstitial fluid and from there through the cell membranes into the cells themselves. Venous blood leaving the tissues is in equilibrium with the tissues. The blood from the tissues returns to the lungs, still carrying some of its original content of anaesthetic, and is again equilibrated with alveolar gas which now contains a slightly higher tension of the anaesthetic. It is in this manner that the alveolar (or arterial) and venous (or tissue) tensions of the anaesthetic in question gradually, and in that order, rise towards eventual equilibrium with the inspired tension.

As this complex process proceeds, the tension of the anaesthetic in the alveolar air increases continuously, but not at a uniform rate. Plotted against time, alveolar tension rises in a curve that, in general, is the same for every inert gas (Fig. 129). In Kety's terminology this curve has an initial rise (which is steep), a knee, and a tail which slopes gradually upwards until, after several hours or even days, depending on the anaesthetic in question, complete equilibrium is reached. The steep initial rise represents the phase in which ventilation is moving anaesthetic into the lungs, i.e. the so-called 'pulmonary washout' phase. The slowly rising tail represents the more gradual

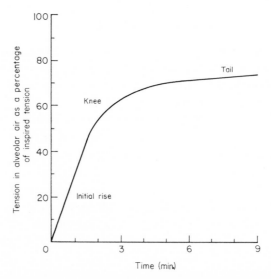

FIG. 129.—Typical alveolar tension curve for an inert gas inhaled at a constant tension from a non-rebreathing system.

process of tissue saturation. The knee marks the point at which lung washout gives place to tissue saturation as the most important influence. The tail can be very long if the anaesthetic in question has a very high fat/blood partition coefficient.

Effect of Blood Solubility on Alveolar Tension

The shape of the curve obtained with any given anaesthetic depends on a number of factors. These include such things as minute volume of respiration; the functional residual capacity of the lungs; the cardiac output; the blood flows to the main anaesthetic absorbing bulk of the body—the muscles and the fat. However, one single physical property of the anaesthetic itself is considerably more important than all of these factors—the solubility of the anaesthetic in the blood. This is the factor which determines the height of the knee in the alveolar uptake curve. With anaesthetics of low blood solubility the knee is high; with those of high blood solubility the knee is low. This may be illustrated by consideration of the hypothetical extremes of solubility.

A totally insoluble gas would not diffuse into the pulmonary blood and would not be carried in it away from the lungs. If such a gas were inhaled at a constant inspired tension in a non-rebreathing system, its alveolar tension would increase exponentially as lung washout proceeded until, after a very short time, alveolar tension equalled inspired tension. The curve obtained would be all initial rise and, there would be no tail (Fig. 130). Such a gas could

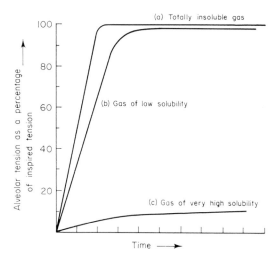

Fig. 130.—Alveolar tension curve for (a) a totally insoluble gas, (b) a gas of low blood solubility, and (c) a gas of extremely high solubility, all breathed at a constant inspired tension from a non-rebreathing circuit.

not, of course, ever be an anaesthetic, since none would ever reach the brain. A gas of extremely low blood solubility (Fig. 130) would give an almost identical curve. The loss into the pulmonary bloodstream of only a minute amount of the gas contained in the lungs at any moment would bring the tension of the gas in the blood into equilibrium with the tension in the al-veolar air. The capacity of the blood for such a gas would be extremely small. Likewise, the capacity of the entire body tissue (with the possible exception of fat) would be small since, as already pointed out, the tissue/blood partition coefficients of most anaesthetics are close to unity. If such an agent, even when given at the highest permissible inspired concentration of 80% with 20% of oxygen, only produced a faint depression of the central nervous system, it could nevertheless be looked upon as a very active agent because it would be deriving its effect through the presence in the brain of only a minute trace. (See discussion of potency, page 333.)

At the other hypothetical extreme would be a gas of very nearly infinite solubility in blood.

All but a very small fraction of the gas in the lungs at any one moment would dissolve in the pulmonary blood as soon as the blood arrived at the alveoli. The capacity of the blood and body tissues for such a gas would be vast. The alveoli tension curve (Fig. 130) would be very flat, with virtually no initial rise, a knee virtually on the base line and a very slow rising tail. Given time enough for full equilibrium, it might be possible to achieve very deep anaesthesia by using a minute inspired tension but, of course, in one sense the gas would be a very weak anaesthetic, since its concentration in the brain would be enormous.

Ranging between these hypothetical extremes of solubility are the gaseous and volatile anaesthetics. Their solubilities in blood and tissues as far as they have been determined (Bourne, 1960; Larson, Eger and Severinghaus, 1962; Mapleson, 1963) are shown in the table below in order of increasing solubility in blood. (Nitrogen, an almost insoluble gas, is included for comparison.)

SOLUBILITIES IN BLOOD AND TISSUES OF THE GASEOUS AND VOLATILE ANAESTHETICS

	Blood/gas	Tissue/blood		Tissue/gas	
Nitrogen	0·01	Brain	1·1	Brain	0·011
		Liver	1·1	Liver	0·011
		Fat	5·2	Fat	0·052
Cyclopropane	0·46	Liver	1·34	Liver	0·616
		Muscle	0·92	Muscle	0·433
		Fat	20·0	Fat	9·2
Nitrous oxide	0·47	Brain	1·0	Brain	0·47
		Heart	1·0	Heart	0·47
		Fat	3·0	Fat	1·41
Halothane	2·3	Brain	2·6	Brain	6·0
		Liver	2·6	Liver	6·0
		Kidney	1·6	Kidney	3·6
		Muscle	3·5	Muscle	8·0
		Fat	60	Fat	138·0
Chloroform	7·3	Brain	1·0	Brain	7·3
		Liver	0·9	Liver	6·57
		Fat	68·5	Fat	500
Trichloroethylene	9·0	Fat	106·7	Fat	960
Methoxyflurane	13·0	Grey matter	1·7	Grey matter	22·1
		White matter	2·34	White matter	30·42
		Muscle	1·34	Muscle	17·42
		Fat	63·5	Fat	825·0
Diethyl ether	15	Brain	1·14	Brain	17·1
		Fat	3·3	Fat	50·0

The effect of the different solubilities on the alveolar tension when the agents are administered at a constant inspired tension is shown in Fig. 131. (It must be appreciated that the curves have not been drawn accurately and are only intended to represent approximate, relative curves. Similar curves, drawn from data computed on an electrical analogue, a device for predicting actual values in man, have been constructed by Mapleson (1963).

The Tension of Anaesthetic Agents in Brain Tissue

In addition to the alveolar tensions, the anaesthetist is also concerned with the tissue tension, and particularly, the tension of anaesthetic agents in the grey matter of the brain. In the lungs (unless pathological changes are present) diffusion from the alveolar air to the blood is almost instantaneous, as has already been pointed out. This means that the tension of the agent in the blood leaving the lungs, that is to say in the arterial blood, may for all practical purposes be regarded as equal to the tension in the alveolar air. Only when the body has become absolutely saturated does the arterial tension equal the tissue

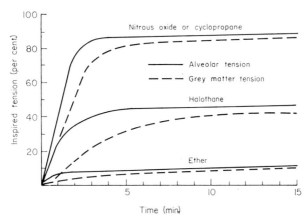

FIG. 131.—Effect of blood solubility on alveolar (and grey matter) tension curves of anaesthetics administered at constant inspired tensions from a non-rebreathing circuit.

tension. During the saturation process, and after the administration is stopped, the tissue tension is accurately represented by the tension of the agent in the venous blood leaving that tissue. This lags behind the arterial tension by an amount which depends mainly upon the blood supply of the tissue. Fatty tissues are exceptions to this rule, for in them the relative solubilities play an important part. In organs with a rich blood supply, such as the brain and heart, the venous tension rises quite quickly to the arterial tension. After about 20 minutes (in man) with anaesthetics whose solubility in grey matter is about equal to that in blood, or perhaps twice that interval in the case of agents like halothane which are a little more soluble in grey matter, arterial and grey matter tensions, during uptake and during elimination, are almost equal (Fig. 131).

It follows from these considerations that if a gas has a low blood solubility, any change in its tension in the alveolar air is quickly reflected in the grey matter in the brain, whereas if the blood solubility is high there will be a considerable delay because the whole body will act as a very large buffer. Thus, with an inhalation anaesthetic, the speed with which induction of anaesthesia can be carried out (when the inspired tension is kept constant) is governed by the solubility of the anaesthetic in the blood. Low solubility (nitrous oxide and cyclopropane) favours rapid induction, whereas high blood solubility (ether) leads to slow induction. The important point to note here is, of course, that so far all arguments have been based on the assumption that the inspired concentration is maintained constant. In fact, alteration of the inspired tension can do much to overcome the slow induction with agents of high blood solubility. For example, if, in man, ether were given at the concentration which would give satisfactory anaesthesia after full equilibration, induction might take as long as 24 hours. It would be a very long time before the patient even lost consciousness. The difficulty is, of course, in practice, overcome by starting the administration not with this concentration, but with one which is much higher and which would if administered indefinitely kill the patient. As the desired level of anaesthesia is approached the inspired concentration is gradually reduced. Even so, induction with this very soluble agent is slow. In dogs, light anaesthesia is produced by tensions of ether in the brain of the order of 23 mm of mercury, while tensions of about 30 mm of mercury produce deep anaesthesia, yet Haggard (1924) had to administer this anaesthetic for about 20 minutes at more than 5 times these concentrations before these brain tensions were obtained.

It is in fact standard practice to hasten induction of inhalation anaesthesia in this way. However, the maximum concentration which can be administered is limited by the volatility of the anaesthetic, and its pungency. Many anaesthetics are so pungent or irritant that they cannot be inhaled in high concentrations.

Recovery from an inhalation anaesthetic cannot be subjected to the same treatment. When the administration of the anaesthetic is terminated its concentration in the inspired air cannot be reduced to below zero. Although the full buffering effect of the body tissues will not be seen after accelerated inductions and brief administrations (those tissues with a poor blood supply or high tissue/blood partition coefficient will then be only very incompletely saturated), elimination of the more soluble anaesthetics must take time and will be slow. Low blood solubility leads to rapid elimination of nitrous oxide and rapid recovery from anaesthesia. Fink (1955) studied the elimination of this gas from the lungs at the end of anaesthesia and found that the volume eliminated was such that the minute volume of expiration exceeded the inspired volume by as much as 10% in the first 10 minutes. This outpouring of nitrous oxide diluted the alveolar oxygen and if the patient was breathing room air, the alveolar oxygen tension fell to levels as low as 85 mm of mercury, resulting in arterial oxygen saturations of only 92%. This phenomenon, which has been named 'diffusion hypoxia', can also happen if nitrous oxide is cut off during anaesthesia. Theoretically, it can happen with any agent, but it is unlikely to have any ill effects with ether, because of the small volumes involved and the slow excretion of ether. The danger will be greatest if two insoluble agents such as nitrous oxide and cyclopropane are administered together.

Potency of an Inhalation Anaesthetic

The potency of an inhalation anaesthetic can be expressed in various ways and this subject has been discussed very clearly by Bourne (1964).

The perhaps most obvious definition of potency is to describe it as the grey matter tension needed to produce a certain, specified and definable level of anaesthesia, i.e. the inspired tension that will, after full equilibration, give that level. However, this potency is very difficult to determine, for although inspired tensions or concentrations may be known, full equilibration may take several hours or even days. Estimations based on administrations which had not allowed sufficient time for full equilibration between grey matter and inspired tension would be misleading. Nevertheless, it is probably this concept of potency which is generally envisaged when the relative potencies of anaesthetics are discussed. Obviously, this concept has practical advantages, because the anaesthetist naturally thinks in terms of inspired concentration and the effect to be obtained.

However, the definition of potency in terms of grey matter tension ignores the wide differences in solubilities of the different anaesthetics in the grey matter of the brain and, therefore, takes no account of the concentrations (mass of anaesthetic per unit mass of brain tissue) in the brain which are producing the effect. In other words, two anaesthetics might be judged on the basis of equal potency as far as brain tensions were concerned, but yet be producing their equal effects with very different grey matter concentrations if their solubilities happened to differ greatly. Thus, an alternative definition of potency offers itself for consideration—the concentration needed in the grey matter to produce a specified level of anaesthesia. To allow comparison between anaesthetics of different molecular weights their concentrations would, of course, have to be expressed in terms of molarity. However, the effect of solubility is slightly more subtle than it might at first appear. An agent may be so insoluble in the grey matter that it could never reach the grey matter concentration easily attained with an agent which is extremely soluble, and thus the two agents could not be compared on a basis of concentrations in the grey matter needed to produce equal levels of anaesthesia. Any comparison based on grey matter concentration must, therefore, include a factor to account for solubility.

Both the above definitions of potency lead to an exaggerated estimate of the potentiality of any inhalation anaesthetic. They imply that all anaesthetics can be given at the same maximum inspired concentration of 80% and ignore the limitations imposed by differences in volatility. For example, methoxy-flurane with a saturated vapour pressure of 25 mm of mercury at 25°C cannot be given, at this temperature, at concentrations of more than about 3%. Clearly, when the potentiality of an inhalation anaesthetic is considered a volatility factor must be taken into account.

All these considerations lead to the conclusion that no really satisfactory definition of potency can be given. Most anaesthetists have their own standards by which, clinically, they appraise the potency of an inhalation anaesthetic and even if their criteria do not stand up very well to critical scrutiny, these criteria must not be lightly dismissed.

The Safety of an Inhalation Anaesthetic

Blood solubility is not only important as a factor influencing the speed of induction and recovery. It has wider implications; it determines (in an inverse manner) the extent to which tissue tension keeps pace with alterations in inspired tension and thus it controls the rate at which anaesthesia can be deepened or lightened. With a very soluble agent such as ether no sudden change in tissue tension is possible; if gross overdosage is given the anaesthetist has plenty of time in which to observe the signs of deepening anaesthesia and reduce the strength of the inhaled mixture. With an anaesthetic of low blood solubility such as cyclopropane, however, increase in tissue tension follows very quickly on the heels of an increase in the inspired tension; anaesthesia may deepen rapidly and a gross overdose may be almost instantly fatal. It is, therefore, very important with the less soluble anaesthetics to consider carefully the factors that favour the giving of an overdose, the chief of which must be volatility and potency.

Volatility governs the potential strength of the inspired mixture for obviously the more volatile the anaesthetic the greater the risk of its being administered at a high concentration. Gaseous anaesthetics and liquid anaesthetics which have low boiling points are, therefore, potentially very dangerous. Because gases are passed through flowmeters the danger is, in their case, rather less, since the anaesthetist has an accuracy of control not possible with volatile liquids except by the use of special, often expensive, apparatus.

Potency determines the magnitude of a possible overdose. With a weak anaesthetic such as nitrous oxide overdose is impossible; if it were not for lack of oxygen, nitrous oxide could be given at 100% concentration without danger. However, a concentration of 80% of an agent which was fully effective when given at a concentration of say 5% would constitute a gross overdose. This is, of course, self-evident, but as has been pointed out by Bourne (1964), anaesthetists have in the past paid insufficient attention to the precise meaning and measurement of potency, so that there is much confusion. An acceptable definition of potency would do much to clarify thought relating to the safety of inhalation anaesthetics.

Uptake and Elimination of Inhalation Anaesthetics in Clinical Practice

The various assumptions made for the purpose of theoretical or mathematical predictions of anaesthetic uptake and elimination cannot, of course, be made in everyday anaesthetic practice. Many of the factors which have to be regarded as constant if any mathematical prediction is to be made, do, in fact, vary considerably during the course of anaesthesia. Such factors include the tidal volume; the physiological dead-space; the functional residual capacity (i.e. that volume of gas in the lungs which dilutes each single breath of anaesthetic); the thickness and permeability of the alveolar-capillary membrane; the cardiac output and pulmonary blood flow (which may be different, especially in pathological conditions of the lungs); regional variations in ventilation-perfusion relationships in the lungs; the blood flow through the tissues of the body; the partition coefficients of the anaesthetic between the gaseous (or vapour) state, and lung tissue or blood, and between blood and the body tissues; and the blood flow, diffusion coefficient and diffusion distance for each of the tissues of the body.

In addition, it must be remembered that the anaesthetics themselves may modify many of the variables as administration proceeds. For example, most anaesthetics depress breathing and decrease the cardiac output.

Considerations such as these indicate only too clearly why it is not yet possible to give a complete account of the uptake and elimination of inhalation anaesthetics as encountered in clinical practice.

Gas Pockets in the Body

The study of the pulmonary exchange of gases has led to an explanation of certain complications of nitrous oxide anaesthesia. Severe abdominal distension may occur in animals suffering from intestinal obstruction when they are anaesthetized with nitrous oxide, and the subarachnoid injection of air for pneumoencephalography may, during nitrous oxide anaesthesia, cause a marked rise in cerebrospinal fluid pressure (Eger and Saidman, 1965; Saidman and Eger, 1965). Intrathoracic pressure in cases of pneumothorax is increased by the administration of nitrous oxide and so is middle ear pressure (Hunter, 1955; Thomsen, Terkildsen and Arnfeld, 1965). The volume of air which must be injected intravenously into rabbits to cause death during nitrous oxide anaesthesia is much less than the lethal volume in rabbits anaesthetized with halothane (Munsen and Merrick, 1966). These hazards of nitrous oxide are explained by the fact that nitrous oxide is 35 times more soluble in blood than is nitrogen. If an air pocket exists anywhere in the body nitrous oxide will diffuse into the pocket as the nitrogen is reabsorbed during the denitrogenation of the body. While the amount of nitrogen reabsorbed is negligible, because of its low solubility, the amount of nitrous oxide diffusing into the pocket will be far from negligible. It can be demonstrated that at equilibrium, which is virtually complete in 10 to 20 minutes, the volume of any gas pocket which existed is doubled if 50% and quadrupled if 75% nitrous oxide is administered. Thus, when nitrous oxide is used, air embolism and the presence of air pockets in the body (e.g. in pneumothorax and paralytic ileus) may constitute major hazards.

Biotransformation of Anaesthetic Gases and Vapours

Until quite recently anaesthetic gases and vapours, with the exception of trichloroethylene, have generally been thought to be chemically inert and to be mainly excreted unchanged through the lungs. However, the studies of Van Dyke, Chenoweth and their colleagues in 1965 showed that both cyclopropane and ethylene undergo metabolic change and since that time considerable work has been done on the metabolism of anaesthetic vapours, particularly the halogenated hydrocarbons and ethers. Chloroform has been shown to give rise to unidentified metabolites. Ether is thought to be broken down first into ethanol and acetylaldehyde, which are subsequently metabolized to form carbon dioxide (Greene, 1968). Metabolism of halothane has been demonstrated in animals and in man, and *in vitro* studies show that hepatic enzyme systems can metabolize it by dechlorination. Repeated exposures to halothane increase the hepatic drug metabolizing enzyme activity. Schimassek, Kunz and Gallwitz (1966) showed that for halothane the induced increase in enzyme activity involves mitochondrial enzymes rather than the microsomal enzyme system. Methoxyflurane is also metabolized by hepatic enzyme systems (Van Dyke and Chenoweth, 1965).

The clinical significance of this metabolism of inhalation anaesthetics is not clear. Certainly, it is of little significance in the maintenance of surgical anaesthesia. Although the end products for halothane and methoxyflurane have been identified and shown to be non-toxic in animals, the intermediary metabolites are largely unknown. Their biologic life and their possible toxic actions in the body are also inknown. Clearly, further studies are desirable.

REFERENCES

BOURNE, J. G. (1960). *Nitrous Oxide in Dentistry*. London: Lloyd-Luke
——— (1964). *Anaesthesia*, **19**, 12
BUTLER, R. A. (1964). *Br. J. Anaesth.* **36** 193
EGER, E. I. (1964). *Br. J. Anaesth.* **36**, 140
——— and SAIDMAN, L. J. (1965). *Anaesthesiology*, **26**, 61
EPSTEIN, R. H. (1964). *Br. J. Anaesth.* **36**, 172
FINK, B. R. (1955). *Anesthesiology*, **16**, 511
GREENE, N. M. (1968). *Anesthesiology*, **29**, 123 and 327
HAGGARD, H. W. (1924). *J. biol. Chem.* **59**, 737
HUNTER, A. R. (1955). *Proc. R. Soc. Med.* **48**, 765
KETY, S. S. (1950). *Anesthesiology*, **11**, 517
——— (1951). *Pharmac. Rev.* **3**, 1
LARSON, C. P., EGER, E. I. and SEVERINGHAUS, J. W. (1962). *Anaesthesiology*, **23**, 349
MAPLESON, W. W. (1963). *Uptake and Distribution of Anaesthetic Agents*. New York: McGraw-Hill
——— (1964). *Br. J. Anaesth.* **36**, 129
MUNSEN, E. S. and MERRICK, H. C. (1966). *Anesthesiology*, **27**, 78
PAPPER, E. M. (1964). *Anesthesiology*, **36**, 124
SAIDMAN, L. J. and EGER, E. I. (1965). *Anesthesiology*, **26**, 67
SCHIMASSEK, H., KUNZ, W. and GALLOWITZ, D. (1966). *Biochem. Pharmac.* **15**, 1957
THOMSEN, K. A., TERHILDSEN, K. and ARNFRED, I. (1965). *Archs Otolar.* **82**, 609
VAN DYKE, R. A. and CHENOWETH, M. B. (1965). *Anesthesiology*, **26**, 384

17

Inhalation Anaesthesia in Horses and Farm Animals

The horse is a good subject for inhalation anaesthesia and in equine practice this type of anaesthesia can offer distinct advantages over intravenous anaesthesia. Cattle are by no means good subjects for any form of general anaesthesia and today the problems involved in the use of general anaesthesia in these animals are well known. Most of them are associated with the danger of regurgitation and inhalation of the contents of the rumen, or the inhalation of saliva. In addition, fermentation of the ingesta and the absence of normal eructation result in distension of the rumen, and gross distension of this organ is another hazard which may be met if anaesthesia is prolonged. Furthermore, when the animal is recumbent, the weight of the abdominal viscera and their contents prevents the diaphragm from moving freely on inspiration and respiration tends to become shallow, rapid and inefficient for the purpose of gaseous exchange in the lungs.

The inhalation agents are, in general, safer in cattle than the intravenous drugs, for their elimination from the body is more rapid and recovery of the righting, swallowing, coughing and eructation reflexes after anaesthesia is, consequently, also more rapid. Experience has shown that provided certain precautions are taken, and that due care is exercised, adult cattle can be subjected, quite safely, to periods of at least 2 hours of inhalation anaesthesia.

The danger of regurgitation and inhalation of ingesta is always present but the likelihood of it occurring can be minimized by:

1. Withholding water for at least 6 hours before anaesthesia.
2. Withholding green foodstuffs and other easily fermentable food for at least 24 hours before anaesthesia.
3. When the animal is to be in lateral recumbency during anaesthesia arranging that the occiput is above the general body level and that the

head slopes so that saliva and any regurgitated material runs freely from the mouth (Fig. 132).

Regurgitation occurs both during light and during deep anaesthesia so that it is probable that two mechanisms are involved in the process. It would appear that during light anaesthesia ingesta may pass up the oesophagus into the pharnyx as a result of an active, but uncontrolled, reflex mechanism. It is then a matter of chance whether or not the protective reflexes, e.g. laryngeal closure, coughing, etc., are active, and can or cannot prevent aspiration. The order in which the reflexes of laryngeal closure, coughing, swallowing and regurgitation disappear as anaesthesia is deepened may well differ from one

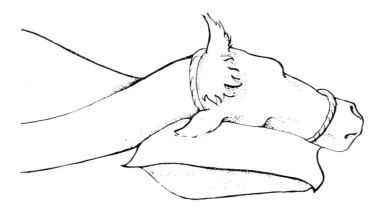

FIG. 132.—Cow's head inclined over a straw-filled sack to allow saliva to drain out of the mouth.

anaesthetic agent to another but the relative safety of the various agents in this respect cannot, at the present moment, be assessed. During deep anaesthesia, on the other hand, regurgitation is a passive process. The striated muscle of the oesophagus loses its tone and any increase in the intraruminal pressure—whether from pressure on the abdominal wall or from fermentation in the rumen itself—may force ingesta up into the pharynx. The protective reflexes are not active and aspiration occurs all too easily. For complete safety, the following procedure should always be adopted to prevent regurgitation and aspiration regardless of the method of general anaesthesia employed.

A narrow-bore stomach tube which has a rubber balloon vulcanized on to its tip so that air blown down the tube inflates the balloon, is passed through one nostril down to the stomach in the fully conscious animal immediately before anaesthesia is induced. The balloon is inflated and the tube withdrawn until the inflated balloon engages in the cardia and it is maintained inflated in this position while anaesthesia is induced. As soon as the animal is anaesthetized it is intubated with a cuffed endotracheal tube, the balloon on the stomach tube is deflated and the stomach tube withdrawn.

Although this procedure prevents regurgitation during light anaesthesia and overcomes the risk of aspiration during deep anaesthesia there are several reasons why it is not often employed. First, it necessitates the use of oesophageal blockers and cuffed endotracheal tubes which are often not readily available. Second, it is often impossible to maintain the balloon in position at the cardia while anaesthesia is induced. Some anaesthetists attempt to overcome this difficulty by simply inflating the balloon in the oesophagus and making no effort to block the cardia. However, when a balloon in the oesophagus is inflated to a degree sufficient to block the passage of ingesta many animals show the signs of marked discomfort seen in cases of acute oesophageal obstruction. Furthermore, it is perhaps simpler in every case to dispense with the use of the oesophageal blocker. Should regurgitation occur during the induction of anaesthesia after the protective reflexes have been subdued but before endotracheal intubation has been performed, the endotracheal tube may be immediately passed into the oesophagus and its cuff inflated so that the regurgitated material passes down the tube. Aspiration is then impossible and the trachea can be intubated with a second tube.

During general anaesthesia salivation also presents a problem in cattle for the copious flow does not cease when the animal is anaesthetized. Antisialogogues are not of much use for they make the secretion more viscid in nature and do not significantly reduce its production. Obstruction of the airway by large quantities of saliva is not uncommon in anaesthetized ruminant animals. It is important to arrange the head of the anaesthetized animal so that saliva drains from the mouth and does not accumulate in the pharynx. Once again, intubation with a cuffed endotracheal tube is the only certain way of preventing the inhalation of saliva.

The restriction of diaphragmatic movement by the heavy abdominal contents may have serious consequences if anaesthesia is prolonged. The anaesthetized ruminant animal should, whenever possible, be placed on an incline so that the viscera fall away from the diaphragm.

All of the factors which complicate general anaesthesia in cattle are also encountered in sheep and goats. The anaesthetist must be prepared to deal with copious salivation, the regurgitation of rumen contents and, when anaesthesia is prolonged, the occurrence of ruminal tympany. There are three points which should always be remembered. First, whenever possible sheep and goats should be properly prepared by withholding easily fermentable foodstuffs for 24 hours before anaesthesia is to be induced. Second, for all but the most transient periods of anesthesia, the animal should be intubated with a cuffed endotracheal tube early on in the course of the administration of the anaesthetic. Thirdly, any anaesthetic technique employed should be designed so that recovery from anaesthesia is rapid.

In clinical practice the indications for general anaesthesia in pigs are not numerous. Most of the operations which may necessitate general anaesthesia are rapidly performed and only transient anaesthesia is required. Some, however, such as Caesarean hysterotomy and amputation of the prolapsed uterus, necessitate longer periods of anaesthesia. The frequency with which Caesarean hysterotomy is now being performed and the increasing use of pigs for experimental surgical procedures has focused attention on the need for satisfactory anaesthetic techniques which will serve for the performance of operations of long duration. In general, it has been found that the methods of general anaesthesia which have proved to be satisfactory in dogs and cats are equally satisfactory in pigs.

Chloroform

1. The Horse

In horses chloroform is still widely used. Most horses are cast and restrained before administration but a method of commencing the induction of anaes-thesia with the animal standing has been in vogue for many years. Chloroform may be given by open methods but more often a semi-open method using a mask of canvas and/or leather is adopted. It can also be given by closed or semi-closed methods using either a face-mask or an endotracheal tube. In the past, in order to induce anaesthesia quickly when using the semi-open method, it was customary to administer a large single dose (60 ml or more) and to restrict the air supply by closing the front of the mask or by wrapping the face and mask in a heavy rug. There is no doubt that this method resulted in gross rebreathing and entailed an element of asphyxia, but short periods of unconsciousness were produced without killing the animal. This, however speaks well of the horse rather than the method. Asphyxia is known to increase the susceptibility of the heart to fibrillate under the influence of chloroform and to increase the severity of the liver damage caused by this anaesthetic agent.

Administration by the Open Method

This can be applied only to the recumbent animal and the horse must be cast either with ropes or by inducing anaesthesia in the standing animal with thiopentone sodium. The dose of thiopentone used for this purpose (see page 292) should not exceed 1 g for every 90 kg body weight. To ensure a tranquil recovery from the effects of the barbiturate it is essential to employ a pre-medicant or an intravenous sedative at the end of the period of anaesthesia.

When recumbent the lower nostril is plugged with a gauze-wrapped ball of cotton wool and the skin and mucous membrane of the upper nostril coated with petroleum jelly to prevent blistering by liquid chloroform. The upper nostril is then covered with about four layers of Turkish towelling and 4 or 5 drops of chloroform are poured on to the towelling as each inspiration begins. Induction of anaesthesia usually occupies from 8 to 10 minutes and

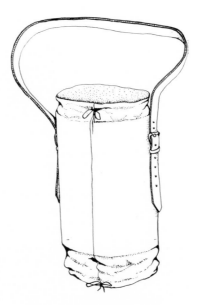

FIG. 133.—Cox's horse mask.

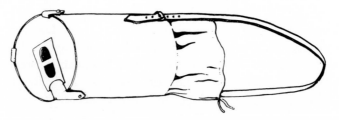

FIG. 134.—Hobday's chloroform mask for the horse.

once a satisfactory plane of anaesthesia has been reached the quantity of chloroform is reduced to the minimum necessary to maintain anaesthesia. To maintain an even plane of anaesthesia over a long period of time requires considerable skill and is much more easily achieved in animals which have received thiopentone than in those which were fully conscious prior to the administration of the chloroform.

Provided due care is exercised and no attempt is made to restrict the free flow of air through the nostril the method is both reasonably safe for the horse and satisfactory for the performance of most surgical or diagnostic procedures. No complicated apparatus is required and this open method of administration can be used under even the most primitive of field conditions.

Administration by the Semi-open Method

For this method a cylindrical mask of canvas and/or leather is applied over the upper or both jaws and the volatile agent is applied to a coarse sponge which is inserted into the distal end of the cylinder.

In the simplest type of mask both the inspired and expired air passes through the sponge so that much of the chloroform is lost to the atmosphere as the animal breathes out. Not all of the exhaled air passes out of the mask and rebreathing occurs. Nasal secretion and saliva often wet the sponge and reduce the volatilization of the chloroform. This simple type of mask, the 'Cox' and 'Hobday' mask (Figs 133 and 134) is not very satisfactory when anaesthesia of more than a transient nature is required. Numerous modifications of the Cox mask have been produced. Many of these allow the amount of air admitted during inspiration to be controlled, i.e. restricted. Such restriction of air entry is, however, most undesirable because it constitutes a mechanical obstruction of the airway. McCunn's mask comprises a canvas-covered leather cylinder, the upper end of which is lined by sorbo rubber which is compressed by pressing against the skin of the horse's face, thus forming an air-tight seal when the mask is correctly applied. At the other end of the cylinder a wire mesh partition serves to prevent the sponge coming into contact with the nostrils and also to carry a rubber disc inlet valve. Two expiratory valves and two small variable extra air holes are also incorporated in the cylinder wall, and a soft leather continuation of the anterior end of the mask serves for the reception of the sponge (Fig. 135). This well-designed mask allows free air entry during inspiration and rebreathing is prevented.

An injector type of mask has been designed by Imrie of Glasgow. This is fitted with inspiratory and expiratory valves and the chloroform is placed in a container from which it drips through a jet (Fig. 136).

The semi-open method of administration is used in both standing and cast horses.

(i) *Administration in the standing position.* This procedure is best carried out in a field where there is space for the animal to move about before it falls down. A strong, well-fitting head collar, which has a rope 8 to 10 feet long attached to the D piece on each side of the face, is applied to the horse. Each rope is held by one or more assistants who stand about 5 feet from the horse and slightly behind its head. It is important that the assistants should be instructed to keep behind the horse's head for if they get in front of the horse and the animal pulls away there is a possibility that the head collar will be pulled off.

A mask is applied and held in position by a poll strap. A Cox type mask is usually employed and in small immature animals both jaws are introduced into the mask, but in large adult horses only the upper jaw is covered. An

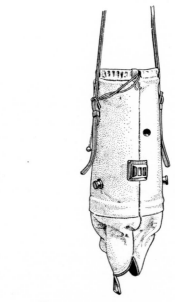

FIG. 135.—McCunn's horse inhaler.

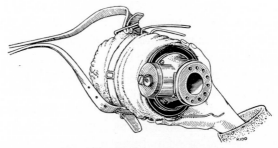

FIG. 136.—Imrie's horse inhaler.

initial dose of 30 to 60 ml of chloroform is poured on to the sponge which is then inserted into the mask, and very often the mask is adjusted so that the air intake is severely curtailed.

The first reaction of most horses is to shake the head in an effort to remove the mask and this is often followed by plunging or rearing. The animal may goose-step or stand with its forelegs widely separated, swaying but refusing to move. Often it is impossible to get beyond this stage with a single dose. The animal is then either cast with ropes or, more commonly, a second dose is given. The front of the mask is opened and a further 15 to 30 ml (i.e. half the initial dose) of chloroform is applied to the sponge. This generally provokes more movement and greater incoordination until finally the animal falls to the ground. An assistant must be ready to pull the animal's head to the ground and maintain it there otherwise vigorous attempts to rise with floundering may occur. From this point induction is completed by the further administration of small (4 to 8 ml) doses of chloroform, allowing a free air supply until the stage of surgical anaesthesia is reached.

This method is chiefly employed for the castration of colts when sufficient help for casting the animal with ropes is not available, or when it is thought that such casting may cause physical injury. It is also used on wild, vicious or unbroken animals. Despite its crudeness the method gives fairly satisfactory results and no ill-effects appear to follow the partial asphyxiation which it entails.

(ii) *Administration to the recumbent animal.* As for the open method the horse is brought to the recumbent state either by forcible casting with ropes or by inducing anaesthesia in the standing animal with thiopentone or methohexitone sodium.

The animal is restrained on its side and its tongue secured in a tape noose. The noose is placed about 7·5 cm behind the tip of the tongue and tied around the lower jaw to prevent the base of the tongue falling back and occluding the pharynx. If the mask to be employed has no partition between the sponge and the nostrils, the nostrils should be anointed with petroleum jelly to prevent blistering by the liquid chloroform. The mask is applied over either the upper jaw alone, or over both jaws and 10 to 30 ml of chloroform poured on the sponge.

The inhalation of chloroform vapour by the conscious but restrained horse usually provokes struggling and the head and neck should be held extended to reduce the force of the struggling. As anaesthesia supervenes the head should be placed in a more natural position. The induction of chloroform anaesthesia in an animal which has received thiopentone sodium is usually smooth for the animal is in a state of basal narcosis.

After a period of 2 to 3 minutes a second dose of half the initial dose of chloroform is given. Additional doses of this amount are given after similar intervals until surgical anaesthesia is attained. Induction of anaesthesia takes about 10 to 15 minutes in an animal which is simply restrained and 5 to 10 minutes in animals which have been given thiopentone sodium to bring them to the recumbent position.

Once surgical anaesthesia has been attained the rate at which the chloroform is administered must be reduced. The anaesthetist must aim at maintaining an even plane of anaesthesia and this is best performed by giving 5 to 10 ml doses of chloroform whenever anaesthesia shows signs of becoming lighter. Good operating conditions with satisfactory muscle relaxation can be obtained when chloroform is administered in this way.

On completion of the operation the mask is removed, the tongue released and the nostrils wiped clean. It is usually safe to remove ropes and hobbles at the same time for anaesthesia is followed by hypnosis, the animal lying quietly in a state of sleep. The sleep usually lasts for about $\frac{1}{2}$ hour and no attempt should be made to induce the animal to get up during this period. As soon as the horse feels able to do so it will get up on its feet—usually in a sluggish manner. There may be considerable incoordination, particularly of the hind-limbs, but provided that the animal has not been made to get up before it was ready to do so, it will be able to maintain the standing position. Very occasionally anaesthesia is followed by a state of vigorous narcotic excitement and if all restraint has been removed the animal may sustain injury. Because of this occasional excitement it is probably wise to maintain control of the head and continue restraint for 10 minutes after completion of the operation in every case. If no struggling occurs during this period, it may be taken as quite certain that recovery will be quiet.

Administration by the Closed Method

In this method the chloroform is vaporized by a stream of oxygen and the horse inhales the oxygen/chloroform mixture from a reservoir bag through a close-fitting face-mask or a cuffed endotracheal tube. A soda-lime canister must be incorporated in the anaesthetic circuit and either the to-and-fro or circle system may be used. Once again, the method can be applied only to the recumbent animal. Anaesthesia is best induced in the standing animal with intravenous thiopentone sodium. The horse is restrained on its side and the endotracheal tube introduced (see page 278) or the face-mask applied. The reservoir bag is half filled with oxygen and connected to the tube or mask. A mild degree of carbon dioxide accumulation assists in the induction of chloroform anaesthesia by stimulating breathing and the soda-lime canister is not introduced into the anaesthetic circuit until full anaesthesia is established.

A flow of 5 litres/minute of oxygen is passed into the anaesthetic system and the expiratory valve is opened. The oxygen stream is used to vaporize the chloroform from a Boyle vaporizer bottle. About 100 ml of liquid chloroform are placed in the bottle, the control lever turned to the full-on mark and the plunger lowered over the J-tube until the oxygen emerges just over the surface of the liquid. It is not usually necessary actually to bubble the oxygen through the chloroform. As soon as second plane anaesthesia is reached the oxygen flow rate is reduced to one just sufficient to supply the animal's basal oxygen requirements (500 to 2000 ml/minute according to the size of the animal), the expiratory valve closed and the soda-lime canister introduced into the circuit. The plunger of the vaporizer bottle is then fully withdrawn and to maintain an even plane of anaesthesia over any length of time it is necessary to reduce progressively the concentration of chloroform entering the circuit by moving the control lever gradually back towards the off position. Throughout anaesthesia the movement of the bag must be carefully watched and any decrease in the tidal volume should be taken to mean that anaesthesia is becoming too deep. If anaesthesia does deepen to the third plane the bag should immediately be half-emptied and re-filled with pure oxygen; this results almost at once in a return to a safe depth of anaesthesia.

It is probable that this is the safest method of administering chloroform. Induction of narcosis with thiopentone sodium avoids the dangers associated with the induction of chloroform anaesthesia. Respiratory depression may be recognized easily and if it occurs respiratory exchange can be assisted by manual compression of the rebreathing bag. The high oxygen content of the respired mixture ensures that oxygenation is adequate throughout anaesthesia and this minimizes the likelihood of the occurrence of cardiac arrest or fibrillation.

Administration by the Semi-closed Method

Theoretically, it should be possible to use a Magill type of attachment (see page 260) for horses but with this type of circuit a very high oxygen flow rate would be necessary to prevent rebreathing. High oxygen flow rates are expensive and, therefore, for economy some degree of rebreathing is desirable so that in practice a circle or to-and-fro carbon dioxide absorption system is used. The expiratory valve is left open and an oxygen flow rate of 4 or 5 litres/minute is used to volatilize the chloroform. Excess of the oxygen/chloroform mixtures issues from the valve.

The method is very similar to the closed one. It can be used only for the recumbent animal and anaesthesia is best induced with thiopentone or methohexitone sodium. Using the semi-closed system the inexperienced anaesthetist will find it easier to maintain an even plane of anaesthesia than when a completely closed system is employed.

Less chloroform is needed if a nitrous oxide–oxygen mixture is used to volatilize the chloroform, but care must be taken to ensure that the proportion of oxygen in the mixture never falls below 35%. The nitrous oxide contributes significantly to the production of anaesthesia and lower concentrations of chloroform are required.

The Place of Chloroform in Anaesthesia for the Horse

Over the years chloroform has acquired the reputation of being the most dangerous of all the anaesthetic agents. However, it seems more than likely that many workers have overestimated the danger associated with the use of chloroform in horses. When in 1911 Levy demonstrated a way in which this drug could, quite unpredictably, produce death in light anaesthesia, it appeared that to use chloroform for any operation in any animal was most unwise. Nevertheless, how often the Levy effect has in fact been a cause of death in horses is open to question. Very many horses have become excited during the induction of chloroform anaesthesia and many more have been subjected to surgical stimuli during light anaesthesia yet only a few have died from ventricular fibrillation at this time. Neither does death during light chloroform anaesthesia appear to occur in man. In a series of over 1100 cases of chloroform anaesthesia in man there were no deaths, but there were four cases of cardiac arrest all of which occurred in deep anaesthesia and one of which is stated, quite bluntly, to have been the result of overdosage (Waters, 1951). Delayed poisoning after chloroform also appears to be a rare occurrence in horses provided there has been no asphyxia during anaesthesia. It must be concluded that provided due care is exercised during its administration chloroform still has a definite place in horse anaesthesia.

Experience teaches several points in the management of chloroform anaesthesia if deaths are to be avoided. First, premedication should be adequate and it is probably wise to use a phenothiazine ataractic drug for this purpose. There is little doubt that this reduces the quantity of chloroform required and protects the heart to some extent from arrhythmia. Whenever possible anaesthesia should be induced with an intravenous agent. In the field circumstances may sometimes dictate that chloroform must be given to an unpremedicated, standing animal, but every step should be taken to ensure that such situations do not often arise.

Second, deep anaesthesia should be avoided: the smallest quantity of chloroform which will suffice is the best dose to use. Deep anaesthesia with chloroform is always accompanied by inadequate ventilation and hypotension; any attempt to use positive pressure respiration will certainly result in a further fall of blood pressure unless anaesthesia be lightened at the same time.

2. The Ox

Until quite recently chloroform was the only inhalation anaesthetic used in cattle. It was usually administered to either standing or recumbent animals by the semi-open method using a canvas and/or leather face-mask of the Cox variety applied over both the upper and lower jaws. The open method of administration was also occasionally used after casting the animal with ropes.

Anaesthesia was seldom carried beyond the light surgical stage and was only maintained for brief periods. Today, chloroform is also given by closed and semi-closed methods and is used to maintain anaesthesia for quite long periods.

The open method of administration can only be applied to the recumbent animal and it is therefore necessary first to cast the animal with ropes or to induce narcosis in the standing animal by some other technique such as the rapid intravenous injection of thiopentone sodium in doses of 0·5 g/estimated 90 kg body weight. In cattle, casting with ropes is a relatively simple matter and is not as hazardous as it may be in horses so that most cattle are cast before general anaesthesia is induced. One nostril must be plugged and the administration of chloroform is carried out in the manner already described for horses.

The semi-open method of administration is also similar to that already described for horses but the induction of anaesthesia is quieter than in horses. An initial dose of about 30 ml of liquid chloroform is placed on the sponge in the face-mask and additional doses of about half that quantity are given from time to time as required. When administered in this way to the standing animal the animal usually falls quietly to the ground as consciousness is lost. For all but the most transient periods of anaesthesia, endotracheal intubation with a cuffed tube should be performed as soon as anaesthesia is induced. The mask is then placed over the open end of the tube and the administration of the chloroform continued in the usual manner by pouring additional quantities on to the sponge as required.

Chloroform may also be administered by the closed method with carbon dioxide absorption as described for horses. Provided that the necessary assistance is available, most cattle are cast with ropes and anaesthesia is induced by the administration of the oxygen/chloroform mixture through a close-fitting face-mask of malleable rubber latex. Endotracheal intubation with a cuffed tube is performed as soon as possible.

Less chloroform is needed if a nitrous oxide/oxygen mixture is used to volatilize the chloroform in a semi-closed system with carbon dioxide absorption. The nitrous oxide contributes significantly to the production of anaesthesia and the inexperienced anaesthetist finds it easier to maintain an even plane of anaesthesia than when a completely closed system is employed.

3. The Sheep and Goat

It is generally agreed that when other agents are available chloroform should not be used as an anaesthetic agent for sheep and goats. However, when used in minimal quantities to supplement nitrous oxide/oxygen anaesthesia it appears to be both useful and relatively harmless.

4. The Pig

Chloroform given by open or semi-open methods of administration is generally agreed to be reasonably safe for transient periods of anaesthesia. It is usually given by semi-open methods and in adults the Cox type of mask is used, doses of 8 to 15 ml of liquid chloroform being applied to the sponge as necessary. Induction of anaesthesia is both quiet and rapid and the mask is removed from the face as soon as anaesthesia is produced. The short period of anaesthesia which follows is adequate for the performance of operations such as castration.

For longer operations anaesthesia may be induced by the rapid intravenous injection of thiopentone sodium and maintained by chloroform. Throughout anaesthesia care must be taken to administer only enough chloroform to produce very light anaesthesia and, in pigs, the ease with which the airway becomes obstructed should be remembered.

Chloroform may also be given by closed or semi-closed circuit methods after volatilization with oxygen or a nitrous oxide/oxygen mixture. In clinical practice there are few indications for endotracheal intubation and when chloroform is given by closed or semi-closed methods it is usually administered through a well fitting rubber latex mask which is moulded to the shape of the face. The tendency towards respiratory obstruction is countered by pulling the tongue of the anaesthetized pig out between the incisor teeth and pushing the lower jaws forwards by applying finger pressure behind the vertical ramus of the mandible.

Halothane

1. The Horse

Because of its great potency, halothane is a most useful inhalation anaesthetic for the horse. It is about twice as potent as chloroform and may be regarded as a much less dangerous anaesthetic agent. Halothane and chloroform both reduce cardiac output and blood pressure but an overdose of halothane causes respiratory failure long before it produces circulatory failure whereas an overdose of chloroform results in almost simultaneous respiratory and circulatory arrest. Furthermore, there is, as yet, no evidence that halothane produces degenerative changes in the liver and kidneys, whereas chemical tests usually demonstrate some degree of damage to these organs after chloroform anaesthesia even when there is no clinical evidence of chloroform poisoning.

Administration

Halothane may be administered to horses by any of the methods described for chloroform. Because of its high cost it is not customary to administer it by open or semi-open methods but very satisfactory anaesthesia can be produced by these. It is usually given by closed or semi-closed methods, oxygen being used to vaporize the liquid halothane. Although this potent drug can be vaporized from any available standard vaporizer bottle, most bottles do not allow of any very fine control of vapour strength. For halothane very fine control is most desirable and consequently special vaporizers which provide this facility are often employed. A simple and comparatively inexpensive

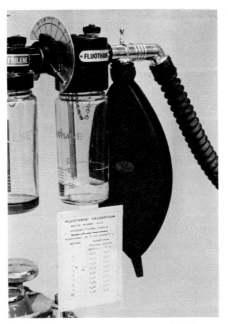

Fig. 137.—Simple vaporizer for halothane.

type of vaporizer bottle is shown in Fig. 137. The temperature and flow compensated vaporizers provide a very fine control of the vapour strength but are more costly pieces of equipment.

Halothane may be given to both standing and recumbent horses by the methods described for the administration of chloroform and both the induction of and recovery from anaesthesia is rapid. Inexperienced anaesthetists may find that the maintenance of smooth anaesthesia is not easy. Small variations in the concentration of the halothane vapour cause marked changes in the depth of anaesthesia so that swinging anaesthesia results unless great care is exercised in the administration of this agent.

During halothane anaesthesia there is usually some slowing of the pulse and occasionally tachypnoea develops. This tachypnoea may be abolished by the intravenous injection of 50 to 100 mg of pethidine hydrochloride. A reasonable degree of muscle relaxation may be obtained during halothane anaesthesia but it is not wise to attempt to produce profound muscle relaxation with this agent because the blood pressure falls as the depth of anaesthesia increases and systolic pressures as low as 30 mm of mercury have been recorded in horses when deep halothane anaesthesia has been induced to obtain relaxation of the abdominal muscles. Recovery of consciousness is rapid after halothane anaesthesia and muscle tremors or frank shivering may be seen in the recovery period. Because horses often try to get up before they are able to maintain the standing position, when a padded recovery box is not available it is usual to restrain the animal with hobbles for about 30 minutes after the administration of the anaesthetic is discontinued.

Halothane is an expensive drug and in veterinary anaesthesia it is essential to keep the quantity used for any one case to within reasonable limits. When halothane is given by semi-open, semi-closed or closed methods of administration, about 30 to 40 ml of the drug are required to induce anaesthesia in horses of about 450 kg body weight. The tissue and fluids of the horse's body continue to absorb halothane after induction and to maintain the concentration in the brain a further quantity of between 35 and 40 ml of the drug has to be administered during the first hour of anaesthesia. During the second and subsequent hours the uptake decreases and eventually equilibrium between the concentration in the body and alveolar air is reached. As may be inferred from these figures, the quantity of halothane required to maintain anaesthesia is small compared to the quantity necessary to induce anaesthesia. Therefore, for economic reasons, it is usual to induce anaesthesia with a drug such as thiopentone sodium and to use halothane simply for the maintenance of the anaesthetic state. After induction of anaesthesia with thiopentone sodium about 30 to 35 ml of halothane are required to maintain anaesthesia for 1 hour in horses of about 450 kg body weight. All that is required in these circumstances is that the inhalation agent shall maintain the depression of the brain as the thiopentone is redistributed in the body.

2. The Ox

Because of its great potency and because it does not appear to have any toxicity, halothane is a most useful inhalation anaesthetic for cattle. It will produce very satisfactory anaesthesia when administered by open, semi-open, closed, or semi-closed methods but because of its high cost it is usually given only by closed or semi-closed circuit methods.

It is also too costly to use for the induction of anaesthesia. Using closed circuit methods between 30 and 40 ml of the liquid must be vaporized to induce anaesthesia in a cow weighing 450 kg and for the maintenance of anaesthesia for 1 hour about a further 30 ml are required. After the induction of anaesthesia with thiopentone sodium in a cow of similar weight anaesthesia can be maintained for 1 hour by the use of 25 to 30 ml of the liquid agent. However, when anaesthesia is induced by a drug such as thiopentone sodium much of the flexibility of halothane anaesthesia is lost and recovery from anaesthesia is, to some extent, delayed.

In cattle, as in horses, halothane is best vaporized from a special vaporizer unit and the inexperienced anaesthetist may find the maintenance of smooth anaesthesia is not easy. The loss of flexibility which occurs when thiopentone is used to induce anaesthesia does to some extent overcome any tendency towards swinging anaesthesia.

It is unwise to attempt to produce marked muscle relaxation with halothane for very low systolic blood pressures have been recorded in cattle under deep halothane anaesthesia.

After anaesthesia recovery of consciousness is rapid and this makes halothane a particularly useful anaesthetic agent for ruminant animals. Most animals can support themselves on the brisket within 6 to 7 minutes from the termination of anaesthesia.

3. The Sheep and Goat

Halothane is an excellent anaesthetic for sheep and goats. It is usually vaporized with oxygen or a nitrous oxide/oxygen mixture and administered by closed or semi-closed circuit methods.

Anaesthesia is induced almost to the point of respiratory failure with a mixture containing 3 to 4% of halothane vapour delivered through a close-fitting face-mask. The mask is removed from the face and endotracheal intubation is performed rapidly as anaesthesia lightens. Anaesthesia is maintained with an inspired mixture containing 1·5 to 2% of halothane vapour and inexperienced anaesthetists find it easier to maintain smooth anaesthesia when a semi-closed rather than a completely closed circuit is used.

Recovery from anaesthesia is rapid even after prolonged administration. As with cyclopropane, induction of anaesthesia with an intravenous agent makes endotracheal intubation easier but prolongs the recovery period.

4. The Pig

Because of its great potency and apparent freedom from toxicity halothane is an excellent anaesthetic for pigs of all ages. When given by open, semi-open, closed or semi-closed methods, induction of anaesthesia is rapid and provided the animal can be effectively restrained there is seldom any need to use an intravenous drug for this purpose before halothane is given. Squealing ceases after as few as 4 or 5 breaths of halothane vapour have been taken and

12

inhalation of the vapour does not provoke salivation or breath-holding. Recovery from anaesthesia is equally smooth and rapid.

Ether

1. The Horse

There is general agreement that using open or semi-open methods of administration it is impossible to anaesthetize adult horses with ether. In 1938 Henkels described an auto-inhalation type of ether vaporizer which enables ether anaesthesia to be induced in horses under chloral hydrate basal narcosis. In this apparatus ether is dripped from a reservoir into the vaporizer bottle which is surrounded by a hot water bath to hasten the volatilization of the ether. During inspiration the inspired air is drawn through the vaporizer bottle while expired gases pass out through an expiratory valve on the face-mask into the atmosphere so that no rebreathing occurs. This type of apparatus has not been used to any extent in Great Britain.

It is now clear that satisfactory anaesthesia can be attained in narcotized horses when ether is given by closed or semi-closed methods. Narcosis is induced by the intravenous injection of thiopentone sodium or chloral hydrate and the ether is administered from a to-and-fro or circle type system with soda lime for the absorption of carbon dioxide. In the circle absorber system a draw over type of ether vaporizer is incorporated on the inspiratory side of the circuit. In the to-and-fro system the fresh gases pass through an ether vaporizer bottle before entering the circuit and it is usually necessary to immerse the bottle in a bath of warm water to secure adequate volatilization of the ether.

In horses ether appears to produce mild respiratory stimulation and the movements of the abdominal wall associated with breathing are more vigorous than during comparable chloroform anaesthesia. Recovery after ether anaesthesia is rapid and horses can usually get up and maintain the standing position 50 to 60 minutes after the administration of the anaesthetic is discontinued.

Since some horses become restless while recovering from ether anaesthesia and when no padded recovery box is available it is customary to apply hobbles and restrain the animal during this period. This post-anaesthetic restlessness may be associated with the use of thiopentone for the induction of anaesthesia rather than with the use of ether. Premedication with the phenothiazine ataractic drugs, or their use in the immediate post-operative period, will overcome any tendency to excitement during recovery.

From time to time ether anaesthesia has been produced by the intravenous injection of a dilute solution of ether in physiological saline. Longley (1950) has reported the use of this method in 6 horses. Working on the figures of Guedel that for surgical anaesthesia the blood concentration of ether should be between 1·1 and 1·4 g/litre Longley estimated that between 75 and 100 ml of ether should be required to produce surgical anaesthesia in horses of 1140 lb body weight. The solution of ether must be prepared immediately before use and Longley dissolved 100 ml of ether in 2 litres of physiological saline at about 30°C and administered this solution to 5 horses which were already narcotized with thiopentone sodium and to 1 horse which was simply cast and restrained. This method of administering ether is really only of academic interest and does not commend itself for use in the field but it should be noted that there were no adverse effects associated with its use in this very small series of cases.

Provided that the necessary apparatus for auto-inhalation or closed or semi-closed administration is available ether has a definite place in equine anaesthesia. It is still the safest of all anaesthetic agents and when used to maintain anaesthesia following an induction dose of thiopentone sodium there is much to commend it.

2. The Ox

It is generally agreed that it is almost impossible to anaesthetize adult cattle by ether when this agent is given by open or semi-open methods. Nevertheless, satisfactory anaesthesia can be maintained in narcotized adult cattle when ether is given by a closed or semi-closed system. Narcosis is usually induced by the intravenous injection of a thiobarbiturate and after endotracheal intubation ether is administered from a to-and-fro or circle type system with soda lime for the absorption of carbon dioxide. In the circle type system a draw-over ether vaporizer is placed on the inspiratory side of the circuit. In the to-and-fro absorption circuit the fresh gases pass through an ether vaporizer bottle before entering the system and it is necessary to immerse the bottle in a warm water bath to obtain adequate volatilization of the ether.

Recovery after ether anaesthesia is quiet and rapid. Provided that the necessary apparatus for closed or semi-closed administration is available, ether is a useful agent for the maintenance of anaesthesia in adult cattle for as in other animals it is a particularly safe drug.

Ether can be used to anaesthetize small calves but its inhalation in the concentrations necessary for the induction of anaesthesia usually produces a profuse outpouring of salivary and bronchial secretion and for this reason even in young animals anaesthesia is usually induced with another agent. The best agent to use for this purpose is debatable but thiopentone sodium given as a 2·5% solution by slow intravenous injection in quantities just sufficient to produce loss of consciousness has given good results.

3. The Sheep and Goat

Although sheep and goats can be forcibly restrained and compelled to breathe the pungent vapour of ether, its inhalation by the conscious animal produces profuse salivation. Furthermore, induction of anaesthesia with ether is a slow process which is most unpleasant for the animal. For these reasons ether is usually only used as an agent for the maintenance of anaesthesia following induction with an intravenous drug. It is either volatilized with oxygen and administered by endotracheal closed circuit methods or used to supplement nitrous oxide/oxygen mixtures given by semi-closed methods.

4. The Pig

Ether should not be given to conscious pigs for its inhalation by the conscious animal provokes copious salivation and bronchial secretion even in animals which have been given atropine premedication. Given by semi-closed or closed methods following the administration of thiopentone and after suitable premedication it provides satisfactory anaesthesia for the performance of operations such as Caesarean hysterotomy.

Trichloroethylene

1. The Sheep and Goat

Trichloroethylene (Trilene) should never be administered as the single anaesthetic agent but it may be used in sheep and goats to supplement the narcotic properties of nitrous oxide/oxygen mixtures. The trichloroethylene/ nitrous oxide/oxygen mixture is administered by endotracheal semi-closed methods (without the use of soda lime for carbon dioxide absorption) following the induction of anaesthesia by an intravenous agent.

For operations such as craniotomies for the removal of tapeworm cysts the sequence of thiopentone sodium induction followed by trichloroethylene/ nitrous oxide/oxygen mixtures for the maintenance of anaesthesia is a very satisfactory technique. The concentration of trichloroethylene in the mixture should never exceed 1% because tachypnoea and cardiac irregularities occur when higher concentrations are used. Very light anaesthesia with excellent suppression of motor reflexes may be produced for long periods with these agents and there is no danger of fire or explosion when electrical apparatus such as diathermy is used. It appears that the use of trichloroethylene in this manner has no effect on the breathing whereas the use of other supplements, such as halothane or methoxyflurane, with the nitrous oxide/oxygen often results in considerable respiratory depression.

2. The Pig

Trichloroethylene has been used by semi-open methods of administration as the sole anaesthetic agent in pigs, but this is not a practice to be recommended. The high concentrations required to produce anaesthesia give rise to tachypnoea and cardiac irregularities.

As in sheep and goats, trichloroethylene is a very useful addition to nitrous oxide/oxygen mixtures.

Methoxyflurane

Methoxyflurane has been used in America (Pitman-Moore Company Reports) and in Glasgow to anaesthetize horses and cattle. The trials in Glasgow showed that this agent can be used not only to maintain anaesthesia following induction with a barbiturate, but that it can also be given for the induction of anaesthesia in both horses and cattle. Vaporized from a vaporizer in a circle absorber circuit, methoxyflurane was capable of maintaining a uniform depth of anaesthesia (Douglas, Jennings, Longstreeth and Weaver, 1964). Nevertheless, it is not a very satisfactory anaesthetic agent for these animals. Its low volatility and high solubility give rise to very slow induction and recovery. Moreover, it is an expensive agent and even when administered in a closed system the cost per hour of anaesthesia is high.

The depth of anaesthesia is difficult to assess, for the respiratory and muscular signs are not correlated as they are with ether; the anaesthetist must aim to produce an absence of response to surgical stimulation while maintaining good respiratory activity.

Cyclopropane

1. The Horse

Cyclopropane has proved to be a most useful anaesthetic agent for horses. Although it is an expensive gas, when used with care in a closed-circuit apparatus the cost is small. For economy, the gas must be used in a completely effective closed-circuit and since it is difficult to achieve a good gas-tight fit between the face and a mask, endotracheal intubation with a cuffed tube must be carried out in every case.

Cyclopropane anaesthesia is very easy to control and recovery from anaesthesia is pleasingly rapid. Attempts to induce anaesthesia with cyclopropane in the standing animal have not been very successful because horses in Stage II —the stage of narcotic excitement—may become very violent. Thus cyclopropane is administered only to recumbent, restrained or narcotized horses.

Administration

1. *To the cast and restrained horse.* For this method the horse is cast with hobbles or ropes in the usual manner and restrained in lateral recumbency. A close-fitting face-mask is applied and connected to the anaesthetic circuit, the rebreathing bag of which is filled with a mixture of approximately equal parts of cyclopropane and oxygen. During the induction of anaesthesia soda lime is not included in the anaesthetic circuit for a mild degree of carbon dioxide accumulation stimulates breathing and hastens the uptake of the anaesthetic gas. The expiratory valve is left open and oxygen and cyclopropane are run into the circuit at equal flow rates so that the concentration of cyclopropane in the rebreathing bag is maintained at about 50%. Either a circle type or to-and-fro type of circuit may be employed.

Administration is usually continued until anaesthesia is deep enough to allow endotracheal intubation to be performed. As an alternative to this, once the animal has lost consciousness a muscle relaxant drug (e.g. suxamethonium chloride in doses of 0·15 mg/kg) may be injected intravenously to abolish swallowing, coughing and the tone of the jaw muscles, so that intubation may be performed without further delay. The mask is removed and a cuffed endotracheal tube introduced (see Chapter 13). The tube is connected to the anaesthetic circuit, the expiratory valve tightly closed and a soda-lime canister introduced into the circuit. Oxygen is run into the circuit at such a rate that the rebreathing bag neither empties nor becomes over full and further cyclopropane is added as required to produce the desired depth of anaesthesia.

Once the administration of the anaesthesia is terminated, recovery is rapid. When a padded recovery box is not available, the animal is restrained in lateral recumbency for about 20 to 30 minutes and is then able to regain its feet without difficulty as soon as the restraint is removed. The rapid recovery makes this a very good way of administering cyclopropane to horses—but the horse has first to be forcibly cast to the ground. Casting of conscious horses is not unassociated with risk of injury to the animal and necessitates the presence of an efficient casting team.

2. *To the narcotized horse.* The usual practice when cyclopropane is to be used is to induce anaesthesia in the standing animal by the rapid intravenous injection of thiopentone or methohexitone sodium after premedication with one of the phenothiazine ataractic drugs. Although the barbiturates and the ataractic drug both undoubtedly delay recovery from anaesthesia the recovery period is not unduly prolonged. The animal can usually regain its feet and maintain the standing position without difficulty within 1 hour of the termination of the anaesthetic. It is certainly much easier to maintain an even plane of anaesthesia with cyclopropane when anaesthesia is induced with thiopentone after suitable premedication than it is when only the gas itself is used

as described in the previous section. Furthermore, premedication and the induction of anaesthesia with thiopentone results in a considerable saving of the rather expensive gas for much less of this is required under these circumstances.

The dose of the ataractic drug used for premedication should be small and no attempt should be made to produce obvious sedation of the animal. The premedication is best given about 1 to $1\frac{1}{2}$ hours before anaesthesia is to be induced, for this will ensure that the animal is not excited when venepuncture is carried out for the injection of the thiopentone. Accurate placing of the needle within the vein is essential before the injection of thiopentone and this is much easier to perform in a tranquillized animal. Premedication can be given by intravenous injection immediately before the induction of anaesthesia but this procedure may itself excite the animal and render the injection of the thiopentone more difficult.

Anaesthesia is induced by the rapid intravenous injection of the usual dose of thiopentone sodium (approximately 11 mg/kg). This dose of thiopentone may not produce sufficient relaxation of the jaw muscles to permit endotracheal intubation to be performed and the usual practice is to follow the injection of the barbiturate with a small dose of a relaxant such as suxamethonium chloride. The syringe which contained the thiopentone is detached from the intravenous needle as soon as the injection is completed and another syringe containing suxamethonium chloride solution attached in its place. The suxamethonium is injected and the needle is withdrawn from the vein. (This procedure is necessary because solutions of thiopentone sodium and suxamethonium chloride will not mix.) The dose of suxamethonium chloride used is of the order of 0·1 to 0·15 mg/kg and does not cause any significant apnoea.

As soon as the horse goes down a cuffed endotracheal tube is introduced into the trachea, the cuff inflated with air and the tube connected to the anaesthetic circuit, the rebreathing bag of which is filled with a mixture of approximately equal parts of cyclopropane and oxygen. Oxygen and cyclopropane are run into the circuit in equal proportions, the expiratory valve is left open and no carbon dioxide absorber is introduced into the circuit until the desired depth of anaesthesia is reached. Once this depth has been attained the expiratory valve is closed, the absorber introduced and the cyclopropane flow turned off. Oxygen is then run into the circuit at such a rate as to keep the rebreathing bag about three-quarters full at the end of each expiration. More cyclopropane may have to be run into the circuit from time to time to maintain an even plane of anaesthesia. Should anaesthesia become too deep respiration fails long before the circulatory system is depressed and all that need be done is to dilute the mixture in the rebreathing bag with oxygen and squeeze the bag to inflate the lungs a few times with the diluted mixture. This results in a rapid lightening of anaesthesia and the return of spontaneous respiration.

At the end of anaesthesia the mouth and pharynx are cleared of any accumulated saliva or mucoid material from the sinuses and the endotracheal tube removed. The horse should be allowed to recover in a padded recovery box or restrained for the first 30 minutes of the recovery period. After this time most animals lie quietly and exhibit no excitement. Unless the horse is lying in a very confined space restraint need not be maintained for longer than this initial part of the recovery period. Most horses make no attempt to stand after the removal of the restraint until they are quite capable of doing so in a completely controlled manner.

The Role of Cyclopropane in Anaesthesia for the Horse

Cyclopropane is a non-irritant gas, so potent that it can be given with high concentrations of oxygen, and it is relatively non-toxic to the cells of the body. Recovery after cyclopropane is rapid and the depth of anaesthesia is under direct and easy control. These advantages, however, are not unaccompanied by disadvantages. Depression of respiration is often severe and the occurrence of apnoea is an embarrassment alike to the horse and to the anaesthetist. The depth of anaesthesia is often difficult to assess for the respiratory signs and muscular signs are not correlated as they are with ether and other volatile agents. Attempts to produce muscular relaxation with cyclopropane may result in apnoea before the required relaxation is attained.

In addition, cyclopropane has many displeasing features. It is explosive and inflammable, and the closed-circuit method of administration calls for a fairly high degree of skill and more or less elaborate and well designed apparatus if good results are to be achieved.

For these reasons it is unlikely that cyclopropane will displace such agents as chloroform, halothane or even ether, from their place in equine anaesthesia. Nevertheless, when the necessary apparatus is available, skilled administration of the gas can provide very smooth well controlled anaesthesia.

2. The Ox

Cyclopropane has proved to be a most useful anaesthetic agent for cattle of all ages and although it is an expensive gas the cost per anaesthetic when it is used in a closed circuit is small. Anaesthesia is easily controlled and recovery is rapid. Best results are achieved when the gas is administered directly to conscious, cast and restrained animals, but it can, of course, also be used as a maintenance agent following the induction of anaesthesia by an intravenous drug. In general, the use of intravenous agents for the induction of anaesthesia in ruminant animals before the administration of cyclopropane is undesirable for they increase the duration of the recovery period. Cattle show no objection to breathing cyclopropane/oxygen mixtures through a face-mask and the induction period is quiet and free from excitement.

The animal is usually restrained in lateral recumbency and a close-fitting face-mask applied. Face-masks designed for dogs are suitable for small calves but a special large malleable rubber latex mask is used in adult animals. The rebreathing bag of the apparatus (circle or to-and-fro absorber system) is filled with a mixture of approximately equal parts of cyclopropane and oxygen and the apparatus connected to the face-mask. The carbon dioxide absorber is not included in the anaesthetic circuit for the induction period and the expiratory valve is left open. Oxygen and cyclopropane are run into the circuit at equal flow rates and no attempt is made to hasten the induction of anaesthesia by increasing the flow rate of the cyclopropane to above that of the oxygen. In calves endotracheal intubation can usually be performed after 4 to 5 minutes, but in adults induction of anaesthesia sufficiently deep to allow intubation usually takes 8 to 10 minutes. During the induction process the animal is observed carefully and if regurgitation occurs the appropriate measures are immediately adopted to prevent aspiration. The cough and laryngeal closure reflexes are usually found to be active when regurgitation occurs during the induction of cyclopropane anaesthesia and all that need be done is to clear the mouth, pharynx and posterior nares of the regurgitated material as quickly as possible before proceeding with the administration of the anaesthetic.

After intubation the tube is connected to the anaesthetic apparatus, the expiratory valve closed and the carbon dioxide absorber introduced into the circuit. The oxygen flow rate is reduced to one which ensures that the rebreathing bag neither empties nor becomes over full and further cyclopropane is added as required to produce the desired depth of anaesthesia.

If prolonged anaesthesia is contemplated no time should be lost in puncturing the rumen through the left body wall with a trochar and cannula. The trochar is withdrawn and the cannula left in the rumen. It is better to perform this operation early on in the anaesthestic rather than be forced to carry it out as an emergency measure later on for the relief of an established tympany.

Once the administration of the anaesthetic is terminated, recovery is rapid. The endotracheal tube is left in the trachea with the cuff still inflated and manipulated at intervals until its manipulation causes the animal to cough. As soon as coughing is provoked by this manoeuvre the tube is withdrawn without prior deflation of the cuff.

In cattle, as in other animals, the depth of cyclopropane anaesthesia is often difficult to assess, for the respiratory signs and muscular signs are not corre-lated as they are with ether and the other volatile anaesthetic agents. Further-more, when anaesthesia is induced with an intravenous barbiturate the respira-tion is sometimes so depressed by small concentrations of cyclopropane that adequate anaesthesia is difficult to obtain. In spite of these disadvantages, however, the gas is a most useful anaesthetic for cattle. The quiet induction and rapid recovery associated with this gas make it a most desirable agent for bovine anaesthesia. In particular, the smooth quiet respiratory movements which are characteristic features of well administered cyclopropane anaes-thesia result in good operating conditions for intra-abdominal surgery. The only real contra-indication to the use of cyclopropane when the necessary apparatus is available is where diathermy or other electrical apparatus is to be used during the anaesthetic period.

3. The Sheep and Goat

In recent years cyclopropane has become a popular anaesthetic for sheep and goats of all ages. In these animals induction of anaesthesia is quiet, the depth of anaesthesia can be varied with ease, and recovery is rapid. Most sheep and goats are easily restrained; they do not resent the application of a face-mask nor do they object to breathing mixtures of cyclopropane and oxygen. Thus in the majority of instances there is no need to induce anaesthesia by the administration of an intravenous agent such as thiopentone sodium before cyclopropane is given.

The animal is restrained on its side and oxygen and cyclopropane are administered from a closed-circuit apparatus through a well fitting face-mask. Either a to-and-fro or a circle type apparatus may be used and during the induction of anaesthesia the absorber is excluded from the anaesthetic circuit and the expiratory valve is left open. Anaesthesia is induced with a mixture of equal parts of cyclopropane and oxygen and as soon as consciousness is lost the animal is turned on to its back in preparation for the performance of endotracheal intubation. Anaesthesia is deepened almost to the point of respiratory failure, the face-mask removed, the pharynx cleared of saliva and any regurgitated ingesta, and endotracheal intubation performed with a cuffed tube. The cuff of the tube is inflated with air, the tube connected to the anaesthetic apparatus and the flow of cyclopropane turned off. The expiratory valve is closed and the carbon dioxide absorber introduced into the circuit. The oxygen flow rate is adjusted so that the rebreathing bag neither empties nor becomes overdistended. Further cyclopropane is run into the circuit as required to produce and maintain the desired plane of anaesthesia. The animal should be positioned so that the head slopes downward to allow saliva to run out of the mouth.

Anaesthesia can be maintained almost indefinitely and it will be found that as time passes further small additions of cyclopropane will be required. Chewing or swallowing movements indicate that anaesthesia is too light while if anaesthesia becomes too deep respiration ceases. Should respiration cease the mixture in the rebreathing bag is diluted with oxygen and the bag gently compressed to produce rhythmical inflation of the lungs; breathing soon recommences.

Anaesthesia is terminated by disconnecting the endotracheal tube from the anaesthetic circuit. The tube is left with its cuff inflated in the trachea until the animal shows signs of coughing and swallowing. As soon as vigorous coughing is seen the tube is withdrawn from the trachea with its cuff still inflated. Even after prolonged anaesthesia the animal will be fully conscious within 15 minutes of the termination of the anaesthetic.

When anaesthesia has been induced with cyclopropane, endotracheal intubation must be performed rapidly for anaesthesia lightens very quickly once the mask is removed from the face. In these circumstances inexperienced anaesthetists may find intubation difficult and those who are not familiar with endotracheal intubation in sheep and goats may be well advised to induce anaesthesia with an intravenous agent such as thiopentone sodium or even pentobarbitone sodium. The use of such intravenous agents allows endotracheal intubation to be performed at leisure *but* it also prolongs the recovery from anaesthesia.

4. The Pig

In pigs cyclopropane anaesthesia presents no special features and, as always, it is given by closed-circuit methods. In small pigs the usual procedure is to induce anaesthesia with the gas, delivering it through a face-mask, but in large pigs anaesthesia is usually induced with an intravenous agent. Although the gas can be administered through a face-mask throughout the period of anaesthesia it is perhaps easier if the pig is intubated and the gas given through the endotracheal tube. The presence of the endotracheal tube protects the patency of the airway but its introduction requires some skill.

Recovery is rapid but some pigs vomit after cyclopropane anaesthesia. No pig should be left unattended until it has regained consciousness.

Nitrous Oxide

1. The Horse

Although nitrous oxide is a very weak agent it can be used in horses to maintain anaesthesia. The anaesthetic state is induced after suitable premedication by the rapid intravenous injection of a small dose of thiopentone sodium, and nitrous oxide and oxygen are then administered through a close-fitting face-mask or endotracheal tube. For the best results the gas has to be used in such a way that nitrogen is eliminated from the body and anaesthetic circuit and the animal is saturated with the anaesthetic agent. In order to produce this elimination of nitrogen the inspired mixture must not be diluted with air and rebreathing must be prevented by the use of non-return expiratory valves and high gas flow rates (equal to, or greater than, the minute volume of respiration) for about the first 20 minutes of the anaesthetic period.

Horses have a large respiratory minute volume and the quantity of nitrous oxide which has to be used to produce denitrogenation and saturation of the animal is correspondingly large. Since even quite small horses have respiratory minute volumes of 50 litres, if a mixture containing 70% of nitrous oxide and 30% of oxygen is to be given, the anaesthetic apparatus used must be capable of delivering at least 35 litres/minute of nitrous oxide and 15 litres/minute of oxygen. There is no standard apparatus which will deliver these gases at these high flow rates and thus if nitrous oxide is to be used really effectively in horses special apparatus must be used. Such apparatus not being readily available the usual practice is to use a nitrous oxide/oxygen mixture to volatilize one of the volatile anaesthetic agents and utilize a semi-closed system with carbon dioxide absorption to allow rebreathing of the mixture and, therefore, lower flow rates to be used. The volatile agents reinforce the anaesthetic action of nitrous oxide and denitrogenation of the animal is not so important.

Nitrous oxide/oxygen mixtures may be used to volatilize chloroform or halothane when these volatile agents are given by semi-closed methods of administration (see page 260). The nitrous oxide makes a significant contribution to the production of anaesthesia and less of the volatile drug is needed than when oxygen alone is used as the volatilizing agent. Trichloroethylene (Trilene) must not be used with nitrous oxide in this manner for it decomposes when it comes into contact with warm moist soda lime in a carbon dioxide absorber and toxic products are formed.

In horses, as indeed in all animals, the disadvantage of nitrous oxide are its lack of potency, its inability to produce muscle relaxation, its tendency to be associated with asphyxia in the hands of the unskilled, and the necessity of expensive and more or less elaborate apparatus for its administration. Nevertheless, when used in horses with skill and discretion, nitrous oxide has many advantages. It is non-explosive, non-inflammable and, in the absence of asphyxia, non-toxic. The judicious use of thiopentone sodium and other agents in combination with nitrous oxide can provide excellent operating conditions in horses with minimal post-anaesthetic effects.

2. The Ox

Anaesthesia can be induced in cattle of all ages with nitrous oxide/oxygen mixtures but denitrogenation of the animal is essential (see page 368) and induction of light surgical anaesthesia in adult animals takes some 8 to 10 minutes. Usually, nitrous oxide/oxygen mixtures are only used to maintain anaesthesia following induction with an intravenous agent such as a barbiturate.

Anaesthesia is induced, the animal intubated with a cuffed endotracheal tube and the nitrous oxide/oxygen mixture administered by a semi-closed method with carbon dioxide absorption. Maintenance of satisfactory anaesthesia with nitrous oxide/oxygen alone requires some skill and the judicious introduction of small quantities of ether, chloroform, halothane or cyclopropane into the anaesthetic circuit makes the task much more easily accomplished. Provided that only minimal quantities of the intravenous drug and supplementary agents have been used recovery is smooth and extremely rapid. When anaesthesia has been induced with nitrous oxide the animal usually regains its feet within 10 minutes of the termination of the anaesthetic.

3. The Sheep and Goat

In sheep and goats nitrous oxide is often used to maintain anaesthesia induced by an intravenous barbiturate drug. Anaesthesia is induced, the animal intubated with a cuffed endotracheal tube and a mixture of nitrous oxide and oxygen administered from a semi-closed circuit. Either a Magill attachment or a semi-closed system with carbon dioxide absorption may be used. Nitrous oxide is run into the circuit at a rate of 6 litres/minute and oxygen at the rate of 3 litres/minute.

Quite commonly the mixture is supplemented by the addition of minimal quantities of halothane, ether, trichloroethylene, methoxyflurane or even chloroform. (N.B.—Trichloroethylene should not be used when the anaesthetic circuit contains soda lime.)

4. The Pig

The sequence of premedication, induction with thiopentone sodium, endotracheal intubation under a relaxant, and the maintenance of anaesthesia by endotracheal semi-closed administration of nitrous oxide has proved to be a very satisfactory method for lengthy experimental surgical procedures in pigs of all ages. By this system very light anaesthesia is maintained and relaxation is produced as required by the administration of relaxant drugs. Recovery from anaesthesia is rapid.

Obviously this technique is not designed for use in the field and it can only be properly applied by a skilled, experienced anaesthetist.

REFERENCES

DOUGLAS, T. A., JENNINGS, S., LONGSTREETH, J. and WEAVER, A. D. (1964). *Vet. Rec.* **76**, 615
GUEDEL, A. E. (1937). *Inhalation Anaesthesia.* London: Macmillan
HENKELS, P. (1938). *Dt. tierärztl. Wschr.* **46**, 801.
LONGLEY, E. O. (1950). *Vet. Rec.* **62**, 30
WATERS, R. M. (1951). *Chloroform. A Study after 100 Years.* Madison: Univ. Wisconsin Press

18

Inhalation Anaesthesia in the Dog and Cat

In dogs and cats the chief disadvantage of the inhalation anaesthetic agents is the unpleasant induction period which may be associated with their use. In the early days of canine anaesthesia attempts were made to overcome this disadvantage by the use of heavy sedation with morphine but in spite of this sedation the induction of anaesthesia often remained an unpleasant, prolonged and dangerous procedure. Today, this disadvantage may be completely mitigated by inducing anaesthesia with very small quantities of intravenous drugs such as the thiobarbiturates. With these intravenous drugs induction of anaesthesia is rapid, pleasant and safe for the animal. The contra-indications to the use of very small doses of intravenous drugs in this manner are very few and there is seldom any need to subject domestic pets to what may become an unpleasant and dangerous experience of induction by an inhalation anaesthetic agent.

A wide variety of inhalation agents is used in canine and feline anaesthesia and all are reasonably safe and satisfactory if used correctly. The choice of agent or agents in any particular case is largely governed by the anaesthetist's knowledge of the limitations of each agent and, of course, by the apparatus, assistance and drugs available at the time.

Nitrous Oxide

It is generally agreed that dogs and cats cannot be anaesthetized with un-supplemented mixtures of nitrous oxide and oxygen without invoking the aid of hypoxia. Thus in canine and feline anaesthesia nitrous oxide is employed only for major surgical procedures where it can be used with other agents and where adequate oxygenation can be assured.

Nitrous oxide is used in a semi-closed system either:

(i) As a vehicle for the vaporization and delivery of ether, trichloro-ethylene and other volatile anaesthetic agents. The proportion of oxygen in the mixture—provided it is at least 30%—is unimportant, because the maintenance of anaesthesia does not depend on the potency of nitrous oxide.

or:

(ii) In conjunction with thiopentone, pethidine and other analgesic supplements, and with muscle relaxants, for maintaining a light plane of anaesthesia. In these circumstances the proportion of oxygen in the nitrous oxide/oxygen mixture delivered to the animal becomes of great importance and two factors must be considered.

To make the most of the advantages offered by nitrous oxide it must not be diluted with nitrogen or oxygen, and the oxygen concentration in the respired mixture must only be sufficient to satisfy the animal's metabolic requirements. The animal must be saturated with nitrous oxide; this can only occur after nitrogen has been eliminated from the body and the time needed for this to occur depends upon five factors:

(a) the degree of ventilation of the lungs,
(b) the solubility of nitrous oxide in the blood, brain and tissues,
(c) the flow of gases delivered to the animal,
(d) the percentage of nitrous oxide in the respired mixture,
(e) the tension of nitrogen in the respired mixture.

In practice, for economy, nitrous oxide/oxygen mixtures are usually given in a semi-closed system with carbon dioxide absorption and satisfactory de-nitrogenation of dogs can be achieved in under 4 minutes using a total gas flow rate of 4 litres/minute.

The second factor which must be considered is that although the percentage of oxygen in the mixture leaving the anaesthetic machine may appear to be adequate, the actual concentration inhaled by the animal may fall below the minimum required. This is because even when the animal is fully saturated with nitrous oxide it still requires oxygen for its metabolic processes. This point may be illustrated by considering a hypothetical example of an animal which is fully saturated with nitrous oxide breathing into a closed system. If this animal consumes oxygen at the rate of 200 ml/minute and oxygen and nitrous oxide are both fed into the circuit at the rate of 250 ml/minute then the oxygen content of the gases actually respired will be

$$\frac{250-200}{250+(250-200)} \times 100$$

or approximately 16·6% although the flowmeter readings indicate that a mixture containing 50% oxygen is being supplied to the animal. The smaller the total gas flow from the machine, the larger must be the proportion of oxygen in the mixture.

The Administration of Nitrous Oxide and Oxygen

Nitrous oxide is always administered in a semi-closed system and it is important that the mixtures of nitrous oxide and oxygen should not be diluted with air. In dogs such dilution is usually prevented by delivering the mixture through a cuffed endotracheal tube for it is not often possible to obtain an airtight fit between the face and a mask. Masks are usually quite adequate in cats for a good fit between the mask and the face is easily achieved.

Satisfactory results may be obtained when nitrous oxide/oxygen mixtures are used to maintain anaesthesia which has been induced by the intravenous injection of thiopentone sodium following well chosen premedication. In many cases, however, the degree of surgical stimulation produced by the operative procedure is sufficiently marked as to make the animal restless when nitrous oxide and oxygen alone are employed. This restlessness often proves to be an embarrassment both to the surgeon and the anaesthetist. In these circumstances the anaesthetist is often tempted to introduce a degree of hypoxia into the administration of the anaesthetic, but this temptation should always be resisted. Better methods are available which provide smooth anaesthesia without sacrificing the benefits of nitrous oxide.

The simplest and safest method of obtaining smooth anaesthesia is to supplement the basal nitrous oxide/oxygen mixture with ether vapour. Since this vapour is pungent and tends to make animals cough, it is better to employ it from the beginning rather than try to introduce it in the middle of an operation. As soon as the animal has been connected to the anaesthetic circuit the gases are made to flow through the ether bottle in such a way that the concentration of ether is minimal. After a few breaths the concentration of ether is steadily increased until first-plane anaesthesia is reached. If the operation does not necessitate the production of muscle relaxation the ether is then turned off and only added again if necessary to control movement of the animal. If, on the other hand, muscle relaxation is required, the administration of the ether is continued until deep second-plane anaesthesia is reached. The ether concentration is then reduced but the ether is not turned off. The degree of muscle relaxation is altered as indicated by the requirements of the operative procedure by varying the concentration of ether delivered to the animal.

Methoxyflurane is also a useful supplement. It is both non-explosive and non-inflammable and by its use reasonably good muscle relaxation can be obtained. It is extremely difficult to administer an overdose of methoxyflurane, so supplementation of nitrous/oxide with this agent is a particularly safe procedure.

Trichloroethylene (Trilene) may be used in a similar way. It has the advantage of being non-explosive and non-inflammable but it cannot be used to produce muscle relaxation. When given in concentrations of over 1% trichloroethylene produces tachypnoea and cardiac irregularities but when given in minimal quantities as an adjuvant to nitrous oxide/oxygen mixtures it seldom causes these undesirable effects.

During nitrous oxide/oxygen anaesthesia small quantities of thiopentone sodium may be injected intravenously to control movement of the animal. In order to prevent the injection of greater quantities than are necessary to achieve the desired object, a $2\frac{1}{2}\%$ solution of the drug should be employed. Carefully and intelligently used this technique is most effective but because thiopentone can be shown to have an anti-analgesic effect some anaesthetists prefer to use pethidine. In dogs, the technique of induction with thiopentone sodium, followed by nitrous oxide/oxygen (allowing at least 30% oxygen in the respired mixture) supplemented by the intravenous injection of 20 to 30 mg of pethidine hydrochloride as required is very satisfactory. A muscle relaxant may be used with this technique if abdominal section is to be performed or the thorax opened. Recovery is rapid when this technique is used and there seems to be the minimum of post-anaesthetic nausea and hang-over for if their surgical condition allows it most dogs will eat a normal meal soon after regaining consciousness.

A mild condition of anoxic anoxia may occur in the period immediately following prolonged nitrous oxide/oxygen anaesthesia. It is due to the outward diffusion of nitrous oxide from the pulmonary blood lowering the partial pressure of oxygen in the alveolar air. Although this type of anoxia is rarely severe its clinical significance may well be important in ill animals. It can be simply prevented by administering oxygen to the animal for 5 to 10 minutes from the time that anaesthesia ceases.

Cyclopropane

Cyclopropane with oxygen is a satisfactory alternative to nitrous oxide and oxygen for all canine and feline surgery. Its advantages are an increased potency, with consequently better surgical conditions in the absence of any suggestion of hypoxia, and greater ease of administration. To set against these advantages there is the occurrence of vomiting after anaesthesia, slow recovery if the administration is protracted, and the risk of explosions in certain circumstances.

In view of the high cost of the gas it is always used in a closed system with carbon dioxide absorption for operations of more than brief duration. The various planes and stages of anaesthesia (see page 195) cannot be satisfactorily applied to cyclopropane anaesthesia because even in small concentrations it is a potent respiratory depressant. As anaesthesia deepens so the respiratory exchange diminishes. The amount of premedication, the dose of the agent used for induction and the efficiency of the carbon dioxide absorption will influence the progress of anaesthesia. If the premedication has been unduly heavy, or the dose of the drug used for induction unduly large, cyclopropane will produce apnoea without adequately suppressing reflexes, so that even minor surgery will be impossible.

If anaesthesia of a depth sufficient to produce reasonable muscular relaxation is to be induced a gradually increasing concentration of cyclopropane must be given to avoid early respiratory depression. The inhalation of high concentrations leads to rapid accumulation in the brain without any marked effect on the other tissues of the body. If, at this point, the cyclopropane is turned off, then redistribution gradually takes place between the brain and tissues; thus anaesthesia becomes light again.

In most instances cyclopropane is administered to animals only after anaesthesia has been induced with a thiobarbiturate given by intravenous injection. However, in cats and in small or very ill dogs anaesthesia may be induced with cyclopropane. The animal is restrained in the prone position and the rebreathing bag of the anaesthetic circuit half-filled with oxygen. The face-mask is applied and with 200 ml/minute of oxygen entering the circuit, cyclopropane is administered at a rate of 500 to 750 ml/minute until anaesthesia is established. The flow of cyclopropane is then stopped completely. The oxygen flow rate is adjusted so that the rebreathing bag neither empties nor becomes over distended and further cyclopropane is only added as necessary to maintain the desired plane of anaesthesia. For short operations endotracheal intubation is unnecessary but the face-mask must fit sufficiently well to prevent leakage around its edges. For longer operations a cuffed endotracheal tube is passed as soon as possible and the gas administered through the tube. Induction of anaesthesia is usually quiet apart from a very short period of narcotic excitement once consciousness is lost. This simple technique is, of course, applicable whichever of the two systems of carbon dioxide absorption is used.

Increased capillary bleeding, or oozing, is a well-known feature of cyclopropane anaesthesia in man and it also appears to occur in dogs and cats. There is a strong clinical impression that oozing is more severe under light than under deep anaesthesia. The mechanism involved is not understood but the oozing may be due to a direct action of the gas on the blood vessels or to the liberation of a humoral vasodilator.

Cardiac arrhythmias are commonplace during cyclopropane anaesthesia, particularly if high concentrations are given rapidly. They are usually ventricular in origin and occur as isolated or multifocal extrasystoles. The exact mechanism by which these disturbances are produced is not clearly understood but it is believed that cyclopropane may act in a number of ways. It is postulated that cyclopropane has some specific action on the myocardium bringing about a displacement of the pacemaker, interference with conduction in the bundle of His and an increased local excitability in the ventricles. Ectopic beats may be initiated by the injection of adrenaline or by adrenaline liberated within the body. However, it is generally agreed today that the appearance of cardiac irregularities during cyclopropane anaesthesia is most commonly due to the accumulation of carbon dioxide in the body as a result of respiratory depression. Restoration of adequate pulmonary ventilation by intermittent pressure on the rebreathing bag usually results in a prompt return to normal cardiac rhythm.

The accumulation of carbon dioxide in the body as a result of the respiratory depression caused by cyclopropane is probably also responsible for a condition known as cyclopropane shock. This condition is sometimes seen after a long operation under cyclopropane anaesthesia. The animal becomes cold with pale mucous membranes and a weak, slow pulse. The use of an absorption technique during anaesthesia will not result in the elimination of carbon dioxide from the body when breathing is shallow. At the end of operation when anaesthesia is terminated, the breathing increases in depth so that the carbon dioxide tension in the body falls rapidly and the circulation, hitherto artificially stimulated, collapses. Adequate artificial respiration to counter any respiratory depression can prevent the occurrence of this type of shock.

In dogs and cats cyclopropane is sometimes used to enable the anaesthetist to control the respiration for intrathoracic surgery. The essential features of the technique are the abolition of natural respiratory movements, and their substitution by rhythmic manual compression of the rebreathing bag sufficiently frequently and vigorously enough to maintain a good tidal exchange. The animal's spontaneous respiration is depressed primarily by the premedication, the induction dose of thiopentone or similar agent (if one has been used for this purpose) and the cyclopropane acting upon the respiratory centre. Apnoea is produced by lowering the tension of carbon dioxide in the blood to a level where it no longer excites the depressed respiratory centre. The tension of carbon dioxide in the blood is reduced by manual compression of the rebreathing bag as the animal breathes in. This manoeuvre augments the tidal volume, and the corresponding exhalations which follow wash out carbon dioxide which is then absorbed by the soda lime. When the lungs are hyperventilated in this way the alveolar tension of carbon dioxide is lowered until a point is reached when the tension of this gas in the blood no longer excites the respiratory centre. Respiration is then under the full control of the anaesthetist. At the end of the operation the absorber is removed from the anaesthetic circuit, carbon dioxide accumulates and spontaneous breathing soon returns.

The accidental production of respiratory arrest is not uncommon during cyclopropane anaesthesia in dogs and cats. When it occurs, the expiratory valve should be opened, any flow of cyclopropane which may be entering the circuit turned off and the oxygen flow rate increased to 1·5 to 2 litres/minute. Rhythmical manual compression of the rebreathing bag at a rate of 12 to 15 times/minute quickly results in a lowering of the cyclopropane content of the body and spontaneous breathing returns. As soon as adequate spontaneous respiration is re-established the circuit may be closed again, the oxygen reduced to the basal flow and if, as frequently happens, the level of anaesthesia has become too light, a small flow of cyclopropane may be run into the circuit until the necessary depth has been reached.

After deep and prolonged anaesthesia dogs and cats may on regaining consciousness vomit several times. There appear to be no other undesirable sequelae. A minor practical point regarding operations under cyclopropane is that administration must be continued until completion, for recovery may be so rapid that even the insertion of the last few sutures can cause embarrassment if the anaesthetic has been discontinued.

Ether

A dog or cat can be anaesthetized with ether by any of the four standard methods, namely open, semi-open, semi-closed and closed with carbon dioxide absorption.

Open ether is not a powerful anaesthetic method, and in practice the semi-open method is almost invariably used in preference to the completely open one. This is because some 16 to 18% of ether vapour is required to induce anaesthesia, while it is not easy to obtain more than 14% from an open mask.

When ether is dropped on to a gauze stretched over a wire-frame face-mask it is vaporized not only by the inspirations but also by the expirations of the animal; indeed, more is vaporized by the latter than by the former, since the expired air is warmer than that inspired. The resulting vapour does not rise to any great distance from the surface of the gauze, nor does it mix rapidly with the air of the room; its density causes it to flow down on to the floor. By various devices a large part of this vapour of expiration can be retained around the mask so that it is inhaled with the next inspiration thus reducing the quantity of ether which has to be used. One method of conserving ether vapour is by means of a folded towel, pinned at one corner, so as to form a cone. The cone is applied over the mask and face and the ether is dropped through its upper aperture on to the gauze of the face-mask. A more common practice is to convert the system to a semi-open one in another way, i.e. by covering the top of the mask with a square of Gamgee tissue which has a hole in the centre, so that ether can be dropped on to the underlying mask. (See Fig. 93, page 251.)

The following points may be made about the administration of ether by semi-open methods:

(a) Ether may be safely given to animals after premedication with any of the drugs mentioned in Chapter 9, and after the induction of unconsciousness by the use of any intravenous agent.

(b) After placing the face cover of Gamgee in position (Fig. 93) the mask should be held 2 or 3 inches away from the face and 1 or 2 drops of ether allowed to fall on the mask. This accustoms the animal to the smell of mild ether vapour and is not a waste of time—it often saves time.

(c) Administration is begun with a drop rate of 1 drop every 3 or 4 seconds and the mask lowered on to the face. If there is any reaction such as coughing or breath-holding the mask is raised off the Gamgee for a few seconds and then reapplied. Ether should be dropped over the whole surface of the mask, not only on one part of it. This prevents freezing. The drop rate is increased to about 1 drop/second and should any reflex stimulation occur the mask is raised from the Gamgee and reapplied as necessary until reflex stimulation ceases.

(d) After about 3 minutes the second piece of Gamgee is applied to diminish air entry and so concentrate the ether vapour.

If the foregoing instructions are followed, the amount of ether employed will not be excessive. Induction will be fairly smooth but all animals will need to be adequately restrained unless unconsciousness is induced with an intravenous agent before ether is exhibited. The attainment of full surgical anaesthesia is often announced audibly, particularly in cats, by the commencement of gentle blowing noises on expiration.

When ether is given by semi-closed methods the vapour is carried over to the dog or cat by a stream of oxygen or nitrous oxide and oxygen. As vaporization of the ether proceeds so the temperature of the liquid ether falls, which in turn slows the rate of vaporization. If, therefore, the control of the vaporizer bottle is set to deliver a strong concentration of ether there is a steady reduction in the vapour concentration as time passes. Visible evidence of this is the formation of ice on the outside of the ether container, due to freezing of moisture from the air in the immediate vicinity. For semi-closed administration the ether vapour may be delivered through a Magill attachment or an absorber unit.

The vaporization of ether in a closed system depends on the particular type of apparatus used. When it is to-and-fro vaporization is exactly as in the semi-closed system, but owing to the small basal flow of oxygen only low concentrations of ether can be obtained. In the circle system the whole of the respired gases can be passed through an ether bottle so that high concentrations of ether can be built up relatively quickly.

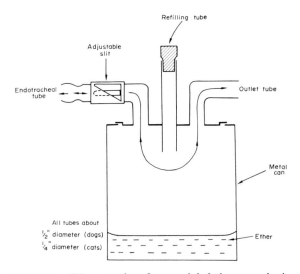

Fig. 138.—Ether container for auto-inhalation anaesthesia.

A simple auto-inhalation method for the administration of ether to dogs and cats was introduced by Hardenburgh and Mann in 1927, and has since been extensively employed for physiological experiments, especially when prolonged anaesthesia is required. The ether container comprises a metal can of 250 to 500 ml capacity closed by an airtight lid (glass containers are unsatisfactory because they are bad conductors of heat). The lid is fitted with three tubes which do not project into the interior (Fig. 138). One tube serves for the addition of ether while the other two are inlet and outlet tubes. The tube conducting the anaesthetic to the animal carries an adjustable slit so that the amount of inspired air drawn from the container can be regulated as required. For cats an ether container of 50 ml capacity should be used. Light anaesthesia is induced by the rapid intravenous injection of a barbiturate and the animal is then intubated with a cuffed endotracheal tube. The endotracheal tube is connected to the apparatus and the slit adjusted until the desired depth of anaesthesia is achieved and maintained. This method is simple and almost foolproof but vaporization of the ether decreases as the temperature of the container falls. This can be overcome by placing the ether can in a hot water bath but it must be borne in mind that by so doing the amount of ether vapour being inhaled is immediately increased and provision made accordingly. Although this technique of auto-inhalation of ether will provide satisfactory anaesthesia, better results are obtained by semi-closed or closed methods of administration, for unless a non-return valve is incorporated in the system auto-inhalation entails a considerable degree of rebreathing which results in hypoxia and carbon dioxide retention.

The Role of Ether in Canine and Feline Anaesthesia

For very many years ether has been administered to dogs and cats both by simple, rather crude, methods and by more refined techniques and has proved itself to be a very useful anaesthetic agent for these animals. The objective in the administration of any anaesthetic is not only to produce unconsciousness but also to suppress the reflex activity of the animal to just a sufficient degree to enable a particular operation to be performed. Modern anaesthetic techniques often go far beyond this, but ether remains the safest and most effective means of gradually producing suppression of reflexes in dogs and cats. As with any other agent, the success of any method of administration depends largely on the ability of the anaesthetist. An experienced anaesthetist can safely administer ether by various means.

Chloroform

It is generally agreed that chloroform is not a safe anaesthetic agent for dogs although no figures are available as to the mortality resulting from chloroform anaesthesia. In cats the use of chloroform is usually regarded as being even more dangerous than in dogs.

The main advantages of chloroform are a sweet-smelling, non-irritant, potent vapour, portability and non-inflammability. Low volatility and a high potency make it particularly valuable in tropical climates, while the fact that an experienced administrator can produce excellent surgical conditions using only a small bottle and a handkerchief or piece of gauze has done much to recommend it in the past. Nevertheless, despite all these advantages chloroform has fallen into disuse. Today most, if not all, of the advantages of chloroform can be obtained by the use of a combination of other agents with less risk to the life of the animal. Only on an occasion where there is no possible alternative, such as may occur unexpectedly in the field, should chloroform now be used as an anaesthetic agent for dogs and cats.

Halothane

Halothane may be administered to dogs and cats by any one of the four standard methods, namely open, semi-open, semi-closed and closed with carbon dioxide absorption. However, it is rather costly and in practice only semi-closed or closed methods are employed.

Because of its potency and because it is well tolerated by the respiratory tract halothane is often used alone as an anaesthetic agent for dogs and cats. The animal is restrained and anaesthesia induced using a face-mask, the halothane being vaporized and delivered to the animal by a stream of oxygen or nitrous oxide–oxygen mixture. In small dogs and in cats induction of anaesthesia is rapid and the duration of the period of narcotic excitement is

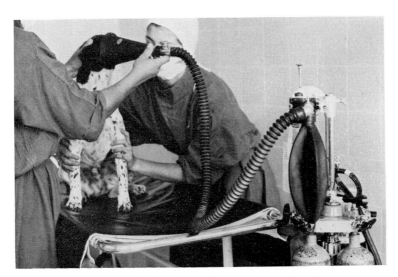

Fig. 139.—Induction of halothane anaesthesia in a dog.
Only the minimum of restraint is usually required.

brief. In larger dogs induction and the narcotic excitement stage are more prolonged and it is usually advisable to give a minimal sleep dose of thiopentone sodium by intravenous injection before halothane is used.

Halothane is extremely potent and anaesthesia is often difficult to control, for small alterations in the concentration of the vapour being respired result in quite gross alterations in the depth of anaesthesia. Even experienced anaesthetists find it difficult to control anaesthesia when halothane is given by completely closed circuit methods. No attempt should be made to produce profound muscle relaxation by increasing the depth of halothane anaesthesia for this results in a severe fall in blood pressure and marked respiratory depression. Because of the respiratory depressant properties of the drug only minimal premedication and the smallest possible quantity of thiopentone should be given prior to the use of halothane.

Cardiac arrhythmias occur quite frequently in cats under halothane anaesthesia (Fig. 140) but much less commonly in dogs. When they occur they can usually be abolished and normal rhythm restored by the performance of artificial respiration to increase the gaseous exchange in the lungs. It appears that the respiratory depressant activity of halothane allows carbon dioxide to accumulate in the body and once the concentration of carbon dioxide exceeds

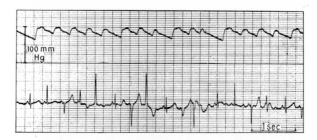

FIG. 140.—Cardiac irregularity in a cat under halothane anaesthesia.
Upper tracing: Arterial blood pressure.
Lower tracing: Lead II E.C.G.

a certain threshold value arrhythmias occur. Lowering the carbon dioxide content of the body by artificial respiration is followed by a return to normal cardiac rhythm.

Halothane lends itself to supplementation of the thiopentone/nitrous oxide/oxygen sequence, particularly when spontaneous respiration is desirable, since very small concentrations produce a good result without marked side-effects. When deeper anaesthesia or more marked muscle relaxation is required it is probably better to substitute ether or use a muscle relaxant drug rather than increase the inspired concentration of halothane to above 3%. Gallamine, aleuronium, pancuronium and suxamethonium may be used with halothane but d-tubocurarine must not be used as it accentuates the hypotensive properties of halothane.

Like any other potent volatile anaesthetic agent, halothane is best administered from a calibrated vaporizer (see page 273) so that the approximate concentration delivered to the animal is known. In any case it is important that the anaesthetist should be fully acquainted with the actual concentrations delivered by any vaporizer which is used. Most ether vaporizers are unsuitable for use with halothane as there is great difficulty in obtaining a constant vapour concentration from them. (See page 272.) Much more accurate control of anaesthesia is obtained by the use of an end-tidal sampling device in conjunction with a rapid analyser such as a Hook and Tucker halothane meter, and the type of vaporizer used, provided it will deliver an adequate concentration of halothane, is then unimportant. However, although these rather expensive items of equipment may be justified for research purposes, it seems highly unlikely that they will ever feature in routine veterinary anaesthesia.

Dogs and cats recover quickly after halothane anaesthesia and at the present time halothane seems the best agent for anaesthetizing animals which have to be returned as soon as possible to their owners.

Trichloroethylene

The fact that trichloroethylene is non-inflammable, almost non-irritant to the respiratory tract, and produces only minimal side-effects, has made it popular as a supplement to the sequence thiopentone/nitrous oxide/oxygen in dogs and cats. Used in this way for the maintenance of light anaesthesia its analgesic properties are most valuable. Its chief disadvantage in general surgery is that it is unsuitable for the production of muscle relaxation, since when any attempt is made to achieve this tachypnoea and cardiac irregularities are quickly encountered. Nevertheless, within the safe limits of its application it is a useful agent.

Almost every known form of cardiac irregularity has been observed in dogs and cats during trichloroethylene anaesthesia but only when high concentrations of the vapour have been employed. Cardiac arrhythmias are also likely to be encountered if adrenaline is used during anaesthesia so that ischaemia of the surgical field should not be produced by the infiltration of dilute solutions of adrenaline.

A strong caution must be given against the use of trichloroethylene in any form of anaesthetic circuit which incorporates an absorber unit. In the presence of alkali the heat generated in the absorber causes the breakdown of trichloroethylene to toxic products such as dichloroacetylene.

Trichloroethylene is usually administered from a Boyle type vaporizer bottle. It is volatilized and delivered to the animal by a stream of oxygen or nitrous oxide–oxygen mixture. When the plunger of the vaporizing bottle is fully withdrawn and the control tap is set to full on, a total gas flow rate of 6 to 8 litres/minute will deliver a concentration of 0·8 to 1·0% of trichloroethylene vapour. No attempt should be made to obtain a greater concentration by lowering the plunger over the J-tube and if deeper anaesthesia is required resort should be made to another agent, for concentrations of trichloroethylene over 1·0% are not safe. The onset of tachypnoea during anaesthesia is not a sign of awakening; it is usually an indication for reducing the inspired concentration of trichloroethylene.

Divinyl Ether

Divinyl ether has a relatively low stability and when it is chemically pure it is so volatile that it is difficult to use for anaesthesia. For this reason 3·5% of absolute alcohol is added to diminish volatility. A non-volatile organic base, phenyl-alpha-naphthylamine, in a concentration of 0·01% is also added to improve the stability. In the United Kingdom the commercial product is known as Vinesthene (May & Baker Ltd.). It is best purchased in ampoules of 3 ml or 5 ml.

Vinesthene has a more rapid action than ethyl ether; it is a useful agent for the induction of anaesthesia and as a supplement to nitrous oxide and oxygen. It does not irritate the respiratory tract and the change over from Vinesthene to ethyl ether, after the former has been used for induction, is very easy.

Vinesthene is both very volatile and expensive, so that its clinical use is restricted. It is usually only employed as an induction agent which, because of its rapidity of action and ease of administration may often advantageously precede general anaesthesia with ether in cats. In any case, divinyl ether can cause central lobular necrosis of the liver if used in high concentrations for prolonged periods so that it should never be used for more than 20 to 30 minutes at one administration.

The important advantages of Vinesthene include a rapid induction of anaesthesia without marked excitement, the production of muscle relaxation equal to that obtained with ether much more rapidly, absence of post-anaesthetic vomiting and a quick recovery. Certain of the properties of vinyl ether, however, are such that they must be regarded as disadvantages. Because of its potency overdosage is easily given; this disadvantage, however, is soon overcome by practice. Maintenance of anaesthesia over long periods requires skill and practice. The explosive and fire risks of Vinesthene are approximately the same as those of other inflammable agents such as ether, cyclopropane and ethyl chloride. The same precautions are necessary with Vinesthene as with these other agents.

Vinesthene may be given by open or semi-open methods but because of its volatility it is difficult to maintain an even plane of anaesthesia and the quantity required makes the procedure uneconomical. These disadvantages have been overcome by the employment of a mixture containing 1 part of vinyl ether to 3 parts of ethyl ether. The use of this mixture also overcomes the disadvantages of ether when used alone, particularly when a large dog has to be anaesthetized. This mixture is sold under the name of Vam (May &

Baker Ltd.). Although Vam is primarily intended for open or semi-open administration it may also be used by closed or semi-closed circuit methods. The mixture is stronger though less irritating than ether, but not so strong as to be dangerous, even in inexperienced hands.

Ethyl Chloride

Inhalation of ethyl chloride causes the rapid onset of anaesthesia and concentrations of about 50% in the inspired air will produce loss of consciousness in about 1 minute in dogs and cats. However, concentrations of this order cause breath-holding and it is better to use concentrations of 10 to 20%.

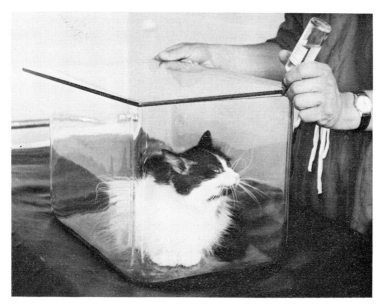

FIG. 141.—Induction of anaesthesia with ethyl chloride.

Anaesthesia may be induced either by spraying ethyl chloride from its container on to an open mask, or the animal may be placed into a tank and a measured quantity of the drug added to the air in the tank (Fig. 141).

Longley (1950) recommended the use of a rectangular glass chamber such as an all-glass battery jar. For computing the quantity of anaesthetic to be used he quoted the following simple formula: the capacity of the chamber in cubic inches divided by 100 gives the volume in millilitres of liquid ethyl chloride necessary for a vapour concentration of 20%. The animal is placed in the container and the liquid ethyl chloride introduced. The top of the vessel is covered and the behaviour of the animal observed. After about 2 minutes the animal loses consciousness and collapses in a state of light anaesthesia. From this point anaesthesia rapidly deepens and in a further period of 30 to 60 seconds has attained the maximum depth consistent with safety. The animal is removed from the container before respiration fails and anaesthesia lasts for a further 2 to 5 minutes.

The more usual way of administering ethyl chloride is to introduce 3 to 5 ml of the liquid in the vaporizer bottle of a semi-closed system. The vapour is delivered to the restrained animal through a face-mask by a stream of oxygen or nitrous oxide and oxygen.

Ethyl chloride is essentially a single dose anaesthetic. Most authorities view coldly attempts to prolong anaesthesia by continuous or by repeated administration. The mortality rate in dogs and cats is high if doses sufficient in themselves to produce anaesthesia are used; the margin between the minimal lethal dose and the amount required for anaesthesia is narrow.

Methoxyflurane

Although methoxyflurane can be administered to dogs and cats by any method, in practice it is best vaporized in a vaporizer and given by semi-closed methods, with or without carbon dioxide absorption. Since the maximum concentration of the vapour which can be obtained from a vaporizer is only about 4% (see page 224), this agent is of little use in the induction of unconsciousness. However, it is a very useful agent for the maintenance of anaesthesia in both dogs and cats once loss of consciousness has been induced by the intravenous injection of a barbiturate. Only a very small dose of the barbiturate should be administered and full anaesthesia should then be produced by the administration of the greatest obtainable concentration of methoxyflurane. Once the desired level of anaesthesia has been reached, the concentration of the vapour is usually decreased but even the continued administration of the high concentration will be tolerated by the animal for a considerable period of time provided that breathing is spontaneous and no attempt is made to augment the lung ventilation. In dogs breathing spontaneously, the mean arterial pressure falls as the inspired vapour concentration increases, but at normal levels of methoxyflurane anaesthesia there is no significant hypotension. Respiratory depression is about equivalent to that produced by halothane. Methoxyflurane is a very safe agent and one which is, perhaps, ideal for the situation where anaesthesia is induced by the veterinary surgeon but a lay assistant or nurse is left to supervise its maintenance. The signs of methoxyflurane anaesthesia differ from those seen with other agents. It is believed that the muscular relaxation during methoxyflurane anaesthesia is due to the depression of spinal cord reflexes and muscle relaxation is present with inspired concentrations less than those required for surgical anaesthesia (Ngai, Hanks and Brody, 1962). The anaesthetist must, as always when breathing is spontaneous, aim at suppressing motor responses to surgical stimulation while preserving the maximum possible respiratory activity.

At one time it was believed that the administration of methoxyflurane–air mixtures using a simple device known as an 'Inhalator' would provide a very easy technique of anaesthesia for use in situations where oxygen cylinders and vaporizers were not available. However, early on in a clinical trial carried out at the Cambridge School it was observed that the dogs breathing methoxy-flurane through the 'Inhalator' often became cyanotic. During the course of a subsequent experimental investigation it became clear that the oxygen content of room air was too low to prevent the development of severe hypoxia when the animal's breathing became depressed by the methoxy-flurane. There was no evidence of hypoxia when ether (a respiratory stimu-lant) was administered in a similar manner through the 'Inhalator' device.

Although methoxyflurane can be administered with oxygen alone, this mixture may not provide satisfactory operating conditions in large dogs and it is probable that methoxyflurane is best used as a supplement to nitrous oxide–oxygen mixtures (Hall, 1964). It seems that the nitrous oxide con-tributes significantly to the anaesthesia so that less methoxyflurane need be given and this results in a more rapid recovery from anaesthesia than when the volatile agent is used with oxygen alone. Nitrous oxide–oxygen–methoxy-flurane mixtures can provide reasonable relaxation of the abdominal muscles and the conditions provided for abdominal surgery by the use of such mix-tures are at least equal to those encountered in animals under barbiturate anaesthesia.

Recently, trials using a cylinder of pre-mixed nitrous oxide and oxygen with a demand valve regulator and a draw-over vaporizer for methoxyflurane have demonstrated that it is possible to produce very satisfactory anaesthesia for canine surgery with simple inexpensive apparatus (Clarke, 1970).

Because of the relatively prolonged recovery period after its use, methoxy-flurane should only be used for major surgery where rapid recovery to full consciousness is not essential and where the apparent post-operative analgesia provided by this agent is an advantage.

REFERENCES

CLARKE, K. W. (1970). Personal communication
HALL, L. W. (1964). *Vet. Rec.* **76**, 650
HARDENBURGH, J. G. and MANN, F. C. (1927). *J. Am. vet. med. Ass.* **71**, 493
LONGLEY, E. O. (1950). *Vet. Rec.* **62**, 152
NGAI, S. H., HANKS, E. C. and BRODY, D. C. (1962). *Proc. First Europ. Congr. Anesthesiol.*, Paper 147

19

Relaxation of the Skeletal Muscles during Anaesthesia

On many occasions, not the least of the purposes of anaesthesia is the production of muscular relaxation to facilitate the performance of some operative or diagnostic procedure. To produce this relaxation of skeletal muscles it is necessary to abolish voluntary muscle contractions and to modify the condition of slight tension which is the normal state of skeletal muscle (its 'tone' or 'tonus'). This tone is maintained by many complex mechanisms but, briefly, it can be said that all these mechanisms result in the slow asynchronous discharge of impulses from cells in the ventral horn region of the spinal cord. This discharge gives rise to impulses in the α-motor neurones which cause the muscle fibres to contract. The activity of these ventral horn cells is controlled by impulses from the higher centres (cerebrum, cerebellum, or medulla oblongata) exciting the α-motor neurone direct, or by impulses through the small motor nerve fibre system (the γ-efferents) which activate them indirectly via the stretch reflex arc.

It has been shown that voluntary movement is controlled to a very important degree by the activity of this small motor nerve fibre system (Hammond, Merton and Sutton, 1956). This system consists peripherally of small myelinated fibres (called γ-fibres to distinguish them from the α-fibres which innervate the skeletal voluntary muscle itself), which leave the spinal cord in the ventral roots and innervate the contractile poles of the muscle spindles. In doing so they 'bias' the muscle spindles, so that their sensory discharge to stretch occurs more readily and is of greater frequency for a given stretch of the muscle. If the stretch reflex arc is intact, increased activity in the afferent fibres from the muscle spindles results in discharge of impulses in the large motor fibres, producing a movement. Thus, it is possible for muscular movement to be brought about entirely by the small motor nerve fibre system.

The importance of this system has become more apparent from work on the cerebellum which has shown that one of the functions of this region of the brain is to control the activity of the γ-fibres system so that it acts as a servo mechanism for controlled activity in the muscle. Movements produced through the voluntary motor nerve system have different characteristics. Movements controlled by the γ-fibre system are essentially directed towards governing the length of the muscle. Voluntary movement, on the other hand, involving direct activity in the α-fibres, results in muscle tension of a given magnitude. The difference between the two pathways is demonstrated by the result of lesions in the cerebellum in which the force of muscle contraction may not be reduced, but the movements are characteristically clumsy. In these cases it appears the ability to control the length at which the muscle is acting is impaired.

The relevance of all this to anaesthesia lies in the fact that the small motor nerve fibre system, like the motor fibres to the skeletal muscles themselves, is a cholinergic one. This means that any drug which can affect the neuro-muscular junction may also interfere with the effect of the γ-fibres on the muscle spindles. A paralysis of the γ-fibre/muscle spindle junction will have, as a major consequence, a reduction in the afferent inflow from the muscle spindles. The mere reduction of such a flow to the brain stem may have subtle effects. Experiments have shown (Bremer, 1953) that if the cat's brain is sectioned at about the junction between the mesencephalon and the di-encephalon (*cerveau isolé*) so that all the sensory inflow except that from the eyes and nose is removed, then the forepart of the brain falls into a state indistinguishable from sleep. A section made a little more posteriorly so that the trigeminal nerve is active, gives signs of wakefulness. It would seem to be a possibility that by the action of a drug which paralyses the γ-fibres and so reduces muscle spindle discharge, a reduction of proprioceptive inflow to the higher centres might actually contribute to a prolonged sleep-like state.

Methods of abolishing Muscle Tone and Ability to Contract

During anaesthesia abolition of muscle tone and ability to contract can be brought about in 3 ways. The first of these is by the use of drugs such as ether, chloroform, chloral hydrate, the barbiturates, etc., which act centrally. The second and third methods utilize drugs which have a peripheral rather than a central action.

1. The centrally acting drugs, by producing a depression of the central nervous system, cause decreased activity of the ventral horn cells in the spinal cord and, thus, muscle relaxation. A profound degree of muscle relaxation can be obtained when a potent narcotic drug is administered in doses which

13

produce a deep generalized depression of the whole central nervous system. However, the consequences of such a generalized depression are widespread. For example, depression of the medullary vasomotor centre contributes to the advent of circulatory failure during an operation, for in deeply narcotized animals severe hypotension is caused by the loss of relatively small quantities of blood. Furthermore, the deeply narcotized animal lacks the ability to compensate for circulatory disturbances caused by sudden changes of posture. Deep narcosis impairs or even abolishes the activity of the medullary respiratory centre and although this may be of little significance during an operation when respiration can be maintained by artificial means, should it persist post-operatively it can have serious consequences. Finally, after deep narcosis there is likely to be a period of depression and immobility which can predispose to complications such as pneumonia in horses and the aspiration of regurgitated ingesta in ruminants.

2. The second method of producing muscle relaxation utilizes drugs which have a peripheral, rather than a central, action. When local analgesics are injected directly into a muscle mass, or around nerve fibres or nerve-endings, the transmission of impulses is blocked and the muscle fibres are effectively isolated from nervous influences. This is strikingly demonstrated by para-vertebral nerve block in cattle. At the same time this method also has its disadvantages. The temperament of some animals is such as to render them unsuitable subjects for the use of local analgesics alone, especially when limb muscles are involved, and even in docile animals immobility of the whole body can only be assured when local analgesia is combined with a state of light narcosis. The injection of local analgesics is a time-consuming procedure and even after the simplest of injection techniques there is a delay before the full degree of relaxation is obtained. Finally, in addition to these disadvantages, techniques such as anterior epidural and subarachnoid blocks cause a loss of control of much of the circulatory system as a result of paralysis of sympathetic nerves.

3. The third way of producing muscle relaxation is by utilizing certain drugs which have an effect at the neuromuscular junction itself. These drugs are known as 'muscle relaxants' or more simply, as 'relaxants'. A relaxant may be defined as a drug other than a general anaesthetic or local analgesic agent which is used to produce relaxation or paralysis of voluntary striated muscle. With the exception of mephanesin and glycerol-guaiacol-ether, which act upon the synapses in the spinal cord, all muscle relaxants exert their effects upon the neuromuscular junction. In general it may be said that they have no significant action in the body other than at the neuromuscular junction, and by their use it is possible to produce instantly, and with cer-tainty, any degree of muscular relaxation without influencing the excitability

and functioning of the central nervous and cardiovascular systems. In order that their mode of action be understood it is essential that the phenomena which occur at the neuromuscular junction upon the arrival of an impulse in the motor nerve should be appreciated. The following brief review of the mechanism of neuromuscular transmission is concerned with such details of the process as are of importance in anaesthesia. For a detailed study of these phenomena reference should be made to the standard works on physiology.

The Anatomy of the Neuromuscular Junction

As the nerve approaches its junction with the muscle fibre it loses its myelin sheath and divides into fine terminals. Electron microscopy shows that, particularly towards the neuromuscular junction area, these terminals contain a large number of vesicles. It is believed that the vesicles contain accumulations of acetylcholine molecules ('quanta' of acetylcholine). At the junction area (the 'endplate' region) the muscle fibre surface is shaped into a gutter which receives the nerve ending. Within the gutter are deep folds, the surface of which can be shown histochemically to be lined with cholinesterase. Around the endplate region the neurolemma is continuous with the sarcolemma and these membranes bind the nerve and muscle fibres together. There is a gap of 200 to 300 Å, partly occupied by basement membrane material, between the nerve ending and the post-synaptic surface.

Theory of Neuromuscular Transmission

The original evidence for the theory of chemical transmission by acetylcholine at the vertebrate neuromuscular junction was provided by Sir Henry Dale and his colleagues (Dale and Feldberg, 1934; Dale, Feldberg and Vogt, 1936). Studies by Eccles, Katz and Kuffler (1941), and others, of the electrical effects accompanying transmission threw further light on the process. It was established that acetylcholine is synthesized and stored in the motor nerve and is released as a result of a propagated impulse in the nerve fibre. Acetylcholine specifically depolarizes the endplate region, leading to a propagated action potential and muscle contraction. Curare, long known to block transmission, was shown also to antagonize these actions and to exert competitive antagonism against acetylcholine on striated muscle *in vitro*. The anticholinesterases reverse curare block, and this was satisfactorily interpreted as causing an increase in the effective local concentration of acetylcholine at the endplate, thus shifting the competitive balance between curare and acetylcholine in favour of the latter.

To understand the transmission process more completely, it is necessary to consider in more detail: (1) the control of the ionic permeability of the muscle membrane; (2) the action of acetylcholine at the motor endplate; (3) the acetylcholine receptors; and (4) acetylcholine synthesis and release. The whole subject is still bedevilled by speculation and hypothesis in regard to finer details but sufficient is known to have considerable bearing on the clinical use and application of neuromuscular blocking drugs.

The Normal Muscle Membrane

The normal muscle membrane, like the limiting membrane of all excitable cells, may be regarded as a lipid partition containing discrete sites or systems at which lipid–insoluble groups can cross. At least three groups of sites can be distinguished: (*a*) Active transport systems such as the sodium pump in which sodium is transported either alone or in exchange for a coupled potassium movement. (*b*) Specific carrier systems involved in facilitated transport handling organic acids, bases such as choline, or uncharged particles such as glucose. (*c*) The third of the channels is believed to be the hydrophilic systems through which ions can move. Here ions move according to both their concentration gradients and electrical potential gradient; the term 'electrochemical potential gradient' represents the resultant. The main ions concerned for striated muscle are sodium, potassium and chloride.

Opening or closing of these channels influences the ionic distribution between the cell and its surroundings. Three main factors govern this distribution. First, in the resting state the membrane is relatively impermeable to sodium (i.e. P_{Na} is low), whereas it permits much freer passage of potassium and chloride (i.e. P_K and P_{Cl} are high). Secondly, the cellular content of sodium is kept low by the active transport mechanism for this ion. Thirdly, the presence within the cell of large non-permeant anions (e.g. proteins and nucleic acids) together with the high external concentration of weakly permeant sodium ions produces an asymmetry of distribution of the permeant ions. According to the Gibbs–Donnan rule, under resting conditions the potassium and chloride ions will become distributed so that their concentration will bear the relationship:

$$\frac{[K^+] \text{ inside the cell}}{[K^+] \text{ outside the cell}} = \frac{[Cl^-] \text{ outside the cell}}{[Cl^-] \text{ inside the cell}}.$$

The net result is that potassium ions are about 50 times more concentrated inside than outside muscle fibres and thus there is a tendency for potassium ions to migrate out of the cells in accordance with the concentration gradient. However, because sodium ions cannot readily move into the cell in exchange, the process stops when, as the result of the movement of a minute number of potassium ions, the outside has become sufficiently positively charged relative to the inside. In general, if the permeability to potassium is much greater than to sodium, the membrane potential is given by the expression:

$$\text{Membrane potential } (E_m) = K + \log_e \frac{K^+ \text{ outside}}{K^+ \text{ inside}}$$

where K is a constant. It can be calculated and shown that the inside is approximately 90 mV negative with respect to the outside of a muscle cell. The membrane is also freely permeable to chloride which will be distributed according to a similar relationship, but because of its opposite electrical charge it will be concentrated outside the cell. If there is a change in membrane permeability so that it becomes much more permeable to sodium than to potassium, E_m will change to:

$$K + \log_e \frac{[Na^+] \text{ outside the cell}}{[Na^+] \text{ inside the cell}}$$

i.e. it will approximate 60 mV, inside positive. Permeability to chloride is always fairly constant and the only effect of the chloride ion seems to be to damp down changes in E_m.

Another way of regarding the membrane is as an electrical resistance which has a capacitance in parallel. By convention, the potential at any point of a resistance falls in the direction of the current flow. Thus, if a current is passed outwards through the muscle membrane the outside is less positive, and the membrane is said to be 'depolarized'. If a cathode is placed at one point on a muscle and an anode is placed at another, the membrane becomes depolarized under the cathode and hyperpolarized under the anode. Because the membrane is not passive, such changes in the membrane potential alter the sodium and potassium permeabilities. It is, perhaps, simpler to talk of conductances for these ions (G_{Na} and G_K) rather than permeabilities, for conductance is merely the reciprocal of resistance and represents the ratio between current flowing and the applied potential difference. The conductance can be measured and, given certain assumptions, taken as an estimate of the number of channels open to a particular ion.

Depolarizing a membrane affects the values of G_{Na} and G_K as follows. There is an initial increase (activation) followed by a slower decline (inactivation). These changes take place faster for G_{Na} than for G_K so that during depolarization a point can be reached (the threshold) at which the current carried in by the sodium ions becomes greater than that carried outwards by potassium ions, giving a net inward movement of positive charge which depolarizes the membrane still further. This gives rise to what is known as the 'action potential', which is terminated partly by a rise in G_K and partly by inactivation of G_{Na}. The result of the whole process is that a small triggering depolarization at one point can lead to a regenerative depolarization at that point. But this is not all. The lipid nature of the membrane gives it capacitance (i.e. ability to hold an electrical charge). The local depolarization, therefore, spreads a short distance along the fibre and falls to $1/e$ of its value at a distance called the space constant (about 1 mm in mammalian muscle fibre). The neighbouring areas, that are slightly depolarized in this way, in turn produce a regenerative response and as a result the action potential propagates along the whole length of the muscle fibre.

A normal action potential lasts for only a few milliseconds and its peak, when P_{Na} greatly exceeds P_K, approaches the sodium 'equilibrium potential'. Drugs which interfere with movement through sodium and potassium channels alter the time course of the action potential. Low concentrations of tetrodotoxin block sodium channels (Kao, 1966; Hille, 1968) and lower the height of the action potential. Conversely, tetraethylammonium ions block potassium channels (Armstrong and Binstock, 1965; Nakajima, 1966; Hille, 1967), thus reducing the rise in G_K during depolarization and prolonging the action potential. The falling phase of the action potential can in fact become so prolonged as to lead to the production of a second action potential, giving rise to the repetitive firing associated with the action of tetraethyammonium ions. Drugs such as procaine affect both sodium and potassium channels, but because the action potential is more sensitive to the action on sodium channels, it is reduced in height or abolished.

The Action of Acetylcholine at the Motor Endplate

Acetylcholine released by the arrival of an impulse in a motor nerve opens sodium and potassium channels so that the conductance to each of these ions increases and the post-synaptic membrane is depolarized. It is believed that acetylcholine produces this effect by interacting with specific receptor sites which control the channels. These channels in the endplate region are different from those involved in the action potential and they are not affected by tetro- dotoxin. Because G_K is already high the most important effect of these in- creases in conductance is to allow sodium ions to enter. The positive charge carried by these sodium ions reduces the inner negativity of the membrane, i.e. depolarizes it. Thus acetylcholine acts rather like a cathode applied to the muscle fibre and the depolarization it produces will lead to the usual changes in G_{Na} and G_K of the surrounding membrane. Normally this depolarization is sufficient to exceed the threshold for the propagation of an action potential. If this threshold is not reached, all that occurs is a so-called 'endplate po- tential' (Fatt and Katz, 1951). The time course of the endplate potential depends on the electrical characteristics of the membrane and on the activity of the cholinesterase of the endplate region. If a microelectrode is inserted at an endplate to record the post-synaptic membrane potential, small (1 mV) depolarizations are seen with an average frequency of about 1/second, occurring at random intervals (Fatt and Katz, 1952). These are due to the spontaneous release of 'quanta' of many thousands of acetylcholine molecules from the nerve terminals and are called 'miniature endplate potentials' (MEPP's); they provide a way of monitoring acetylcholine release. An end-plate potential results normally from a synchronized release of about 300 of these quanta and it consists of a transient acceleration of MEPP's occurring shortly after the action potential reaches the nerve terminal. The MEPP's frequency is very sensitive to presynaptic depolarization and the relationship between the presynaptic membrane potential and the amount of transmitter released is, in fact, related to the presynaptic action potential height and duration and to the resting level of membrane potential.

Another factor influencing the release of acetylcholine by depolarization of the nerve terminals is the concentration of extracellular cations, especially calcium and magnesium. Very little can be released in the absence of calcium. Magnesium antagonizes the action of calcium and the two ions behave as though competing for some reactive site in the membrane.

If the endplate potentials are recorded while tetanic stimulation is applied to the nerve, their size is found to fall from an initial maximum towards a plateau level. The fall appears to be due to a reduced output of the transmitter substance (Martin, 1966). This may be the result of deletion either of pre-synaptic acetylcholine stores or of a component of the system producing release. The process of quantal release may be described by the equation $m = np$; where m is the number of quanta of acetylcholine released by an action potential in the nerve fibre and constitutes a fraction (p) of an available supply (n). After tetanic stimulation of the motor nerve there is a period of post-tetanic potentiation during which the output of transmitter, m, is raised by an increase in p that lasts longer than the reduction in n (Liley and North, 1953; Martin, 1966).

The Acetylcholine Receptor

Conductance changes are mediated at a receptor located on the outside of the muscle membrane. Receptors can be detected, by the electrophoretic application of acetylcholine, not only under the nerve endings but beyond this immediate region to as far as 1 mm away. Thus sensitivity to acetyl-choline extends beyond the region where cholinesterase is located and when a muscle is denervated, new receptors appear and ultimately cover the whole of the fibre (Axelsson and Thesleff, 1959; Miledi, 1960). This contributes to the hypersensitivity of denervated muscle to acetylcholine and other drugs.

Attempts have been made to investigate the properties of receptors and even to isolate the receptor material. Waser (1967) has shown that curare alkaloids become localized at the endplate region to the extent of about 5×10^6 molecules/endplate. But a similar localization did not occur in the region of new receptors in denervated muscle. It is possible, therefore, that some of the uptake of curare may be due to its affinity for mucopolysaccharides which are present in the basement membrane at the endplate region, rather than to uptake by physiological acetylcholine receptors. From the chemical structure of potent blocking agents attempts have been made to deduce the structure of the receptor; but apart from the fact that an anionic group must be present in the receptor, the arguments remain speculative. It has been suggested that the anionic group could be phosphate (Nastuk, 1967).

The action of acetylcholine at the endplate is increased at lower temperatures. This may be due to the effect of temperature on the reaction of acetylcholine with receptor or binding sites, on membrane potential and conductance, and/or on cholinesterase activity.

A remarkable property known as 'desensitization' is displayed by the acetylcholine receptor of striated muscle and its associated systems. This appears as the waning of a stimulant effect or the development of repolarization (usually partial but under some circumstances complete) in the continued presence of acetylcholine or some other depolarizing substance. The rate of this repolarization increases with the concentration of the drug (Fatt, 1950; Katz and Thesleff, 1957). It has been proposed that receptors can exist either in their normal state or in some conformationally different desensitized state. Katz and Thesleff concluded from a kinetic analysis that a model such as

$$\begin{array}{ccc} D+R & \leftrightharpoons & DR \\ \updownarrow & & \updownarrow \\ D+R^1 & \leftrightharpoons & DR^1 \end{array}$$

was applicable where D is the drug, R the normal receptor, R^1 the desensitized receptor and DR or DR^1 the drug–receptor complexes of each kind. The extent of desensitization appears to vary both between species and between individuals of any one species. Repolarization occurs faster when the extracellular concentration of calcium is high and acetylcholine has been shown to change the affinity of the receptor for certain blocking agents in a way which may be connected with the desensitization process.

Acetylcholine Synthesis

A supply of choline is necessary for the synthesis of acetylcholine in nerve endings and this supply may be rate-limiting, since choline is not synthesized locally, but is derived from plasma. Uptake into the nerve ending occurs mainly by a saturable transport system. Choline acetylation by choline acetyl-yase occurs chiefly in the soluble cytoplasm, followed by concentration of acetylcholine in the vesicles of the nerve ending (Fonnum, 1967). Any substance which competes with choline for the transport carrier system will produce a deficiency of choline in the nerve endings and the use of one such substance, hemicholinium, has thrown light on acetylcholine metabolism (Birks and MacIntosh, 1961).

Neuromuscular Block

Consideration of the mechanisms of neuromuscular transmission outlined above suggests many ways in which the process may be modified to produce failure or block of transmission. However, only 3 mechanisms of block are of importance to the anaesthetist. These are: (1) interference with acetylcholine release; (2) change of sensitivity of the endplate to released acetylcholine; (3) change of the threshold for propagation from the endplate to the rest of the muscle fibre.

Interference with Acetylcholine Release

Hemicholinium, which competes with choline for the 'carrier' system to the inside of the nerve cell, can produce neuromuscular block. Onset of block is always slow because the existing stores of acetylcholine must be used up before block appears and the importance of this type of paralysis in anaesthesia is probably greater as a contributory factor than as a primary cause. Blocking agents with a curare-like action begin to show, after a fairly prolonged exposure with repeated stimulation of the motor nerves, a hemicholinium-like effect. It seems likely that most quaternary blocking substances can interfere with choline transport to some extent. This effect has been demonstrated on choline transport into red cells for tubocurarine, dimethyl-tubocurarine, decamethonium and suxamethonium (Askari, 1966). In man, MacIntosh (1963) has shown that abdominal operations combined with prolonged use of relaxants are associated with a fall in blood choline levels, a condition which favours hemicholinium-like action. A functional choline deficiency may, therefore, be involved in cases where the restoration of full muscle power proves difficult after abdominal operations.

The original evidence for the theory of chemical transmission at the neuromuscular junction did not suggest a presynaptic action by substances such as acetylcholine, tubocurarine or anticholinesterases. By 1940, however, there was evidence that, in the presence of an anticholinesterase, a single motor nerve volley, or the injection of acetylcholine, evokes a repetitive antidromic discharge in the motor nerve (Masland and Wigton, 1940). Hubbard and other workers (1965, 1968) have studied these actions in rat muscles using microelectrodes. Acetylcholine was found to increase the excitability of the nerve endings and this was associated with a reduction in transmitter output as judged by the quantal content of endplate potentials. Hubbard interprets this to mean that acetylcholine can act directly to depolarize the nerve, probably at the nearest node of Ranvier. The presence of presynaptic receptors for acetylcholine would make some of the original evidence for chemical transmission open to more than one interpretation but Hubbard's findings suggest that, while presynaptic actions of depolarizing drugs are of pharmacological interest, their physiological importance is uncertain.

The administration of an anticholinesterase produces a very confusing situation at the neuromuscular junction. The drug itself may act on the nerve terminal, or the acetylcholine released by the nerve ending and preserved through cholinesterase inhibition may do so. The post-synaptic region may be depolarized either directly or by accumulating acetylcholine so that the nerve ending lies in an electrical potential gradient. Depolarization of the muscle fibre may result in the accumulation of potassium ions in the region and some anticholinesterases may have tetraethylammonium ion-like actions on the presynaptic action potential. Antidromic activity at one terminal may lead through an axon reflex to orthodromic activity in another branch of the same motor unit, leading to 'reverberation' between endplate regions. Few would disagree with Blaber and Bowman (1963) that the situation is difficult to disentangle!

Since a fall in the ratio of ionized calcium to ionized magnesium in the extracellular fluid depresses acetylcholine release, it is possible that drugs may act by upsetting this ratio. For example, they might interfere with the binding of calcium ions to some negatively charged molecule at the membrane surface or interfere with the effect of the complex in causing an enhanced quantal release.

The output of acetylcholine is reduced by botulinus toxin which neither interferes with nerve impulse conduction nor reduces the size of the acetylcholine quanta. This toxin reduces the resting and evoked release of normal quanta in some unknown way. Noradrenaline increases transmitter output in skeletal muscle. The catecholamine effect on the motor nerve endings is thought to be an α-effect (Bowman and Nott, 1969) contributing to an anticurare action; it contrasts with a β-effect on the post-synaptic membrane which leads to hyperpolarization and a deepening of curare block. These results, together with the effect of catecholamines on muscle contraction, account for the very diverse results recorded following the administration of catecholamines.

Change of Sensitivity to Acetylcholine

The depolarizing effect of acetylcholine may be blocked by the administration of drugs which, having a molecular configuration similar to acetylcholine, compete for the receptors on the endplate region and occupy them without producing depolarization. Such substances may be classified as 'antidepolarizing' in that they prevent the depolarization of the membrane by acetylcholine, and they may be said to act by 'competitive inhibition' of acetylcholine. This type of neuromuscular block is obviously dependent on the presence of molecules of the drug and, when these leave the endplate region, the membrane is unaltered and reacts normally to acetylcholine.

The classical conception that tubocurarine and similar substances act in this way has been amply supported by recent work.

Change of Propagation Threshold

It is now well known that some drugs will produce depolarization and then prevent the passage of excitation from motor nerve to muscle fibre. Such drugs have been termed 'depolarizing agents' and the analysis of their actions brought to light a variety of stimulant effects analogous to those of acetylcholine itself, and attributable to endplate depolarization. In themselves, however, these effects do not explain how synaptic block is produced, nor even why the overt signs of stimulation (such as fasciculations and limb movements) are quite transient, although the depolarization persists. In 1951 Burns and Paton found that during the block of cat's gracilis muscle produced by a depolarizing agent, (1) the endplate region provided a barrier to the passage of a directly evoked muscle action potential; (2) the size of the endplate potential required to propagate was unusually large; and (3) the endplate region itself was electrically less excitable. From these results it was concluded that a new mechanism of neuromuscular block was present, namely a decrease of electrical excitability of the membrane of the endplate region as a result of the persisting depolarization. Further evidence for this was provided by the finding that the block was reduced by passing current through an anode placed on the depolarized endplate, a procedure which will intensify block due to a competitive inhibitor such as curare.

This type of action at the endplate has been likened to cathodal block in other tissues, in which the block is known to be largely due to an inactivation of the sodium conductance by the depolarization (Hodgkin, 1964) Theoretically, the rise in potassium conductance associated with depolarization will also reduce excitability, but the effect may be much smaller (Adrian, Chandler and Hodgkin, 1966). The depolarization also produces an output of potassium ions which will accumulate in the tissue spaces and contribute to the spread of depolarization. This will lead to further sodium inactivation and thus an increase in the area of inexcitability.

Depolarization block may be followed by an alteration of the threshold of the endplate region to depolarization by acetylcholine. This 'raised threshold block' was originally described by Zaimis (1952) as 'dual block'. Foldes, Wnuck, Hamer Hodges, Thesleff and de Beer (1957) suggested the term 'phase 2 block' to indicate that it follows 'phase 1' which is the depolarizing activity of the drug. One possible explanation for this phenomenon may be the occurrence of desensitization during the block by the depolarizing drug reducing the depolarization and hence the contribution by cathodal block to the interference with transmission; at the same time the desensitization itself will contribute to the block. Gibberd (1966) found that potassium loss from rat diaphragm was associated with an increased liability to phase 2 block.

The Safety Factor of Neuromuscular Transmission

It is relatively easy to suggest mechanisms of neuromuscular block, more difficult to prove their existence and to define their characteristics, and very difficult indeed to determine the contribution to block by the various mechanisms in any given situation. Consideration of the 'safety factor' of transmission provides a useful general approach (Paton and Waud, 1967).

It is known that acetylcholine output is lower at high than at slow rates of motor nerve stimulation. It is also known that normal transmission does not begin to fail until quite high rates of stimulation are applied. It follows that at slow rates of stimulation considerably more acetylcholine is released per volley than is required for successful transmission. In other words, there is a substantial 'safety factor'. This is not easily measured by direct determination of transmitter release but it can be estimated by pharmacological means. This entails measurement of the extent to which a depolarizing drug is antagonized by a given dose of tubocurarine. By such a method it has been shown that under certain conditions in cat tibialis muscle 4 to 5 times as much acetylcholine is released as is needed for threshold action. Expressed in terms of receptors this means that 75 to 80% of the receptors must be occluded before the threshold is reached.

The existence of a safety factor has obvious practical significance. It means, for example, that the action of a drug is far from terminated at the time when transmission is apparently normal. There is likely to be considerable 'subthreshold action' which is only detectable when a tetanic stimulus is applied to the motor nerve or when some other drug is potentiated. In addition it explains the properties of muscles partially blocked by competitive drugs, such as the fall of tension during a tetanus, the sensitivity of the depth of block to anticholinesterases, catecholamines, previous tetanization, anaesthesia and a wide range of drugs.

The situation may be illustrated by considering a muscle whose fibres vary in their safety factor from 5 to 20. A dose of tubocurarine occupying 90% of receptors will block transmission to those fibres with a safety factor of less than 10. Any procedure which halves the safety factor will deepen the block to include even those fibres with a safety factor of 20, whereas doubling the safety factor will relieve block in all fibres with a normal safety factor of 5 or more. During a tetanus applied to the motor nerve, the output of transmitter per volley may be half that during a slow rate of stimulation and consequently the first of a series of stimuli will be transmitted to many more fibres than the last stimulus and the tension developed in the muscle will fade from an early maximum. Once a partial block has been produced by competitive blocking drugs the effect of various procedures on the block will depend on the variation of safety factor between the different individual fibres. If the variation is small, then small changes of safety factor have a large effect. On the other hand, if the variation is very large, then a partial block will appear relatively insensitive to procedures modifying the safety factor.

Depolarizing drugs will increase the variation of safety factor. Slightly depolarized fibres become more excitable, i.e. their safety factor becomes greater than normal. Conversely, deeply depolarized fibres become less excitable; if the depolarization is sufficient, the propagation threshold may rise above the maximum depolarization which can be achieved by acetylcholine and the safety factor becomes zero. It is likely that this underlies the general insensitivity of partial depolarization block.

In the past, neuromuscular block has been classified as 'depolarizing' or 'competitive' solely on characteristics such as the response to an anticholinesterase, the behaviour during and after the application of a tetanic stimulus, and interaction with other drugs. This now seems a dangerous outlook. Erosion of the safety factor from some cause makes it possible for a block to arise from quite a small rise in propagation threshold produced by a depolarizing drug without greatly increasing the variation in safety factor; such a block would show many of the characteristics of a competitive block. When it is realized that some neuromuscular blocking agents may be 'partial agonists' (i.e. possessing limited ability themselves to depolarize as well as an ability to compete) and that drugs may act presynaptically as well as post-synaptically, it becomes clear that under clinical conditions many situations will arise where the underlying mechanisms can only, at the moment, be guessed. To interpret the effect of neuromuscular blocking drugs clinically it is necessary to assess contributions due to depolarization, competitive antagonism, desensitization and presynaptic action produced by the various drugs used and to be aware of the safety factors of transmission in the absence of such drugs.

The Pattern of Neuromuscular Block

The one feature of neuromuscular block which appears to be common to all species of animal and all types of relaxant drugs is the sequence of events as each muscle group becomes involved (Fig. 142).

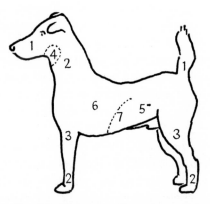

FIG. 142.—Sequence of muscle paralysis.
(1) The muscles of expression, the jaw muscles and tail muscles. (2) The neck muscles and distal limb muscles. (3) The proximal limb muscles. (4) The swallowing and phonatory muscles. (5) The muscles of the abdominal wall. (6) The intercostal muscles. (7) The diaphragm.

The muscles of facial expression, the jaw and the tail become paralysed within 30 to 60 seconds of the intravenous injection of the drug. Paralysis of the limb and neck muscles follows next and then the swallowing and phonatory muscles are affected. Soon after this the abdominal muscles become involved, then the intercostals fail and finally the diaphragm becomes paralysed. Although this is the commonly accepted sequence of the paralysis, individual animals have been observed to be able to make chewing movements or to move a limb although 'curarized' to the point of respiratory arrest. The sequence of events on recovery is an almost exact reversal of that of paralysis. The reasons for this relatively consistent pattern of response to neuromuscular blocking drugs are largely unknown.

In the past attempts were made to take advantage of this pattern of response by giving doses of relaxants which were just enough to paralyse the abdominal muscles without involvement of the intercostal muscles and diaphragm. However, useful relaxation of the abdominal muscles is invariably associated with a marked diminution in the tidal volume of respiration. The animal may compensate for this respiratory impairment, when it is of a minor degree, by an increase in respiratory rate. The breathing which results is characterized by a pause between inspiration and expiration, which produces a rectangular pattern when recorded spirometrically. The increased respiratory rate is accompanied by overactivity of the diaphragm producing very turbulent conditions for intra-abdominal surgery. Larger doses of the relaxant will result in respiratory depression which cannot be compensated for by an increase in rate. Although hypoxia may not result, because of the oxygen-rich mixtures which are commonly used in breathing circuits, nevertheless the decreased minute volume of respiration will lead to an inefficient elimination of carbon dioxide. The results of this are likely to be a rising blood pressure, an increased oozing from cut cutaneous vessels and distressed respiratory efforts. Thus, it is now generally agreed that if the abdominal muscles are to be relaxed some form of artificial respiration will be required. Consequently, for abdominal surgery there is little point in attempting to assess the exact dose of relaxant in any individual animal, for any spontaneous respiratory movements may interfere with efficient intermittent positive pressure ventilation of the lungs, and all that is required is to ensure that the dose given is sufficiently large to produce complete respiratory arrest. On the other hand it is sometimes useful to produce paresis of the *limb* muscles with a dose of relaxant which produces no significant reduction in tidal volume so that intermittent positive pressure ventilation is not required. The use of small doses of muscle relaxants in this way enables many operations to be performed on the extremities of lightly narcotized animals but the anaesthetist must always be prepared to assist the ventilation if spontaneous breathing becomes too shallow.

Agents which produce Competitive Block

The characteristics of myoneural block produced by agents which act by competitive inhibition, the 'antidepolarizing agents' or 'true curarizing drugs', may be summarized as follows:

1. They paralyse voluntary striated muscle by preventing the transmission of the motor nerve impulse across the myoneural junction.
2. Both the nerve and muscle fibre remain excitable by direct stimulation throughout the duration of the block.
3. During the block acetylcholine is produced in normal quantities at the endplate region by stimulation of the motor nerve.
4. Anticholinesterase drugs, such as neostigmine and edrophonium, have an antagonistic effect.

Certain representatives of this group of compounds must be considered in some detail because they have great clinical importance.

d-Tubocurarine Chloride

The quaternary alkaloid, d-tubocurarine, first prepared in a pure form by King (1935) in London, is the most important of the substances which have yet been isolated from curare, the crude arrow poison of the South American natives. Reports of this poison first appeared about 1516 and during the next $2\frac{1}{2}$ centuries various missionaries gave imaginative and lurid descriptions of its effects, but it was only at the beginning of the nineteenth century that any really accurate information was forthcoming. Charles Waterton (1825), after a journey to South America in 1812, described accurately the progression of paralysis following the injection of curare and showed that a curarized animal could be resuscitated if its lungs were artificially ventilated by means of a bellows.

During the middle of the nineteenth century Claude Bernard (1857) elucidated the characteristics of the paralysis, but curare, to all intents and purposes, because of the impurity of the preparations available, remained an experimental tool of the physiologists and pharmacologists. A purified, biologically standardized preparation of curare (Intocostrin) was used by Bennett (1940) to soften the convulsions of psychiatric convulsive therapy in human patients, and later by Griffith and Johnson (1942) in anaesthesia. It was, however, a relatively crude substance, and only in 1944 was the pure quaternary alkaloid d-tubocurarine used in anaesthesia (Gray and Halton, 1946).

Chemically, d-tubocurarine chloride is a bis-benzyl-isoquinoline derivative, which is a white powder, fairly soluble in water but more so in normal saline solution. In most preparations a neutral solution is used, containing 10 mg of the pure alkaloid per ml and pharmacologically inactive preservatives.

d-Tubocurarine chloride is readily absorbed from subcutaneous, intraperitoneal and intramuscular sites but it is only slowly absorbed from the alimentary tract. For d-tubocurarine chloride to be effective when given orally, 50 to 70 times the dose which is lethal when administered by injection must be used. In anaesthesia the drug is almost always given by intravenous injection and following this 30 to 40% of the dose is excreted unchanged in the urine within 3 to 4 hours. The fate of the remainder is uncertain. Experimental results indicate that, at least in the dog, the liver plays little part in the detoxication of the drug (Rothberger and Winterberg, 1905; Stead and Andrews, 1957). There is evidence that, as in the case of many compounds containing amine groups, plasma proteins have the power of binding d-tubocurarine chloride (Aladjemoff, Dikstein and Shafrir, 1958) and a great deal of attention has been paid to this aspect of deactivation. A full discussion of the fate of tubocurarine has been given by Kalow (1959), who describes 3 phases in the distribution of this drug. The first phase consists of a selective distribution of the drug to endplate receptors, protein binding in the serum and distribution between blood and extracellular fluid. The second phase consists of the very gradual disappearance of the drug from the serum after its equilibrium with the extracellular fluid. This must mean a diminishing concentration also in the extracellular fluid. The slope of the curve of disappearance from the serum is in line with the calculated disappearance from the serum of that fraction of the injected dose which appears in the urine, and the approximate two-thirds which move into some, as yet unknown, compartment. It is possible that this compartment might be the intracellular water of some tissues, but the drug is likely to bind to proteins, e.g. muscle proteins. The third phase consists of destruction of d-tubocurarine, according to Kalow probably in that unknown space to which two-thirds of the injected dose has been redistributed in the second phase.

Utting (1963) demonstrated in dogs that the blood concentration of tubocurarine is low in alkalaemia and high in acidaemia. The change in reaction of the blood from acid to alkaline will apparently drive tubocurarine out of the blood, presumably to specific and non-specific receptors.

The most important pharmacological activity of d-tubocurarine chloride is its ability to produce paralysis of voluntary striated muscle. The nature of this paralysis and the mechanism by which it is produced have been discussed earlier in this chapter. After intravenous injection the maximum activity is apparent within 2 to 3 minutes and lasts for 30 to 35 minutes in most species of animal.

d-Tubocurarine chloride is used most extensively in man and has proved to be a safe and reliable relaxant drug. In veterinary anaesthesia it is, perhaps, not so useful. In 1951 Pickett reported the use of doses of the order of 0·12 mg/kg body weight in 250 dogs, but it soon became apparent that this dose is inadequate for the production of really useful relaxation and the effective dose for the dogs is approximately 0·4 mg/kg. Use of this effective dose showed that in dogs d-tubocurarine chloride has actions other than at the neuro-muscular junction for it causes a severe fall in blood pressure. This fall in arterial blood pressure appears to be due to (a) the blocking by the drug of impulse transmission across autonomic ganglia, and (b) the release of histamine. Even large doses of the drug do not affect the canine myocardium (Gray and Gregory, 1948). A similar severe fall in arterial blood pressure occurs when the drug is administered intravenously to cats and in clinical practice it is now generally agreed that it is unwise to use d-tubocurarine chloride as a relaxant in canine and feline anaesthesia.

In pigs, doses of the order of 0·3 mg/kg cause complete relaxation with respiratory paralysis without at the same time causing any marked fall in arterial blood pressure. Although unlikely to be of use in clinical porcine anaesthesia, d-tubocurarine chloride has proved to be a useful agent for the production of the profound relaxation required for experimental surgery carried out in pigs.

Little is known about the action of d-tubocurarine chloride in ruminant animals. Young lambs and calves appear very sensitive to the paralysing action of the drug but doses of up to 0·06 mg/kg have been given to these animals without harmful effects being noted. In adult ruminants the administration of very small doses has caused the death of the animal. The cause of death in these instances is unknown, but it is not due to asphyxia or to the inhalation of ruminal contents.

Booth and Rankin (1953) studied the action of a crude curare preparation in horses during chloral hydrate narcosis and came to the conclusion that this combination of drugs had no value in equine anaesthesia. However, once again it is apparent that the dose of curare used (about 0·12 mg/kg when expressed in terms of the pure alkaloid d-tubocurarine) was much less than what is today regarded as the minimal effective dose. Doses of the order of 0·22 to 0·25 mg/kg produce good relaxation with respiratory arrest in anaesthetized horses breathing 0·8 to 1% halothane or 0·4 to 0·6% methoxyflurane, and no significant hypotension is encountered. Unless complete relaxation is achieved horses are extremely difficult to ventilate adequately, and the use of high airway pressures in attempts to overcome this difficulty may result in marked circulatory depression. The use of d-tubocurarine in horses suffering from asthma or alveolar emphysema may be associated with the production of bronchospasm, presumably due to histamine release.

d-Tubocurarine chloride has few actions in the body other than at the neuromuscular junction. It is without any action on the liver and kidneys. Although hyperglycaemia has been reported in animals by many authors it is likely that it was due to an increased secretion of adrenaline consequent to fright and apprehension. It can be employed in the presence of liver or kidney disease, because, although in part it is excreted by the kidneys, the body seems to have some other method of elimination of this substance. It has been used in animals suffering from complete anuria without any prolongation of its effects. It does not have any effect on the electrocardiogram.

There is a considerable diversity of opinion as to the action of d-tubocurarine on the central nervous system. It is certain that the drug has no influence on the passage of sensory nerve impulses, yet it has been maintained, on the basis of animal experiments, that curare is a central nervous depressant. In these experiments the electro-encephalogram showed signs of decreased cortical activity after the administration of the drug (Feitelberg and Pick, 1942; Pick and Klaus, 1945; McIntyre, 1947). The electro-encephalogram, however, is notoriously difficult to interpret and there is a great deal of other experimental evidence to suggest that d-tubocurarine has a stimulant action on the central nervous system (Martin-Magron and Buisson, 1859; Tillie, 1890; von Euler and Wahlund, 1941; Cohnberg, 1946; Salama and Wright, 1950). It would appear to have been definitely established that, at least initially, d-tubocurarine has a stimulant action on the central nervous system although later on depression may be seen. The stimulating effect may explain the terror experienced by emotionally detached scientific workers subjected to intravenous doses of curare under experimental conditions. This terror is said to be quite out of proportion to any discomfort which the subjects may experience.

Certain antibiotics, notably neomycin and streptomycin, may produce neuromuscular block and animals receiving these drugs may exhibit some increased sensitivity to d-tubocurarine chloride. It is a wise precaution always to give a small quantity of the relaxant as a test dose, and a great deal of information regarding an individual animal's reaction to the drug can be obtained when this is done.

Gallamine Triethiodide (Flaxedil)

Following the introduction of d-tubocurarine into anaesthesia, pharmacologists throughout the world sought for synthetic drugs with a similar action. In 1947, Bovet and his co-workers described the neuromuscular blocking properties of a synthetic product—gallamine triethiodide.

This drug is a white amorphous powder which is supplied commercially as a clear, colourless solution containing 40 mg/ml. Ampoules of 80 mg (2 ml) and 120 mg (3 ml) and multidose containers are available. It is relatively stable and can be mixed with thiopentone solutions.

Gallamine triethiodide acts at the neuromuscular junction by competitive inhibition in a manner similar to d-tubocurarine. It does not appear to have any direct action on the myocardium although it has been suggested that it reduces the incidence of cardiac arrhythmias during cyclopropane anaesthesia (Ricker and Wescoe, 1951). It has well marked vagal blocking activity and this is useful during halothane anaesthesia since halothane tends to stimulate the vagus nerves. Tachycardia occurs within 1 to $1\frac{1}{2}$ minutes after the intravenous injection of gallamine and in dogs and pigs the heart rate increases by 10 to 20%. The rise in heart rate is sometimes accompanied by a rise in the arterial blood pressure. There is no clear evidence that clinical doses of the drug have any action on the central nervous system and it has no direct action on the liver or kidneys. It may, however, have a weak inhibitory effect on cholinesterase produced by the liver and this action is believed to be responsible for a transient fall in arterial blood pressure which is sometimes seen in cats after the intravenous injection of the drug. The injection of gallamine does not appear to give rise to histamine release in dogs so that this compound is a useful non-depolarizing relaxant in these animals.

The agent is not detoxicated in the body and it is excreted unchanged in the urine. In cats 30 to 100% of the total dose injected can be recovered from the urine within 2 hours (Mushin, Wien, Mason and Langston, 1949). It is obvious that gallamine should not be given to animals suffering from renal failure, but chronic nephritis does not seem to constitute a contra-indication to the use of the drug. Another contra-indication to the use of gallamine is where shock is present, for this condition results in impaired renal blood flow.

In dogs doses of 1·0 mg/kg by intravenous injection usually cause complete relaxation within 2 minutes. Apnoea persists for 15 to 20 minutes. Apart from causing a slight tachycardia, the drug appears to produce no side effects in the majority of dogs, but occasionally hypertension follows its administration. In cats 1·0 mg/kg provokes apnoea of 10 to 20 minutes' duration and as already mentioned the intravenous administration of the drug may cause a transient period of hypotension. This fall in blood pressure appears to have no clinical significance. Pigs are very resistant to the effects of gallamine and doses of 4 mg/kg are needed to produce complete relaxation with apnoea. Gallamine may also be used in horses in doses of 0·5 to 1·0 mg/kg and these produce complete paralysis with apnoea of 10 to 20 minutes' duration. Young lambs and calves have been given doses of 0·4 mg/kg without harmful effect but in these animals apnoea may be prolonged.

Harthoorn (1962) reported on the effects produced in conscious cattle by the intramuscular injection of gallamine in doses of approximately 1·1 to 2·2 mg/kg. Doses of more than 1·5 mg/kg produced respiratory paralysis. Neostigmine was found to be an effective antidote. (It is likely that smaller doses of gallamine given by intravenous injection during anaesthesia will produce respiratory arrest and necessitate the use of intermittent positive pressure ventilation of the lungs.) The duration of action of gallamine after intramuscular injection was found to be about 30 minutes.

Dimethyl Ether of d-Tubocurarine

The dimethyl ether of d-tubocurarine (Collier, 1950) has been used as a relaxant during anaesthesia in dogs and pigs and appeared to be 2 to 3 times more potent than d-tubocurarine chloride. Its mode of action is similar to that of d-tubocurarine chloride but the duration of neuromuscular blockade is slightly shorter. This agent never gained a wide popularity in anaesthesia and is no longer commercially available.

Laudexium Methyl Sulphate (Laudolissin)

Laudexium is another non-depolarizing relaxant which must be mentioned for the sake of completeness. It is a synthetic substance which, in dogs, has about half the potency of d-tubocurarine. The maximum degree of relaxation is obtained 4 or 5 minutes after intravenous injection and the duration of activity is about twice that of d-tubocurarine. It does not appear to cause the release of histamine or to block transmission at autonomic ganglia. Neostigmine antagonizes the action of laudexium but in view of the long duration of laudexium's action there is the danger that the effect of neostigmine may wane before that of the relaxant wears off, so that the animal becomes paralysed again. Laudexium has failed to gain much popularity as a relaxant drug.

Alcuronium Chloride (Alloferin)

This compound is diallylnor-toxiferine, a derivative of the alkaloid toxiferine which is obtained from calabash curare. It is an antidepolarizing (competitive) neuromuscular blocking agent with a medium duration of action.

Alcuronium has now been used quite extensively in dogs and horses and seems to have no significant histamine liberating or ganglionic blocking effects in these species of animal. During light anaesthesia the dose required to produce complete relaxation with respiratory arrest is 0·1 mg/kg. Intravenous injection produces no change in heart rate, arterial blood pressure or central venous pressure. The return of spontaneous breathing is apparently followed by a prolonged period of partial paresis; because of this, reversal of the myoneural block with an anticholinesterase is advisable in every case. If only one dose of alcuronium chloride has been given during the course of an operation, the block is very readily reversed by neostigmine. However, when more than one dose of alcuronium has been administered, some difficulty has been experienced in antagonizing its effects. It is, therefore, probably advisable to limit the use of alcuronium chloride to anaesthesia for operations which can be completed in the 25 to 30 minute period of relaxation which follows one injection of the drug.

Pancuronium Bromide (Pavulon, NA–97)

Pancuronium bromide is a new potent neuromuscular blocking agent. It is an amino-steroid which has an antidepolarizing (competitive) mode of action and which is free from hormonal action. At the moment it seems that pancuronium fulfils the need for a rapidly acting, non-depolarizing neuromuscular blocker with a rapid onset of action and a duration of activity which is similar to or rather less than d-tubocurarine. It seems to be free from undesirable side effects.

A study of the effects of pancuronium bromide in dogs, cats and horses (Massey, 1970) has shown that the intravenous injection of the drug causes no change in heart rate, central venous pressure or electrocardiogram. During light anaesthesia doses of 0·06 mg/kg have been found to produce complete relaxation with apnoea of about 20 minutes' duration, and a short-lived rise in arterial blood pressure. A similar period of apnoea follows a second dose of about 0·03 mg/kg. The delay in achieving maximum effect after intravenous administration is much less than is found with d-tubo-curarine or alcuronium. Complete antagonism with neostigmine (always given with atropine) is readily obtained and no cases of relapse into neuro-muscular block have been encountered. The lack of histamine release makes this drug of value in cases where the administration of d-tubocurarine might be dangerous. It seems that care should be taken in dogs suffering from chronic nephritis and other conditions which impair kidney function, because pancuronium is, in part, excreted unchanged in the urine.

Agents which produce Depolarization Block

Muscle paralysis due to depolarization differs from that caused by non-depolarizing drugs in the following respects:

1. The paralysis is preceded by the transient stimulation of muscle fibres, probably caused by the initial depolarization. The muscle twitching which results from this is visible in animal subjects.

2. Substances which antagonize the non-depolarizing agents tend to potentiate the depolarizing drugs and thus in clinical practice it is im-portant to note that drugs such as neostigmine may actually prolong the action of depolarizing relaxants.

3. In a nerve–muscle preparation it can be demonstrated that after partial paralysis with a non-depolarizing drug there is a rapid decay of an induced tetanus, whereas after a corresponding degree of paralysis caused by a depolarizing agent an induced tetanus is sustained.

4. It is unlikely that the depolarizing agents ever produce a pure type of neuromuscular block. For example in dogs they cause both depolariz-ation and desensitization. The true competitive inhibitors always have a pure non-depolarizing action.

5. In the cat, rat and mouse, the depolarizing agents affect the red muscles more than the white, whereas the non-depolarizing agents have the opposite effect.

From a study of the pharmacological properties of a series of polymethy-lene-bis-trimethyl ammonium compounds, Paton and Zaimis (1948) con-sidered that the decane compound, decamethonium iodide, might be a useful substitute for d-tubocurarine in anaesthesia. Organe (1949) reported on the use of this substance in clinical practice on human patients, but although it was used on animals it never made any impact in veterinary anaesthesia. Bovet and his colleagues (1949a, b) and, independently in the United Kingdom, Buttle and Zaimis (1949) found that the esters of choline, notably the succinyl derivatives, caused neuromuscular block of short duration by depolarization. The two compounds concerned were dimethylsuccinylcholine and diethylsuccinylcholine and Edridge (1952) suggested that the former substance should be known as suxamethonium and the latter as suxethonium. The two compounds resemble each other pharmacologically, with the sole difference that the paralysis caused by the suxethonium compound is rather more rapid in onset and of slightly shorter duration. Both compounds form salts with halogens and the dosage required to produce equivalent degrees of paralysis depends on the halogen with which they are combined. For this reason, in pharmacological practice it is customary to state the dosage in terms of active cation. In anaesthetic practice, however, it is more usual to give the dosage in terms of the total weight of the drug. The first of the two compounds to be used in veterinary anaesthesia was suxethonium bromide (Hall, 1952) but the suxamethonium compound is the one more generally employed today. Because the pharmacology of suxethonium and suxamethonium is so comparable, a description of the properties of suxamethonium only will be given.

Suxamethonium (Scoline, Anectine, Brevedil, Celocurin, Sucostrin, Syncurol, Succinylcholine)

The mode of action of suxamethonium at the neuromuscular junction has already been discussed. There is a wide variation in response to suxamethonium throughout the animal kingdom. In each species too there is some slight variation in the response of the various muscle groups but in all species the diaphragmatic muscle is the last to be affected. The exact reason why the diaphragm should be the last muscle to be paralysed and usually the first to recover is still unknown. Suxamethonium causes marked muscle fasciculation and in man these contractions frequently lead to muscle pains which are noticed by the patient on the day after operation. Conscious volunteers given suxamethonium for experimental purposes have reported that the muscle fasciculations are extremely painful. There is evidence to suggest that suxamethonium produces actual muscle injury. Airaksinen and Tammisto (1966) reported myoglobinuria after intermittent administration of the drug and muscle damage is also indicated by the finding that serum creatine kinase levels are raised by the use of suxamethonium during halothane anaesthesia (Tammisto, Leikkonen and Airaksinen, 1967).

There are wide species differences between the various domestic animals in their sensitivity to the neuromuscular blocking action of suxamethonium. The horse, pig and cat are relatively resistant, but dogs, sheep and cattle are paralysed by very small doses of the drug. Like acetylcholine, suxamethonium is hydrolysed by cholinesterases and this hydrolysis is believed to be responsible for recovery from its effects. Because of this, attempts have been made to correlate the sensitivity of an animal to this drug with the levels of cholinesterase present in its blood. Hansson (1957) was unable to demonstrate any such correlation, but it has been shown in dogs that the injection of a purified pseudocholinesterase preparation produces a marked increase in resistance to the effect of the drug (Hall, Lehmann and Silk, 1953).

In man, atypical forms of pseudocholinesterase are recognized. These abnormal forms are active in hydrolysing acetylcholine but not suxamethonium. They can be differentiated from normal pseudocholinesterases by their failure to be inactivated by certain substances which affect the latter enzyme. The local analgesic cinchocaine (proprietary name Dibucaine) is one such substance which inactivates around 80% of normal pseudocholinesterase but less than 20% of one atypical variety. Patients with a normal enzyme are therefore described as having a 'Dibucaine Number' of 80 and those having the atypical variety a Dibucaine Number of 20 or less. There is a third group of individuals with both forms of the enzyme and they will have Dibucaine Numbers of between 40 and 70. It has been demonstrated that atypical cholinesterase is a genetically linked characteristic and the type of enzyme present in an individual is determined by a pair of allelomorphic, non-dominant autosomal genes. Thus it is possible to have homozygotes (atypical enzyme present only) or heterozygotes (mixture of typical and atypical forms present) or normal homozygotes. Determination of the Dibucaine Number clearly identifies the heterozygote and has therefore become a standard technique in the investigation of families and in population surveys (Lehmann and Liddell, 1969). Harris and Whittaker (1961) found that sodium fluoride was a differential inhibitor of the usual and atypical enzyme in a manner similar to Dibucaine. Use of sodium fluoride inhibition detected two additional subgroups of human beings, also due to the presence of a cholinesterase gene, an allele of the others (Harris and Whittaker, 1962, 1963). Liddell, Lehmann and Silk (1962) discovered yet another group with marked sensitivity to suxamethonium and no detectable cholinesterase activity. People with no cholinesterase activity are homozygous for yet another cholinesterase gene.

Atypical pseudocholinesterases have been found in animals but their significance and mode of inheritance have not yet been determined (Lehmann, 1971).

Since suxamethonium is so closely related to acetylcholine it might be expected to have actions in the body in addition to its effects at the neuromuscular junction and this is indeed the case. Injection of suxamethonium causes a rise in blood pressure in all animals, although in some species the rise may be preceded by a fall. In cats there is an immediate marked fall in arterial blood pressure, followed by a slower rise to above the resting level. The fall in blood pressure can be prevented by the prior administration of atropine, and the rise of hexamethonium. The prior administration of both these drugs prevents any blood pressure change. Blood pressure changes are seen after each successive dose of suxamethonium but with progressively diminishing severity. Pulse rate changes are variable, both bradycardia and tachycardia being observed, sometimes in the same animal, and often the heart rate does not change. In horses and dogs the nicotinic response predominates (Adams and Hall, 1962a, b)—very occasionally a fall in blood pressure with bradycardia is seen, but an increase in both blood pressure and heart rate is the usual response.

Cardiac arrhythmias are frequently seen after the intravenous injection of suxamethonium and usually take the form of A–V nodal rhythm. Stevenson (1960) has demonstrated that one injection of suxamethonium causes a rise in the level of serum potassium and since this is not abolished by adrenalectomy, ganglionic blockade, adrenolytic drugs or high epidural block it is likely to be due to the release of potassium ions from muscle. This rise in serum potassium may also be associated with cardiac irregularities. Prolonged administration of suxemethonium, on the other hand, causes a large decrease in serum potassium in dogs, but the reason for this is unknown (Stevenson, 1960).

There is very little evidence either in animals or in man to suggest that suxamethonium has any action on the spinal cord or brain although very large doses have been found to depress the activity of the respiratory centre in cats (Ellis, Morgan and de Beer, 1952). The stimulating effect of suxamethonium on the autonomic ganglia has already been mentioned but very large doses will finally depress conduction through the ganglia. However, enormous doses are required to bring about this block and in this respect the drug compares very favourably with d-tubocurarine where the muscle-paralysing dose may block transmission at autonomic ganglia.

The main value of suxamethonium as a muscle relaxant is that it is hydrolysed *in vivo* by cholinesterases to succinic acid and choline—both normal metabolites. This process occurs in two stages:

1. *Succinyldicholine (suxamethonium) to succinylmonocholine.* This hydrolysis is rapid and is brought about by an enzyme which is found in the plasma. This enzyme has now been named by the Commission on Enzymes of the International Union of Biochemistry as cholinesterase (acetylcholine acylhydrolase, 3.1.1.8) but it is almost universally known in anaesthetic practice as

'pseudocholinesterase'. Other names were butyryl cholinesterase and non-specific cholinesterase.

Acetylcholinesterase (acetylcholine acetyl-hydrolase, 3.1.1.7), formerly known as 'true cholinesterase' which is predominantly found in the red blood cells and also in some other tissues, is not believed to take part in this process.

2. *Succinylmonocholine to succinic acid and choline.* The hydrolysis of the monocholine is a slower process and both cholinesterase and acetylcholinesterase are believed to take part. A small proportion of the suxamethonium administered to an animal is hydrolysed by the alkaline reaction of the blood and this does not require the presence of enzymes. The urinary excretion of suxamethonium is very low because by far the greater part of any dose is hydrolysed in the body.

Suxamethonium is usually administered by intravenous injection but in combination with the enzyme hyaluronidase it can be given intramuscularly with satisfactory results. In horses doses of 0·12 to 0·15 mg/kg usually cause paralysis of the limb, head and neck muscles without producing diaphragmatic paralysis. In most horses double this dose will cause total paralysis but the exact effect produced in any individual animal will depend on the depth of anaesthesia at the time when the relaxant is administered. After a single dose paralysis generally lasts for about 4 to 5 minutes although limb weakness may persist for several more minutes. In cattle doses of about one-sixth of this quantity (0·02 mg/kg) produce paralysis of the body muscles without diaphragmatic paralysis and this relaxation lasts 6 to 8 minutes. Once again, double this dose will cause complete paralysis in most animals. In sheep doses similar to those used in cattle are employed. Pigs require much larger doses; to facilitate endotracheal intubation the dose required is about 2 mg/kg which produces complete paralysis of 2 to 3 minutes' duration. In cats quantities of 3 to 5 mg of suxamethonium chloride (total dose) produce 5 to 6 minutes of complete paralysis. The dog is comparatively sensitive to suxamethonium and doses of 0·3 mg/kg produce total paralysis of 15 to 20 minutes' duration. A single dose may produce dual block in dogs and dual block may also be produced when more than one dose of the drug is given to other animals. It is believed that the response of the motor endplate gradually alters with each successive dose but the precise time and dose relationship is not yet known.

It should be remembered that the enzyme cholinesterase (pseudocholinesterase) is formed in the liver and in the event of the existence of severe liver damage, cachexia, or malnutrition an increased duration of action should be anticipated.

In recent years a number of reports have appeared on the use of suxamethonium by intravenous injection as a method of casting fully conscious horses and cattle. It is the transient nature of the drug's action which makes its use for this purpose feasible, for while the period of paralysis is sufficiently long to allow the application of suitable restraining tackle, the apnoea that accompanies the paralysis is usually not of sufficient duration to endanger the animal's life.

In horses the method has been claimed to be relatively safe for the dose necessary to paralyse the limb muscles is about half that necessary to produce more than very transient respiratory arrest. Moreover, the horse is relatively resistant to the effects of the drug so that the dose used is fairly large and easily measured. Cattle, on the other hand, are very sensitive to the action of suxamethonium and the effective dose is only one-tenth that in horses. This means that although the dose which causes fatal respiratory arrest is again about double that which paralyses the limb muscles, the safety margin is small and very accurate measurement of the dose administered is essential. For this reason, and because the casting of cattle with ropes is relatively simple, the method has only been used to any extent in horses.

A dose of 9 mg/50 kg body weight given by rapid intravenous injection will cast a horse. After a period of some 36 to 60 seconds the animal sinks quietly to the ground and apnoea occurs. The apnoea seldom lasts for more than 1 to 2 minutes, and it is said that cyanosis does not occur unless apnoea lasts longer than this. Following the apnoeic period there is a period of vigorous hyperventilation which lasts about 2 minutes. The animal then lies quietly in a relaxed state for several minutes. Return of motor power to the limbs is often indicated by vigorous coordinated struggling movements. Finally the animal is able to rise to its feet (Stowe, 1955; Hansson, 1957, 1958; Larsen, 1958; Neal and Wright, 1959).

Clearly, a procedure which provokes complete paralysis of the skeletal muscles and in most cases transient respiratory arrest, in a fully conscious animal, is open to criticism on humane grounds. In the absence of evidence to the contrary it seems reasonable to assume that the onset of generalized muscular paralysis has a frightening effect. The degree of distress, however, is impossible to assess for the phonatory, facial and ocular muscles are under the influence of the drug so that the animal is unable to make a noise or to alter its facial expression. It is always unwise to draw too close analogies between the species but the evidence of human volunteers that the muscle fasciculations which precede paralysis are extremely painful would appear to add further grounds for criticism on this score. Thus, whether this method is more or less inhumane than is casting a fully conscious animal with hobbles is a matter of surmise.

This method of casting horses possesses certain attractions. While casting with hobbles or ropes is a safe and practicable procedure under field conditions, it does necessitate considerable assistance and unless some at least of the casting team are experienced in the technique, accidents are liable to occur. By the use of suxamethonium, on the other hand, casting can be accomplished with the assistance of one man at the head and perhaps two others to hold the restraining rope once the animal is on the ground. In contrast to forcible casting the animal sinks quietly to the ground and thus the danger of injury resulting from a heavy fall is eliminated. Perhaps the most useful application of the drug is in unbroken or vicious animals. In these, casting by ropes or hobbles may be more or less impossible owing to the horse kicking violently when anything touches its legs. Neal and Wright (1959) are of the opinion that in such animals the use of suxamethonium is not only a safer and more certain method, but also one which is no more distressing than the conventional methods of casting.

The aspect of the use of suxamethonium which has given rise to most concern is the likelihood of painful interferences being performed while the horse is under the paralysing influence of the drug. One dose may be given to cast the horse and further doses then given to keep it immobile while surgery is performed. A slow intravenous drip infusion of a dilute suxamethonium solution may also be used for maintaining immobility during surgery. However if surgery is to be carried out under this form of restraint effective local analgesia must also be used or the horse will almost certainly move in response to painful stimuli for the dose of suxamethonium used must, in the field, be small enough to permit spontaneous respiration to continue.

Fortunately for the horse, the procedure is now known to be unsafe and there are pharmacological reasons why it should not be adopted. Neal and Wright (1959) drew attention to the tachycardia and cardiac arrythmias encountered in horses submitted to casting with suxamethonium. Tavernor (1959) confirmed these findings and reported 2 instances of cardiac arrest associated with the use of the drug. Larsen (1958) reported 2 deaths due to rupture of the aorta after the administration of the drug and it seems likely that these resulted from the marked rise in blood pressure produced by suxamethonium in horses. Clearly, too, the rise in blood pressure is more likely to be dangerous if a horse has any parasitic lesions of the blood vessels. There is evidence that in horses, as in other animals, the injection of suxamethonium causes the release of adrenaline from the adrenal medulla and stimulation of post-ganglionic sympathetic nerve fibres (Stevenson and Hall, 1959). Since it is generally agreed that the production of these effects by any agent can provoke cardiac irregularities there is probably no need to postulate any direct effect on the myocardium as was suggested by Hansson (1958). It has also been shown that the administration of one dose of the drug causes a rise of as much as 3 mEq/litre in the serum potassium level (Stevenson, 1960) and an increase of this magnitude may well be sufficient to embarrass cardiac function or cause cardiac arrest. When all these factors are considered together a very strong suspicion arises that the use of suxamethonium for casting fully conscious horses is not unassociated with the risk of death even in healthy animals.

Miscellaneous Muscle Relaxants

Mephanesin (Myanesin)

Mephanesin is believed to act on the internuncial neurones of the spinal cord. These neurones pass between the ventral and dorsal horn cells at any segmental level and also connect up neighbouring segments. Reflex pathways involving the spinal cord must pass through these neurones and in the dog and cat the system is capable of diminishing reflex activity.

The drug is a colourless, odourless, crystalline solid soluble in alcohol and propylene glycol and is supplied in 10 ml ampoules containing 1 g of the drug. The intravenous injection of this 10% solution leads to a high incidence of venous thrombosis and also to haemolysis which may cause haemoglobinuria, oliguria, uraemia and death. The drug is partly detoxicated in the liver and partly excreted unchanged in the urine.

Mephanesin enjoyed a brief period of popularity in anaesthesia because it was believed that full abdominal relaxation could be produced without depressing normal respiratory activity. Theoretically, it was argued that although it blocked transmission to the spinal nerves it had no action on phrenic nerve activity so that diaphragmatic movement could continue. In practice, however, abdominal relaxation is rarely satisfactory with mephanesin and it has virtually been abandoned in anaesthesia. The practice of combining small quantities of mephanesin with pentobarbitone for canine and feline anaesthesia has been tried but the combination has not proved to have any significant advantage over pentobarbitone alone.

Guaiacol Glycerine (My 301, Reorganin, GGG, Myocain A)

Guaiacol glycerine ether is a mephanesin-like compound which has been used in Germany for many years (Frey, Göpfert and Raule, 1952; Marcus and Lobermeyer, 1955; Dietz, Krause and Sattler, 1969; Krause and Illing, 1960) and is now being introduced into the United States of America and elsewhere. It is employed as a 5% aqueous solution because stronger solutions have been shown to cause haemolysis and haemoglobinuria. Provided the concentration is kept below that which causes haemolysis, liver and kidney function is unimpaired by the drug which is inactivated in the body by an incompletely understood process before being excreted mainly in the urine as the glycuronide.

In horses under chloral hydrate narcosis, intravenous doses of 3 to 4 g/50 kg of guaiacol glycerine ether produce surgically useful degrees of abdominal relaxation lasting 10 to 15 minutes, without at the same time causing significant respiratory depression (Westhues and Fritsch, 1961). Relaxation of the pharyngeal and laryngeal muscles is sufficient to facilitate endotracheal intubation.

The drug may be used to cast horses and cattle. If these animals are premedicated with tranquillizers and analgesics the necessary dose for casting purposes is 4 to 5 g/50 kg, i.e. about 1 litre of the 5% solution in an animal weighing 500 kg. Towards the end or after the completion of this intravenous injection the animal starts to sway and then falls relaxed. Barbiturates may be mixed with the solution (e.g. 0·25 g of thiobarbiturate per 50 kg body weight) but as the two drugs potentiate each other most animals then fall during the infusion, which is completed in the cast position.

Guaiacol glycerine ether may be used in other species of animal but its administration is rendered difficult by the large volumes of solution which must be infused. Even in horses and cattle this is the main disadvantage associated with its use.

Although the abdominal relaxation obtained with doses of guaiacol glycerine ether which do not interfere with respiratory activity is never as good as can be produced with the proper use of neuromuscular blocking drugs, it may be useful in situations where inhalation anaesthesia cannot be used or the services of a trained anaesthetist are not available.

The Use of Muscle Relaxants in Veterinary Anaesthesia

Indications

The general indications for the use of muscle relaxants during anaesthesia in veterinary clinical practice are as follows:

1. To relax the skeletal muscles for easier surgical access.
2. To facilitate control of respiration during intrathoracic surgery.
3. To assist the reduction of dislocated joints. Clinical experience shows that not only are dislocations more easily reduced if the muscles are paralysed but also that re-luxation is facilitated by the absence of muscle tone. The reduction of fractures, on the other hand, is seldom eased by the administration of relaxants.
4. To limit the amount of general anaesthetic used when muscular relaxation itself is not the prime requisite. For example, in dogs no muscle

relaxation is required during the operation of aural resection but the surgical stimulation is intense and results in head-shaking unless the animal is very deeply anaesthetized. The judicious use of a muscle relaxant prevents head-shaking by weakening the muscles of the neck and so very much smaller quantities of anaesthetic or analgesic can be employed. In these circumstances all that is required of the anaesthetic is to produce unconsciousness, and thus the detrimental effects of deep depression of the central nervous system are avoided.

5. To ease the induction of full inhalation anaesthesia in animals already unconscious from intravenous narcotic drugs. For example, when thiopentone is used to induce loss of consciousness in horses before the administration of an inhalant such as halothane, there is a period when the effect of the thiopentone is waning and the uptake of the inhalation agent is not yet sufficient to prevent movement of the limbs. The careful use of small doses of relaxant can do much to 'smooth out' this transitional period by paralysing the limb muscles.

6. To facilitate the performance of endotracheal intubation and endoscopy. Although animals can be intubated without the use of relaxants the use of these drugs may make atraumatic intubation very much easier, especially in cats and pigs.

Contra-indications

It must be very clearly understood that a relaxant should never be administered unless facilities which enable immediate and sustained artificial respiration to be applied to the animal are available. The administration of even small doses of these drugs may, on occasion, be followed by respiratory paralysis. An animal *cannot* be ventilated efficiently for very long by the application of pressure to the chest wall and artificial respiration must be carried out by the application of intermittent positive pressure to the lungs through an endotracheal tube—the use of a face-mask is not really satisfactory.

In addition, it must be clearly recognized that relaxant drugs have no narcotic or analgesic properties. *It is impossible to overemphasize the importance of ensuring beyond all reasonable doubt that during* ANY SURGICAL OPERATION *an animal is unconscious and incapable of appreciating pain or fear throughout the whole period of action of the relaxant drug which may be employed.* Fortunately, provided due care is taken, it is a relatively simple matter to ensure this, but *any doubt about the maintenance of the unconscious state must constitute an absolute contra-indication to the use of relaxant drugs.*

Experience has shown that caution should be exercised in the use of these drugs in ruminants, and in animals suffering from electrolyte imbalance (e.g. cases of intestinal obstruction) or respiratory obstruction.

Technique of Use

There are several points in the use of relaxants that need emphasis and detailed consideration.

Premedication

The induction of anaesthesia by intravenous medication is simple and pleasant for the animal so that heavy sedation with large doses of narcotic or ataractic drugs is neither necessary for desirable. When, however, the use of an intravenous agent is deemed undesirable and anaesthesia is to be induced with an inhalation agent, somewhat heavier premedication is indicated. In these cases, too, the relaxant may be given as soon as consciousness is lost to avoid the occurrence of narcotic excitement with its associated struggling. Atropine or hyoscine should always be given to avoid the troublesome salivation and increased bronchial secretion which may otherwise follow the administration of relaxant drugs.

Induction and Maintenance of Anaesthesia

Induction of anaesthesia with a barbiturate drug given by intravenous injection has very few contra-indications provided that only minimal doses are employed. The dose used should be only just sufficient to produce loss of consciousness and relaxation of the jaw muscles. Dogs, horses and ruminants may then be intubated. In cats and pigs the injection of the barbiturate is immediately followed by that of the relaxant and the animal allowed to breathe oxygen through a close-fitting face-mask until respiration ceases and atraumatic intubation can be performed. These animals are perhaps best intubated under suxamethonium-induced relaxation and full respiration should be allowed to return before a further dose, or another relaxant, is administered.

Endotracheal intubation is essential when relaxant drugs are to be used because:

(a) A perfectly clear airway is required at all times.

(b) Owing to relaxation of oesophageal muscle, the stomach contents are apt to be regurgitated and their passage into the lungs is facilitated by the absence of the protective reflexes of the pharynx and larynx.

(c) If an endotracheal tube is not used the stomach and even the intestines may be inflated by gases forced down the oesophagus when positive pressure is applied to the airway at the mouth and nostrils. This may be dangerous and is always a nuisance in abdominal surgery.

Maintenance of anaesthesia involves the administration of further doses of the relaxant drug whenever these are indicated, and ensuring that the animal remains lightly anaesthetized throughout the operation.

The indications for supplementary doses of relaxant are relatively easy to state. These drugs are always best given by the intravenous injection of repeated small doses until the desired degree of relaxation is obtained. One exception to this rule is that a dose given prior to endotracheal intubation *must* be large enough to abolish respiratory movements so that the tube may be introduced between completely relaxed vocal cords. During the operation more relaxant is given if muscle relaxation becomes inadequate, or if forceful spontaneous respiratory movements return. When an animal is being maintained in complete apnoea, the dose of relaxant drug used should be such that if given the opportunity (by temporarily suspending intermittent positive pressure ventilation), the animal is just capable of making feeble respiratory efforts. Resistance to inflation of the lungs, in the absence of other obvious causes (e.g. obstruction of the airway), indicates that forceful respiratory efforts are imminent and that a further small dose of relaxant should be given. This sign is readily observable in horses, and in these animals waning relaxation manifests itself by hypoxia and hypercapnia which are easily noted if the blood gases are being monitored. Supplementary doses of relaxants given during the course of an operation should, in general, not exceed half the initial dose.

The maintenance of a light plane of anaesthesia throughout the operation is of very great importance. Allowing the animal to awaken to consciousness during the course of an operation clearly cannot be tolerated, yet deep anaesthesia must be avoided if full benefit is to be derived from the use of any relaxant drug. Probably the best agent with which to maintain a light level of unconsciousness is nitrous oxide since this agent can never, in the absence of hypoxia, produce profound depression of the central nervous system. However, nitrous oxide/oxygen mixtures alone may, sometimes, fail to maintain anaesthesia, and on these occasions some supplementation will be required. The indications for the supplementation of nitrous oxide/oxygen mixtures when relaxants are being used include:

1. The appearance of signs of vasovagal syncope (pallor, hypotension).
2. A rise in pulse rate which cannot be accounted for by such factors as haemorrhage or tachycardia due to gallamine.
3. The occurrence of reflex movements. Contractions of limb or facial muscles either spontaneously, or in response to stimulation, must be regarded as indicating that the animal is awakening. It is most important to note that these movements can always be seen, even when full doses of relaxants have been given, if the depth of unconsciousness becomes

14

too shallow. The reason for this is unknown, but it is tempting to speculate that the γ-fibre endings (see page 384) are more sensitive to the action of relaxant drugs than are the α-fibre endings, for if this is so the drugs might abolish muscle tonus and produce relaxation without entirely preventing contraction of the muscles due to impulses in the α-motor neurones.

The effect of the nitrous oxide/oxygen mixture may be reinforced in 3 ways:

1. *By overventilation of the animal.* It can be demonstrated that when animals are overventilated so that hypocapnia is induced, the requirements of agents such as thiopentone and relaxants are decreased. In clinical practice overventilation certainly seems to provide some reinforcement of the effects of nitrous oxide and is very frequently employed for this purpose in animals and in man. Clutton-Brock (1957) expressed some concern as to the safety of the technique and it has been implied that hypocapnia can produce cerebral hypoxia (which is most undesirable) through the medium of cerebral vaso-constriction (Allen and Morris, 1962; Bollen, 1962). In man, overventilation during thiopentone anaesthesia results in a sharp rise in cerebrovascular resistance, and a decrease in cerebral blood flow and cerebral oxygen consumption (Pierce, Lambertsen, Deutsch, Chase, Linde, Dripps and Price, 1962). The oxygen tension in brain tissue has also been shown to decrease during overventilation (Sugioka and Davis, 1960), while the electro-encephalogram progresses through slowing to flattening, especially if a reduction in blood pressure is produced by systemic hypotension or local interference with blood flow (Meyer and Gotoh, 1960). Despite these suggestive data, however, there has been no report of any deleterious effect of overventilation under controlled clinical conditions. Robinson and Gray (1961) believe that the cerebral and electro-encephalographic effects of overventilation may well be due to the direct effect of carbon dioxide tension and pH changes on the brain, rather than to ischaemia. More recent work (Wilkinson and Browne, 1970) has confirmed that brain ischaemia does not occur under clinical conditions. However, in spite of these findings, the majority of anaesthetists now believe that overventilation should involve simple hyperinflation of the lungs while the arterial carbon dioxide tension is kept as near normal as possible. Separation of lung inflation from the production of hypocapnia is achieved by ventilating at about twice the spontaneous tidal and minute volumes with increased apparatus dead-space, partial bypass of the soda lime or, in non-rebreathing circuits, with the addition of 4 to 5% of carbon dioxide to the inspired gases. Use of this technique has shown that the clinically beneficial effects of hyper-ventilation do not depend on hypocapnia.

2. *By intravenous injections of barbiturates and analgesics* Small intravenous injections of thiopentone or an analgesic such as pethidine may be administered as required, and the anaesthetist is then completely aware of the total amounts of all central nervous depressants which have been given. When vigorous overinflation of the lungs without the induction of hypocapnia is practised only very small quantities of intravenous supplements will be required.

3. *By adding other inhalation agents.* Anaesthesia can always be deepened by adding other inhalation agents to the nitrous oxide/oxygen mixture. However, unless accurately calibrated vaporizers are used, the anaesthetist is unaware of how much of the agent is being administered to the animal. Indeed, even when calibrated vaporizers are available, it must be remembered that their output may be upset by the application of intermittent positive pressure to the airway and, unless due allowance is made for this, serious overdosage may occur. When halothane is added, a halothane meter such as the Hook and Tucker Analyser may be used to monitor the end-tidal halothane concentration, but such meters are not generally available to the veterinary anaesthetist. As a general rule it may be said the use of supplementary inhalation agents with nitrous oxide/oxygen, and the use of more potent agents instead of nitrous oxide to maintain anaesthesia, are both unwise. Much more needs to be known about the rate of uptake of inhalation agents in domestic animals before their forced administration to any animal can be undertaken with safety. Although under certain circumstances the experienced anaesthetist may safely add 0·2 to 0·6% of methoxyflurane, or 0·5 to 1·0% of halothane, to the inspired mixture, this cannot be recommended to the less experienced.

It must be emphasized that the danger of an animal becoming fully awake during an operation when relaxants are being used, although always present, should never be allowed to deter the anaesthetist from making full use of these most useful agents. The danger of awakening is a remote one, for provided due attention is being given to the administration of the anaesthetic, when clinical doses of relaxants are used reflex movements can be observed long before consciousness or awareness return. There should never be any doubt that the animal is unconscious during the whole operation period.

Mixing of Muscle Relaxants

Theoretically, it is unwise to use drugs of differing actions at the myoneural junction in the same animal at any one time. There is some clinical evidence to support this view yet with a proper appreciation of the risks involved and the avoidance of certain sequences, drugs such as suxamethonium and pancuronium can be given with safety to the animal during one operation.

For example, in pigs it is often desirable to produce total paralysis rapidly with suxamethonium so as to obtain the best possible conditions for intubation of the trachea and yet to obtain relaxation throughout the subsequent operation with a competitive inhibitor such as pancuronium or gallamine. Provided the effects of the suxamethonium have worn off (as judged by the respiratory activity) few, if any, harmful effects are seen when the non-depolarizing (competitive) relaxant is given. On the other hand, the use of suxamethonium at the end of a long operation when a non-depolarizing drug has provided the relaxation up to the last few minutes, seems to involve considerable risk of the production of persistent apnoea. The presence of clinically unrecognizable concentrations of non-depolarizing agents at the neuromuscular junction will markedly increase the resistance towards the blocking effects of subsequently administered depolarizing compounds. Under these circumstances, excessive doses of depolarizing relaxants have to be administered before the desired degree of relaxation can be obtained. These large doses of depolarizing agents may cause endplate desensitization and prolonged postoperative apnoea.

Dosage

It is quite impossible to be dogmatic about the dose of any relaxant to be used in any particular case. The dose used will depend on the physical build of the animal, the normality of its neuromuscular junction and transmission, the anaesthetic agents used and the requirements of the operation. Body weight is no more than a guide to the quantity likely to be required. Sex appears to have no influence on the reaction to these drugs. The disease from which the animal is suffering must, however, be taken into consideration. Animals suffering from liver disease are likely to have low plasma cholinesterase levels and thus suxamethonium which depends on this enzyme for hydrolysis, should be used with caution. In conditions where there is likely to be an electrolyte imbalance a hypersensitive reaction to non-depolarizing drugs may be encountered. During any operation cumulative effects should not be forgotten—if it is necessary to administer a second dose of relaxant the quantity given should not exceed half the total dose used initially to secure the desired degree of relaxation. Various antibiotics (e.g. neomycin, streptomycin) may also have an additive effect at the neuromuscular junction with those of the neuromuscular blocking agent used.

The response of young animals to neuromuscular blocking drugs is different from that of adults. Maclagan and Vrbova (1966) found the muscles of a 7-day-old kitten are about 10 times less sensitive to depolarizing drugs than those of a normal adult cat but very sensitive to tubocurarine. Lim, Davenport and Robson (1964) found that the anaesthetic drugs themselves have an age dependent effect upon neuromuscular transmission so that the complementary relaxation provided by some anaesthetics is variable and important.

Changes in muscle temperature affect the action of neuromuscular blocking drugs. For example, in both animals and man, lowered muscle temperature increases the magnitude of the effect of depolarizing drugs and markedly prolongs their duration of action. In contrast, the magnitude of a block produced by d-tubocurarine is reduced (Zaimis, 1956; Bigland, Goetzee, Maclagen and Zaimis, 1958; Cannard and Zaimis, 1959). On rewarming the muscles, these effects are reversed.

Postoperative Complications associated with the Use of Relaxant Drugs

The most important complication is prolonged apnoea. The best prevention of this complication is the avoidance of excessive doses of relaxant drugs. The potentially troublesome desensitization of the postjunctional membrane can be avoided if the anaesthetist does not persist with the administration of increasingly larger doses of depolarizing agents in the face of obvious tachyphylaxis to their blocking effect. In the presence of postoperative apnoea, the animal should be ventilated until the cause of the apnoea can be ascertained and treated. If non-depolarizing agents were used during the operation and the cause of apnoea seems to be due to paralysis of the respiratory muscles, it may be treated by the intravenous injection of atropine and neostigmine. Neostigmine may also be used with caution, in small doses, always with atropine, if the presence of a phase 2 block is suspected after the use of depolarizing relaxants. There is no antidote to the phase 1 block of the depolarizing drugs and the only treatment is ventilation until the return of adequate spontaneous breathing.

When neostigmine is ineffective but the apnoea appears to be due to neuromuscular block caused by non-depolarizing agents, or is due to a phase 2 block, the effects of the intravenous administration of potassium and/or calcium may be tried. In the absence of a urinary output potassium should be given cautiously and if possible myocardial activity should be continuously monitored for incipient electrocardiographic evidence of hyperkalaemia (e.g. high, spiking T-waves, shortening of the S-T segment). If the administration of potassium is not effective and there is reason to believe that the plasma level of ionized calcium has been diminished (e.g. after the transfusion of large quantities of citrated blood), calcium gluconate or calcium chloride solutions may be given. The administration of calcium can also antagonize the neuromuscular block if it is partly or wholly due to antibiotics.

Animals should not be left in the postoperative period with any residual neuromuscular block. Harroun, Beckert and Hathaway (1948) found that if dogs were returned to their cages with any residual curarization pulmonary atelectasis invariably developed. Estimation of the tone of the masseter muscle, by gentle traction on the mandible, has proved to be a useful test for detecting slight degrees of muscular weakness. If the masseter tone is good there is unlikely to be any trouble with respiration.

Use of Antidotes

There are no effective antidotes to those agents which act by depolarization, but neostigmine is an efficient antidote to the non-depolarizing relaxants and to the phase 2 block of depolarizers.

Neostigmine may be used:

1. To restore full respiratory activity at the end of an operation when non-depolarizing agents have been used.
2. To antagonize the effects of non-depolarizing agents in an unexpectedly short operation—e.g. when a prolonged operation is contemplated but is found, on surgical exploration, to be impracticable or unnecessary.
3. To abolish the occasional long-lasting effects of curarization.

Before giving neostigmine care must be taken to ensure that any observed respiratory insufficiency is due to the relaxant and not to central nervous depression. Neostigmine should never be given until there is some sign of spontaneous respiratory activity, otherwise there is no way of assessing its effects and the possibility of passing from a non-depolarization to a depolarization block exists.

Atropine should always be given to counteract the muscarinic effects of neostigmine (bradycardia, salivation, defaecation and urination). Atropine sulphate is best given intravenously to produce obvious cardiac acceleration before the neostigmine is given in small repeated doses until full respiratory activity is established.

Neostigmine, even if it is given after atropine, may cause serious cardiac arrhythmia. This is likely to occur if there has been serious underventilation during anaesthesia or if carbon dioxide has been allowed to accumulate at the end of the operation with a view to ensuring the return of spontaneous respiration. Hypercapnia also increases the neuromuscular block of non-depolarizing agents and so antagonism is likely to be less effective under these conditions. It has been shown that after anaesthesia in which pulmonary ventilation has been used to lower the carbon dioxide tension of the arterial blood, spontaneous breathing returns at low carbon dioxide tensions, provided that no depressant drugs have been used. This is probably due to the effect of stimuli arising in the trachea and bronchi, skin and, perhaps, to the effect of a sudden increase of afferent nerve impulses resulting from the return of proprioceptive activity in muscle, as the muscle tone is restored following the administration of neostigmine. The practical implication of this is that neostigmine may be given while the pulmonary ventilation is continued, provided that there is some evidence of a return of muscle tone (decreasing chest compliance in the absence of respiratory obstruction; attempts at spontaneous breathing; movement in response to stimuli such as movement of the endotracheal tube in the trachea). If the neostigmine is given while the pulmonary ventilation is continued there is no danger of hypoxia or hypercapnia and it is most unlikely that its administration will be followed by any cardiac irregularity. The return of spontaneous breathing can then be encouraged by tracheal aspiration, gentle movement of the endotracheal tube, and lightening the anaesthesia.

It is probable that the dose of neostigmine used should always be supramaximal, in order to be completely sure of full reversal of all the effects of the relaxant drug.

REFERENCES

ADAMS, A. K. and HALL, L. W. (1962a). *Br. J. Anaesth.* **34**, 445
——— ——— (1962b). *Proc. 1st Europ. Cong. Anaesth. Vienna*
ADRIAN, R. H., CHANDLER, W. K. and HODGKIN, A. L. (1966). *J. Physiol.* **186**, 51P
AIRAKSINEN, M. M. and TAMMASTO, T. (1966). *Clin. Pharmac.* **7**, 583
ALADJEMOFF, L., DIKSTEIN, S. and SHAFRIR, E. (1958). *J. Pharmac.* **123**, 43
ALLEN, G. D. and MORRIS, E. (1962). *Br. J. Anaesth.* **34**, 296
ARMSTRONG, C. M. and BINSTOCK, L. (1965). *J. gen. Physiol.* **48**, 859
ASKARI, A. (1966). *J. gen. Physiol.* **49**, 1147
AXELSSON, J. and THESLEFF, S. (1959). *J. Physiol.* **147**, 178
BENNETT, A. E. (1940). *J. Am. med. Ass.* **114**, 322
BERNARD, C. (1857). *Leçons sur les Effets des Substances Toxiques et Medicamenteuses.* Paris: Baillière
BIGLAND, B., GOETZEE, B., MACLAGAN, J. and ZAIMIS, E. J. (1958). *J. Physiol.* **141**, 425
BIRKS, R. and MACINTOSH, F. C. (1961). *Can. J. Biochem. Physiol.* **39**, 787
BLABER, L. C. and BOWMAN, W. C. (1963). *Br. J. Pharmac. Chemother.* **20**, 326
BOLLEN, A. R. (1962). *Br. J. Anaesth.* **34**, 890
BOOTH, N. H. and RANKIN, A. D. (1953). *Am. J. vet. Res.* **14**, 51 and 59
BOVET, D., BOVET-NITTI, F., GUARINO, S., LANGO, V. G. and MAROTTI, M. (1949). *R.C. 1st sup. San.* **12**, 106
——— COURVOISIER, S. and DE LESTRANGE, Y. (1949). *Archs int. Pharmacodyn.* **80**, 172
——— DEPIERRE, F. and DE LESTRANGE, Y. (1947). *C.R. Acad. Sci., Paris*, **225**, 74
BOWMAN, W. C. and NOTT, M. W. (1969). *Pharmac. Rev.* **21**, 27
BREMER, F. (1953). *Some Problems in Neurophysiology.* London: Athlone Press
BURNS, B. D. and PATON, W. D. M. (1951). *J. Physiol.* **115**, 41
BUTTLE, G. A. H. and ZAIMIS, E. J. (1949). *J. Pharm. Lond.* **1**, 991
CANNARD, T. H. and ZAIMIS, E. J. (1959). *J. Physiol.* **149**, 112
CLUTTON-BROCK, J. (1957). *Br. J. Anaesth.* **29**, 111
COHNBERG, R. E. (1946). *J. Lab. clin. Med.* **31**, 866
COLLIER, H. O. J. (1950). *Br. med. J.* i, 1293
DALE, H. H. and FELDBERG, W. (1934). *J. Physiol.* **81**, 39
——— ——— and VOGT, M. (1936). *J. Physiol.* **86**, 353
DIETZ, O., KRAUSE, W. and SATTLER, H. G. (1959). *Mhefte Vet. med.* **14**, 363
ECCLES, J. C., KATZ, B. and KUFFLER, S. W. (1941). *J. Neurophysiol.* **4**, 362
EDRIDGE, A. (1952). *Proc. R. Soc. Med.* **45**, 869

ELLIS, C. H., MORGAN, W. V. and DE BEER, E. J. (1952). *J. Pharmac.* **106**, 353
FATT, P. (1950). *J. Physiol.* **111**, 408
—— and KATZ, B. (1951). *J. Physiol.* **115**, 320
—— —— (1952). *J. Physiol.* **117**, 109
FEITELBERG, S. and PICK, E. P. (1942). *Proc. Soc. exp. Biol.* **49**, 654
FOLDES, F. F., WNUCK, A. L., HAMER HODGES, R. J., THESLEFF, S. and DE BEER, E. J. (1957). *Anesth. Analg. curr. Res.* **36**, 23
FONNUM, F. (1967). *Biochem. J.* **103**, 262
FREY, GÖPFERT and RAULE (1952). *Anaesthetist*, **1**, 33
FRITSCH, R. (1961). *Dt. Tierärztl. Wschr.* **68**, 123
GIBBERD, F. B. (1966). *Br. J. Pharmac. Chemother.* **28**, 128
GRAY, T. C. and GREGORY, R. A. (1948). *Anaesthesia*, **3**, 17
—— and HALTON, J. (1946). *Proc. R. Soc. Med.*, **39**, 400
GRIFFITH, H. R. and JOHNSON, G. ENID (1942). *Anesthesiology*, **3**, 418
HALL, L. W. (1952). *Vet. Rec.* **64**, 491
—— LEHMANN, H. and SILK, E. (1953). *Br. med. J.* i, 134
HAMMOND, P. H., MERTON, P. A. and SUTTON, G. G. (1956). *Br. med. Bull.* **12**, 214
HANSSON, C. H. (1957). *Nord. vet. Med.* **9**, 753
—— (1958). *Nord. vet. Med.* **10**, 201
HARRIS, H. and WHITTAKER, M. (1961). *Nature, Lond.* **191**, 496
—— —— (1962) *Ann. hum. Genet.* **26**, 59
—— —— (1963). *Ann. hum. Genet.* **26**, 359
HARROUN, PHYLLIS, BERKERT, G. E. and HATHAWAY, H. R. (1946). *Anesthesiology*, **7**, 24
HARTHOORN, A. M. (1962). *Vet. Rec.* **74**, 395
HILLE, B. (1967). *J. gen. Physiol.* **50**, 1287
—— (1968). *J. gen. Physiol.* **51**, 199
HODGKIN, A. L. (1964). *The Sherrington Lectures, VII*, Liverpool: Liverpool University Press
HUBBARD, J. I., JONES, S. F. and LANDAU, E. M. (1968). *J. Physiol.* **196**, 75
—— SCHMIDT, R. F. and YOKOTA, T. (1965). *J. Physiol.* **181**, 810
KALOW, W. (1959). *Anesthesiology*, **20**, 505
KAO, C. Y. (1966). *Pharmac. Rev.* **19**, 997
KATZ, B. and THESELEFF, S. (1957). *J. Physiol.* **138**, 63
KING, H. (1935). *J. Chem. Soc.* 1381
KRAUSE, H. and ILLING, K. (1960). *Mhefte Vet. med.* **15**, 22
LARSEN, L. H. (1958). *New Zealand vet. J.* **6**, 61
LEHMANN, H. (1971). Personal communication
—— and LIDDELL, J. (1969). *Br. J. Anaesth.* **41**, 235
LIDDELL, J., LEHMANN, H. and SILK, E. (1962). *Nature, Lond.* **193**, 1561
LILEY, A. W. and NORTH, D. A. K. (1953). *J. Neurophysiol.* **16**, 509
LIM, H. S., DAVENPORT, H. T. and ROBSON, J. G. (1964). *Anesthesiology*, **25**, 161
MACINTOSH, F. C. (1963). *Can. J. Biochem. Physiol.* **41**, 2555
McINTYRE, A. R. (1947). *Curare.* Chicago: Chicago University Press
MACLAGAN, J. and VRBOVA, G. (1966). *J. Physiol.* **182**, 131
MARCUS, G. H. and LOBERMEYER, G. (1955). *Anaesthestist*, **4**, 167
MARTIN, A. R. (1966). *Physiol. Rev.* **46**, 51
MARTIN-MAGRON and BUISSON, (1859). *J. Physiol.* **2**, 647
MASLAND, R. L. and WIGTON, R. S. (1950). *J. Neurophysiol.* **3**, 269
MASSEY, G. M. (1970). In the press
MEYER, J. S. and GOTCH, F. (1960). *Archs Neurol., Chicago*, **3**, 539
MILEDI, R. (1960). *J. Physiol.* **151**, 1
MUSHIN, W. W., WIEN, R. MASON, D. F. J. and LANGSTON, G. T. (1949). *Lancet*, i, 726
NAKAJIMA, S. (1966). *J. gen. Physiol.* **49**, 629
NASTUK, W. L. (1967). *Fedn Proc. Fedn Am. Socs exp. Biol.* **26**, 1639
NEAL, P. A. and WRIGHT, J. G. (1959). *Vet. Rec.* **71**, 731
ORGANE, G. (1949). *Lancet*, i, 773
PATON, W. D. M. and WAUD, D. R. (1967). *J. Physiol.* **191**, 59
—— and ZAIMIS, E. J. (1948). *Nature, Lond.* **162**, 810
PICK, E. P. and KLAUS, U. (1945). *J. Pharmac.* **83**, 59
PICKETT, D. (1951). *J. Am. vet. med. Ass.* **119**, 346
PIERCE, E. C., LAMBERTSEN, C. J., DEUTSCH, S., CHASE, P. E., LINDE, H. W., DRIPPS, R. D. and PRICE, H. L. (1962). *J. clin. Invest.* **41**, 1664
RICKER, W. F. and WESCOE, W. C. (1946). *J. Pharmac. exp. Ther.* **88**, 58
ROBINSON, J. S. and GRAY, T. C. (1961). *Br. J. Anaesth.* **33**, 62
ROTHBERGER, C. J. and WINTERBERG, H. (1905). *Archs int. Pharmacodyn.* **15**, 339
SALAMA, S. and WRIGHT, S. (1950). *Br. J. Pharmac.* **5**, 49

STEAD, A. L. and ANDREWS, W. H. H. (1957). *Br. J. Anaesth.* **29**, 151
STEVENSON, D. E. (1960). *Brit. J. Anaesth.* **32**, 364
—— and HALL, L. W. (1959). *Vet. Rec.* **71**, 818
STOWE, C. M. (1955). *Cornell Vet.* **45**, 193
SUGIOKA, K. and DAVIS, D. A. (1960). *Anesthesiology*, **21**, 135
TAMMISTO, T., LEIKKONEN, P. and AIRAKSINEN, M. (1967). *Acta anaesth. scand.* **11**, 333
TAVERNOR, W. D. (1959). *Vet. Rec.* **71**, 774
TILLIE, J. (1890). *J. Anat.* **24**, 509
UTTING, J. E. (1963). *Br. J. Anaesth.* **35**, 706
VON EULER, U. S. and WAHLUND, H. (1941). *Acta physiol. scand.* **2**, 327
WASER, P. G. (1967). *Ann. N. Y. Acad. Sci.* **144**, 737
WATERTON, C. (1825). *Wanderings in South America*. London: Fellowes
WESTHUES, M. and FRITSCH, R. (1961). *Die Narkose der Tiere: Allgemeinnarkose.* Berlin: Paul Parey
WILKINSON, I. M. S. and BROWN, DOREEN, R. G. (1970). *Br. J. Anaesth.* **42**, 472
ZAIMIS, E. J. (1952). *Nature, Lond.* **170**, 617
—— (1956). *Lectures on the Scientific Basis of Medicine*, Vol. 6. London: Athlone Press

20

Artificial Ventilation of the Lungs

The successful results obtained today in intrathoracic and cardiac surgery are due largely, if not entirely, to the use of special anaesthetic techniques which have been developed within comparatively recent years to provide efficient pulmonary ventilation when a large hole exists in the pleural cavity. These techniques are now also employed to sustain life when the respiratory muscles are paralysed by neuromuscular blocking drugs or, indeed, whenever respiratory failure occurs from any cause. They involve the rhythmical inflation of the lungs by a process termed 'controlled respiration', 'intermittent positive pressure respiration' (IPPR), or 'intermittent positive pressure ventilation' (IPPV). Because controlled respiration techniques were developed for use during intrathoracic surgery, it seems pertinent to consider first the consequences of making a large opening into the pleural cavity and the reasons why these techniques produce efficient pulmonary ventilation under these circumstances. The differences between controlled respiration when the chest is open and when it is closed may then be appreciated.

When a large opening is made into the pleural cavity the exposed lung collapses and the respiratory movements, although vigorous, are not capable of maintaining life. In the past, various measures have been tried to obviate the dire effects of such an opening into the pleural cavity. For example, one method was to keep the opening small enough to be almost completely blocked by the exploring fingers of the surgeon. Another method, known as 'Muller's handgrip', consisted of pulling the lung out through the incision immediately after opening the chest, thus plugging the thoracotomy wound with the lung itself. It was also known that little difficulty was encountered when the lung was found to be adherent to the chest wall, with the result that some surgeons attempted to provoke such adhesions by injecting irritants into the pleural cavity several days before thoracotomy was attempted. In veterinary surgery a number of operations for the relief of diaphragmatic rupture were carried out under pentobarbitone narcosis while rhythmical inflation of the lungs was carried out by some simple pumping apparatus (e.g.

bicycle-tyre pump or Higginson's syringe). O'Shaugnessy used a positive pressure apparatus to inflate the lungs of anaesthetized dogs and more recently Wood devised an apparatus which was used very successfully by Knight to perform artificial respiration during many thoracotomies on dogs under deep pentobarbitone narcosis.

Events which occur when the Pleural Sac is opened

1. Collapse of the Lung

The thoracic cage is a firm, but flexible, air-tight box. Since the alveoli of the lungs are in free communication with the outside air the atmospheric pressure keeps the lungs distended so that their outer surface is in apposition

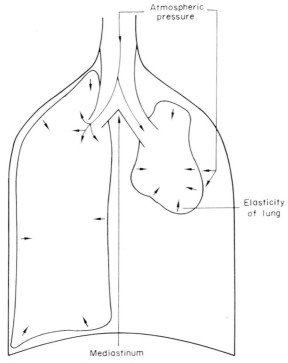

FIG. 143.—Forces responsible for collapse of lung when the chest wall is opened.

with the inner lining of the thoracic cage. The distending force (i.e. atmospheric pressure) is opposed only by the natural elasticity of the lung tissue and the contact between the exterior of the lungs and the chest wall is maintained throughout the rhythmic expansion and contraction of the chest produced by the respiratory muscles. When the chest wall is opened and atmospheric pressure is admitted to act on the outside as well as the inside of the lung, the natural elasticity of the tissues is unopposed and the organ collapses (Fig. 143).

The collapsed lung acts as a venous-arterial shunt and the venous blood leaving the right ventricle is returned unoxygenated to the arterial side of the circulation.

2. Mediastinal Movement

The mediastinal partition which divides the thorax into two halves is by no means rigid in any normal animal. The behaviour of each half of the chest during the respiratory cycle is therefore dependent on the conditions prevailing in the other half. The presence of a pneumothorax on one side causes the flexible mediastinum to move towards the unopened side of the chest during inspiration, while on expiration the reverse movement occurs. The effect of these movements of the mediastinum is first to reduce the volume of air entering the lung on the intact side and secondly to impede the venous return to the heart.

3. Paradoxical Respiration

If an opening is made through the chest wall of an animal which is breathing spontaneously, the exposed lung, although collapsed, will be seen to be moving in a rhythmical manner. The exposed lung becomes smaller on inspiration and larger on expiration—hence the term 'paradoxical respiration'.

On inspiration the whole thorax enlarges and its increased volume is occupied by air which enters the lungs and by blood which enters the heart and great veins. If a thoracotomy opening is present, air enters the thorax not only through the trachea into the interior of the lungs, but also through the thoracotomy wound into the pleural cavity. The volumes of air which enter by each route will depend on the relation between the cross-sectional area of the trachea and that of the thoracotomy opening. With a large thoracotomy opening the greater amount of air enters the thorax through this and the mediastinum is pushed towards the unopened side of the chest.

During inspiration the air pressure in the main bronchus of the exposed lung is greater than in the trachea, since the elastic recoil of this lung is added to the atmospheric pressure (Fig. 144). Thus the increase in volume of the intact half of the thorax during inspiration is filled first by air which comes from the exposed lung and only secondly by air which enters from the trachea and the exterior. Therefore, on inspiration the exposed lung becomes smaller.

The reverse procedure occurs on expiration. The thorax becomes smaller in size and on the open air side is discharged freely through the thoracotomy wound. On the intact side air is discharged partly into the trachea and partly into the exposed lung which then increases in size.

Thus an animal which is breathing spontaneously and has a large opening in its chest wall suffers from increasing asphyxia due to the transfer of air from one lung to the other at each breath. This 'pendulum air' passing from lung to lung is virtually an increase in dead space, making the animal's respiratory efforts very much less effective in the production of gaseous exchange.

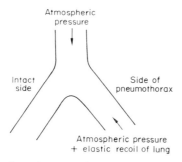

FIG. 144—Effect of unilateral pneumothorax on tracheal and bronchial pressures.

Controlled Respiration

The harmful effects of the events described above can be countered by abolishing spontaneous respiratory movements and maintaining life by rhythmical and controlled inflation of the lungs. If the pressure in the trachea can be raised during inspiration and lowered during expiration air will flow into both lungs during inspiration and from both during expiration. 'Pendulum air' will thus be abolished, and the mediastinum will be stabilized and its movements stopped. This change in pressure in the trachea is most simply accomplished by compressing the reservoir bag of an anaesthetic circuit during inspiration and relaxing the compression during expiration. If this is done while following the animal's own respiratory rhythm it constitutes 'assisted respiration'. The increased volume of tidal air caused by the assistance lowers the carbon dioxide content of the blood below the threshold required to stimulate the respiratory centre, the animal becomes apnoeic and the anaesthetist imposes the respiratory rhythm of choice—'controlled respiration'. Controlled respiration has now been in daily routine use in anaesthesia for some 30 years and many millions of humans and animals have been successfully ventilated by this means with little evidence of harmful result. When the mean pressure in the lungs is not excessive, the gas flows through the respiratory tract are within normal limits, and there is no disease resulting in gross alteration in local areas of compliance and resistance, then the harmful effects, if any, are so small as to be negligible.

Nevertheless, it is essential to understand the basis of the effectiveness of controlled respiration and the mechanisms underlying the harmful effects which may, in certain circumstances, be produced. The meaning of certain terms and the differences between controlled and spontaneous respiration must also be clearly appreciated.

Compliance is the relationship between the volume of gas and its pressure in the alveoli. It may be defined as the volume increase which corresponds with unit increase in alveolar pressure. Normally it is expressed in litres/centimetre of water (litres/cm H_2O). The actual value of the compliance varies considerably in different individuals of one species of animal and in different circumstances in the same individual. The total compliance has two components: that of the chest wall and that of the lungs. When the chest is opened the influence of the thoracic wall becomes very small and the total compliance is virtually equal to the compliance of the lungs alone. In clinical anaesthesia the compliance may be modified considerably from moment to moment by such factors as assistants leaning on the chest, retractors pushing against the lungs and the degree of muscle relaxation.

Airway resistance expresses the relationship between the pressure difference across the airway (between mouth and alveoli), and the rate at which gas is flowing through the airway. It is expressed as pressure difference per unit flow and is usually measured in centimetres of water/litre/second (cm H_2O/litre/second). In addition to airway resistance there is also 'viscous' tissue resistance to expansion of the lungs. The viscous resistance arises from the lung lobes sliding against each other, the mediastinal structures such as the heart and the chest wall. The sum of airway resistance and tissue resistance is referred to as respiratory resistance.

The value of the airway resistance is increased during anaesthesia. This may arise due to both a narrowing and an elongation of the bronchi, and to the presence of an endotracheal tube. The presence of disease may also increase the respiratory resistance. For example, Gillespie, Tyler and Eberly (1966) showed that 'broken-winded' horses have a rapid increase in airway resistance at the end of expiration.

During inflation of the lungs the pressure at the mouth must be greater than the pressure in the alveoli or no gas would flow from one to the other. Conversely, during the expiratory phase the pressure in the alveoli must be greater and there is, therefore, at least an instant of time between the two phases when the pressure is the same throughout the respiratory tract and no gas flows in either direction. The differences in pressure depend on, and are an indication of, the magnitude of the respiratory resistance. During inflation the actual pressure at the mouth at any moment is the sum of the pressure drop across the airway resistance and the alveolar pressure, which corresponds to the volume of gas in the lungs at that moment. A clear distinction must, therefore, always be drawn between the pressure registered at the mouth (the pressure generated in an automatic ventilating machine) and the alveolar pressure. A high gas flow into the lungs, or a high airway resistance, and hence a high pressure difference across the airway, can lead to a peak pressure at the mouth much in excess of the final peak pressure in the alveoli. The biggest difference in pressure between the mouth and alveoli occurs when the flow into the lungs is greatest. As the end of the inspiratory phase is reached the difference becomes smaller until, at the end of the phase, no flow occurs and the pressure is the same throughout the respiratory tract. The peak pressure at the mouth is higher than the peak pressure reached in the alveoli and it occurs some time before the latter, which marks the end of the inspiratory phase. It is possible, by watching a manometer registering the mouth pressure, to note the highest pressure reached there, but the instant at which the mouth pressure and the alveolar pressure become the same cannot be recognized. The anaesthetist must, therefore, exercise caution in translating a manometer reading of pressure at the mouth into volume of gas transferred to the lungs. Figures for compliance relate changes in the volume and pressure in the *alveoli*.

The resistance of an unobstructed airway is small and, with a slow rhythm of ventilation, the pressure at the mouth during the inspiratory phase is little more than 4 to 6 cm H_2O higher than that in the alveoli (at least in dogs). In these circumstances a practical approximation of the volume exchange can be made from the manometer readings if the compliance of the chest is known or assumed. A higher pressure at the mouth then indicates that a correspondingly larger volume has been transferred to the animal, and this may well be in excess of the normal tidal volume and undesirable.

There are other occasions, however, when a high pressure at the mouth may be needed to produce a tidal volume within the normal range. For example, the airway resistance may be high or the compliance low. A fall in tidal exchange resulting from an increase in the airway resistance due to causes such as obstruction by secretions or kinking of an endotracheal tube can be overcome to a large extent by increasing the pressure at the mouth, thereby maintaining a sufficient flow of gas, so that a volume within the desired range is again transferred into the lungs in the required time. In such circumstances the pressure in the alveoli, being determined only by the compliance and volume transferred will, of course, be within normal limits. Since, in such a case, expiration will be impeded by the obstruction and the pressure difference across the airway at the beginning of the expiratory phase is less than that applied at the beginning of the inspiration, either extra time must be allowed for the lungs to empty or negative pressure must be applied at the mouth during this phase to increase the pressure difference between alveoli and mouth and so speed up the flow of gas out of the lungs.

In some mechanical ventilators the reservoir bag is calibrated and there is a temptation to assume that the volume expelled from the bag during the inspiratory phase is the volume which actually reaches the alveoli. Great caution is necessary here for the volume expelled from the bag may, in fact, differ very considerably from the volume entering the animal's lungs. Losses may occur due to the distension of the breathing tubes of the apparatus and also the compression of the gas within them. In addition, the entry and escape of gas into and from the breathing circuit are responsible for further differences between the two volumes. From a clinical point of view, this latter phenomenon occurs in most ventilators in which the reservoir bag of the ventilator takes the place of the reservoir bag of a carbon dioxide absorption apparatus. In these circumstances the volume of gas entering the animal's lungs may be either greater or less than the volume leaving the reservoir bag of the ventilator. Whether it is greater or less, and the magnitude of the difference, depend on the rate of fresh gas supply and the arrangements for admitting fresh gas and disposing of excess. An accurate estimate of the volume transferred to the animal's lungs is only possible after a careful study of the ventilator mechanism and of its physical characteristics, so that the simplest solution is to monitor the expired gas volume with some type of ventilation meter.

The Differences between Controlled and Spontaneous Respiration

During normal spontaneous breathing the size of the thoracic cavity is increased during inspiration by contraction of the diaphragm and other respiratory muscles. As the thorax enlarges the specific volume of the gas within it increases, and the pressure with the thorax falls. The difference between the intrapleural and alveolar pressures overcomes the elasticity of the lungs: the difference between the pressure in the alveoli and the exterior overcomes the airway resistance. The sizes of these two pressure differences differ from each other; that across the airway, even at the height of gas flow, is small so long as the airway is unobstructed, that between pleura and alveoli is larger and is greater at the top than at the bottom of the lungs.

Intrapulmonary Pressure

During spontaneous respiration air flows from the outside atmosphere to the inside of the lungs because a pressure difference is created between the exterior and the alveoli. This pressure difference is of relatively small magnitude since it has only to overcome airway resistance, the main effort of the respiratory muscles being used to overcome the elastic recoil force of the lungs. The pressure difference in a conscious animal breathing quietly is of the order of 1 or 2 centimetres of water and since the mouth pressure is atmospheric, the pressure in the alveoli during inspiration must be sub-atmospheric by this amount. By the end of inspiration the pressure in the alveoli has become atmospheric again. When expiration starts, the pressure in the alveoli rises a few centimetres of water above atmospheric and gradually falls to atmospheric once again as the lungs empty.

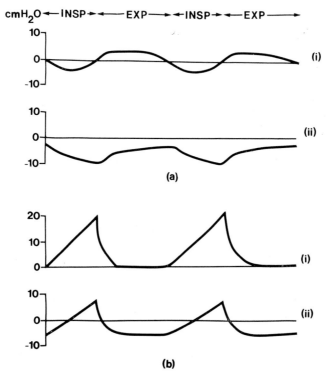

FIG. 145.—Pressure changes (i) at the mouth and (ii) in the pleural cavity during (a) spontaneous and (b) controlled respiration.

During controlled respiration (Fig. 145) with positive pressure alone, the pressure at the mouth rises from atmospheric to a relatively high level and during the expiratory phase falls to atmospheric as the lungs empty.

Intrapleural Pressure

The intrapleural pressure also reflects the considerable difference between the two types of respiration. The differences are illustrated in Fig. 145.

Harmful Effects of Controlled Respiration

In spite of the striking efficacy and safety of controlled respiration the considerations above indicate that the method involves a considerable deviation from the normal physiological mechanism of respiration. When used improperly, or on animals incapable of compensating for the almost inevitable though usually minor upsets which can result from interferences with normal bodily processes, controlled respiration may be harmful to a significant degree.

The connection between the venous return and the intrathoracic pressure was recognized by Valsalva in the seventeenth century. His trick of trying to expire against a closed glottis raises the intrathoracic pressure to a positive level, interfering with the venous return and causing marked distension of the peripheral veins, especially in the head and neck, a fall in arterial pressure and, if the subject is persistent, loss of consciousness due to cerebral ischaemia.

The fall in intrathoracic pressure during spontaneous respiration not only sucks air into the lungs, but also blood from outside the thorax into the thoracic veins and heart. The interference with, and the modification of, the subatmospheric pressure within the chest by controlled respiration disturb this important mechanism. Only during expiration is the negative intrapleural pressure the same in both spontaneous and controlled respiration. During spontaneous breathing the venous return is therefore greatest during inspiration, but during controlled respiration the situation is reversed and the venous return rises during the expiratory phase.

At the end of the inspiratory phase of controlled respiration the central venous pressure is raised and the venous gradient is decreased. The venous return to the heart and hence the cardiac output are reduced and the blood pressure falls. Normally, however, this is rapidly compensated for by a rise in the peripheral venous pressure which restores the venous gradient and so re-establishes the venous return to its former level. The restoration of the venous gradient is essential if an adequate cardiac output is to be maintained during controlled respiration. It is dependent on the ability to adjust the distribution of blood between the vascular compartments by changes in vascular tone, and on the presence of a normal circulating blood volume.

Should either of these factors be interfered with, or the inspiratory phase be unduly prolonged, then the untoward circulatory effects of the positive pressure in the lungs will become marked. For example, severe haemorrhage reduces the circulating blood volume and in this event such extensive vasoconstriction may have taken place that further compensation will be impossible; the effect of controlled respiration may then be disastrous.

During the inspiratory phase of controlled respiration the heart itself may be compressed between the inflating lungs so that cardiac tamponade occurs and the cardiac output falls. The higher the peak pressure and the longer the time during which it acts, the greater is the cardiac tamponade and the interference with cardiac output.

Because the pulmonary capillary blood pressure is only a few centimetres of water the capillaries will suffer compression in part or whole as the alveolar pressure rises above atmospheric. Even pressures as low as 6 cm H_2O in the lungs decrease the pulmonary capillary blood flow and throw an extra burden on the right ventricle. If the animal is on the verge of decompensation, even such low pressures as this may be sufficient to precipitate right heart failure.

In considering the relative importance of these three ways in which controlled respiration may be harmful to the circulatory system, it should be borne in mind that they are probably only of importance in animals with an intact chest wall. Once the chest is opened the thoracic pump mechanism no longer operates, while any cardiac tamponade is likely to be of mainly surgical origin. The interference with pulmonary capillary blood flow is the only factor which can have an adverse effect during controlled respiration with an open chest and this is usually easily minimized by keeping the inflating pressures low and of short duration.

The possibility of rupture of the alveoli is remote in properly conducted controlled respiration, unless a condition such as bullous emphysema is present. Rupture even then is probably no more likely to occur than during normal life. Coughing produces intrapulmonary pressures as high as 80 to 90 cm H_2O, and straining at defaecation may give rise to still higher pressures. The pressure required to rupture the exposed and unsupported lungs of various animals has been found to be about 40 to 80 cm H_2O. When the lungs are supported by the thoracic cage and the abdominal musculature of a living animal a pressure of 80 to 140 cm H_2O is needed. The maximum safe intrapulmonary pressure in the intact mammal is about 70 cm H_2O. The pressure developed by squeezing the thin rubber bag commonly found as the reservoir bag on anaesthetic apparatus can rarely be made to exceed 40 to 60 cm H_2O. In animals rupture of the lungs is usually into the mediastinum with passage of air up the fascial planes into the cervical region. At higher pressures this is sometimes accompanied by air embolism and haemorrhages into the lung tissues.

These considerations make it evident that the risk of rupture of the alveoli during controlled respiration is very small, even in animals which have a high airway resistance and a low lung compliance. However, in many animals the distribution of inflating gas within the lungs is not uniform. When this occurs the normal relationship that must exist between ventilation and perfusion within the lungs is disturbed. The full implications of uneven ventilation are complex and may be exaggerated by inexpert controlled respiration. The most serious result of this is the perfusion of insufficiently ventilated parts of the lung with blood and therefore insufficient oxygenation of this blood. In otherwise healthy animals uneven distribution of ventilation eventually results in a diminution of blood flow through the less well ventilated parts of the lung and any right to left shunting effect is thereby minimized. Another possible effect of importance is the ventilation of poorly perfused parts of the lung; such ventilation is 'wasted' and represents an increase in physiological dead space. In such circumstances a 'normal' total tidal or minute ventilation may result in a raised arterial carbon dioxide tension.

Uneven distribution of inspired gas may also be due to localized changes in elasticity or in the patency of the small airways such as are found in asthma, chronic bronchitis and emphysema. Apart from pathological causes within the animal itself, the lateral posture causes uneven ventilation by decreasing ventilation of the dependent lung. Surgical retractors and packs may also cause uneven ventilation by limiting the expansion of small or even major parts of the lung. The localized accumulation of secretions will also have the same effect.

In any of these circumstances of uneven ventilation, an added risk of alveolar damage exists during controlled respiration. For example, the anaesthetist, unaware that a deterioration in the animal's condition is due to uneven distribution of gas within the lungs, may make vigorous efforts to increase the tidal volume in the belief that increased ventilation is the animal's only requirement. In other cases the high inspiratory flow, which may occur when a short inspiratory period is sought to reduce the mean intrapulmonary pressure, may produce a great difference in pressure between two adjacent alveoli, even when the extent of any concomitant pathology is comparatively minor. Thus, whenever either the inspiratory flow is increased, or the pressure at the mouth is raised to a high level, any tendency to uneven distribution of the tidal gas is exaggerated. It is then that, at some point in the respiratory cycle, differences exist between the pressure in neighbouring alveoli or parts of the lung setting up unequal forces across the alveolar septa and inclining them to rupture.

The possibility of damage to the lungs resulting from maldistribution of gas is, to some extent, speculative and it should not deter from attempts to ventilate adequately. The maintenance of effective alveolar ventilation on which life depends is of paramount importance, though the manner in which this is achieved is often variable.

The acid–base balance of the blood will be disturbed with any deviation from normal alveolar ventilation. There is no lack of evidence of the harmful effects of underventilation. The retention of carbon dioxide due to underventilation leads not only to general depression of the body, including the central nervous system, ending in coma, but also to important undesirable effects on other individual organs. On the heart, for example, it enhances the toxic action of many drugs and of such procedures as hypothermia, giving rise to an increased irritability and liability to arrhythmias, and ultimately to ventricular fibrillation. The sensitivity of the heart and other organs to hypoxia is likewise increased in the presence of carbon dioxide retention.

There is much less certainty of the harm of overventilation. Short periods of overventilation, such as may be encountered during surgery, seem to be harmless from a purely metabolic point of view and inasmuch as overventilation will, in general, ensure good oxygenation of the blood leaving the lungs, it is to be preferred to under-ventilation. However, like under-ventilation it also produces changes in tissue activity. For example, it produces an alteration in activity of various drugs, especially muscle relaxants (see page 401).

Certain other harmful effects may be associated with controlled respiration, especially if it is carried out with a face-mask instead of an endotracheal tube. Inflation through a face-mask may result in inflation of the stomach. When a mask is used the pressure applied should be carefully limited; pressures up to 15 cm H_2O rarely distend the stomach, pressures over 20 cm H_2O invariably do so. If this occurs the stomach dilates and may present a hindrance to the surgeon performing an intra-abdominal operation. In addition, unless the gas in the stomach is removed by means of a stomach tube, its presence may encourage the regurgitation of gastric fluids.

Mean Pressure within the Lungs

Any harmful effects of controlled respiration on the cardiovascular system are basically the result of abnormally high pressures within the lungs eliminating the whole or part of the normal subatmospheric pressure within the thorax. Both the magnitude of the positive pressure and the time during which it acts are of importance; these two factors are combined in the term 'mean pressure'. The lower the mean intrapulmonary pressure during the respiratory cycle, the less marked these cardiovascular effects will be.

The term 'mean pressure' does not, in this context, imply the arithmetical mean between the highest and lowest pressures in the respiratory cycle. It is, in fact, the mean of a very large number of equally-spaced instantaneous readings of pressure within the lung during one respiratory cycle. The ways in which the mean pressure in the lungs may be kept low are:

1. *Short application*: Once the required volume has entered the lungs expiration should be allowed to begin. In healthy lungs it is extremely unlikely that any important additional gaseous exchange with the blood occurs

once the volume exchange has taken place. The maintenance of a plateau in the pressure curve after volume exchange has occurred may assist the more even distribution of gas in animals with pulmonary disease, but it will also embarrass the circulation.

2. *Long expiratory phase*: The inspiratory phase should occupy less than half of the total respiratory cycle. A longer positive pressure phase will tend to cause reduction of cardiac output. A long expiratory phase allows the lungs to deflate so that the intrapulmonary pressure falls to zero. The heart is free from tamponade and its output rises, the intrathoracic pressure falls, and the great veins and heart fill. If the expiratory period is too short these events are curtailed and the next inflation occurs while the lung is still partially inflated; the heart is subjected to continuous tamponade, the venous return is severely hampered and the pulmonary circulation continuously impeded. The mean pressure within the lungs is raised, and, even in a healthy adult animal, a short expiratory period may cause gradually increasing cardiovascular embarrassment.

3. *Rapid gas flows*: The faster the flow of gas into the lungs the shorter the inspiratory period can be. Limits, however, are set by the danger of alveolar rupture in circumstances of uneven ventilation, and even by the development of uneven ventilation itself by virtue of the resultant short inspiratory period. Nevertheless, in general, the tendency should be to use higher rather than lower flows during inspiration.

4. *Low expiratory resistance*: Any resistance to expiration will delay the fall of pressure during the expiratory phase and must be avoided if the mean intrapulmonary pressure is to be kept low.

5. *Minimal dead space*: By reducing the dead space the tidal volume needed to produce a given alveolar ventilation at a given respiratory frequency can be reduced. This will reduce the peak, and hence the mean, intrapulmonary pressure.

6. *Application of negative pressure*: The application of negative (i.e. sub-atmospheric) pressure during the expiratory phase lowers the mean intrapulmonary pressure in two ways:

(*a*) A particular volume exchange during the inspiratory phase requires a certain pressure difference between the mouth and alveoli depending on the compliance and airway resistance. If the inspiratory phase starts with a sub-atmospheric pressure of a few cm H_2O in the lungs, the required pressure difference and hence volume exchange, occurs with a lower peak of positive pressure. This is what occurs in automatic lung ventilators in which a sub-atmospheric pressure is maintained throughout the expiratory part of the respiratory cycle.

(b) A negative pressure phase can also accelerate the fall in pressure in the lungs during expiration.

In clinical practice most or all of these various methods of reducing the mean intrapulmonary pressure and maintaining the venous return are employed at the same time. That the animal suffers least cardiovascular harm if its ventilatory requirements are satisfied with as low as possible mean intrapulmonary pressure, is not in doubt. Whether one factor is more important than another is still not clear.

In addition to reducing the mean intrapulmonary pressure, a negative pressure phase will also have some direct effect in increasing the venous return. This seems to be due to a restoration of a suction effect during the expiratory phase in contradistinction to the natural thoracic pump of spontaneous inspiration. Negative pressure during the expiratory phase is transmitted to the intrathoracic structures, including the great veins, and causes an increased venous pressure gradient during the time it acts. The increased venous return, which occurs when a negative pressure phase is introduced, does not take place when the chest is widely opened and all the intrathoracic structures are exposed to atmospheric pressure, so there is little point in employing a negative pressure phase during thoracic surgery.

In spite of all the apparent advantages of a negative pressure phase in the respiratory cycle there are circumstances in which it may be actually harmful. In emphysema the pathological changes result in a high lung compliance and high airway resistance. In addition the wall structure of the smaller airways becomes weaker and more easily collapsed than normal. As a result, when the pressure difference between the alveoli and mouth exceeds a certain critical value, the well-known 'check-valve' or 'trapping' mechanism comes into play; the small airways collapse and expiration slows down. By increasing the pressure drop across the airway the use of a negative pressure phase in the respiratory cycle actually impedes or even arrests the expiratory gas flow. A negative pressure phase should, therefore, be employed with very great caution, if at all, in emphysematous animals. In extreme cases such an animal can be reduced to a state of asphyxia by the use of a high pressure difference, whether this is the result of a high positive pressure in the alveoli at the end of inspiration without a negative pressure in the expiratory phase, or a lower positive pressure in the alveoli and a negative pressure in the expiratory phase.

A further disadvantage of a negative pressure expiratory phase is that it is accompanied by an increase in physiological dead space. An additional need for caution is during operations on the head and neck in the head-up position, in which large veins may be opened and also in other circumstances where air can enter veins. The increased negative pressure in the thorax as a result of the negative pressure phase may be transmitted through the veins increasing the danger of air embolism.

Management of Controlled Respiration

The institution of controlled respiration entails the abolition of all spontaneous respiratory movements and the main factors are:

1. Depression of the respiratory centre by the premedicant drugs, thiopentone and maintenance anaesthetic agents. These probably act by raising the carbon dioxide threshold level of the centre.
2. Reflex inhibition of the respiratory centre—overstimulation of the Hering-Breuer reflex from regular rhythmical inflation of the lungs by the anaesthetist. Regular stimulation of the stretch receptors results in inhibition of the inspiratory centre of the medulla by afferent impulses in the vagus nerves.
3. Lowering of the carbon dioxide tension of the blood by hyperventilation.
4. Paralysis of the respiratory muscles by the use of relaxant drugs.

In most animals apnoea is established by the use of respiratory depressant and relaxant drugs, but in ruminants the use of relaxants seems, at the moment, to be unwise and should be avoided. In ruminant animals it is safer to induce apnoea by assisting the spontaneous respiratory movements so that hyperventilation is produced—the reservoir bag being squeezed at the end of each spontaneous inspiration to force a little more gas into the lungs. This manoeuvre soon results in the establishment of controlled respiration.

Once spontaneous respiration is abolished the interchange of gases is accomplished by gentle rhythmical compression of the reservoir bag. The rate of compression should, in general, be greater than the normal respiratory rate of the animal and as soon as the desired degree of inflation of the lungs has been effected the bag should be released smartly and the lungs allowed to empty freely. During thoracotomy, excessive inflation of the lungs is shown by expansion of the lung beyond the limits of the thoracotomy opening.

The rhythmical squeezing of the bag for long periods is both a tedious and monotonous procedure. The anaesthetist may also need to have his hands free for such things as setting up an intravenous infusion, sucking out the tracheobronchial tree or otherwise looking after the welfare of the animal. Sometimes too, the anaesthetist may be inexperienced and not have all the skill and knowledge necessary to carry out manually controlled respiration in the proper manner. It has been considerations such as these which have been responsible for the introduction of mechanical devices ('ventilators') for maintaining controlled respiration. However, it must not be imagined that manual squeezing of the breathing bag has no advantages to offer the anaesthetist. Manual squeezing of a reservoir bag is noiseless; there is nothing mechanical to break down and much valuable information can be gained by having a hand in contact with the bag. The effort necessary to produce the desired degree of inflation of the lungs gives the anaesthetist information about the level of anaesthesia or the degree of relaxation of the respiratory muscles; easier inflation means greater relaxation of the respiratory muscles and, therefore, deeper anaesthesia or more complete curarization. The presence or absence of respiratory obstruction may also be indicated in this way. Every flicker of the diaphragm and every attempt at coughing is transmitted to the bag and the anaesthetist's hand. Observation of the bag between compressions shows the volume changes due to the heart beat. Nevertheless, in spite of these considerations, it is now generally agreed that ventilators have a valuable place in veterinary anaesthesia and that the anaesthetist needs to understand their operation.

Ventilators

Ventilators are machines for providing a tidal flow of gases into, and out of, the respiratory tract. Very many of the large number available commercially are suitable for use on small animal patients, but there are very few machines which will ventilate horses and cattle adequately. A description of every available machine is outside the scope of this book and all that can be said is that certain basic features are now established which a ventilator, claiming to be consistently adequate, should possess. If its design and performance do not measure up to these basic requirements, a machine can only be but a poor competitor with manual squeezing of the reservoir bag of a closed or semi-closed circuit.

Very briefly, ventilators can generally be classified as either flow generators or pressure generators. With flow generators the flow pattern during inspiration is *entirely* determined by the ventilator and quite independent of lung characteristics which determine the pressures generated during the inspiratory phase. Examples of flow generator systems are the reducing valves on a cylinder or gas pipeline which give a very high constant pressure, electrically driven compressors, injector pumps and piston pumps. All except the piston pump, which gives a variable flow pattern, yield a constant flow pattern (Fig. 146).

In pressure generator systems the pressure applied to the airway during the inspiratory phase of the respiratory cycle is determined by the ventilator setting. Both the flow and volume delivered will depend on the lung character-

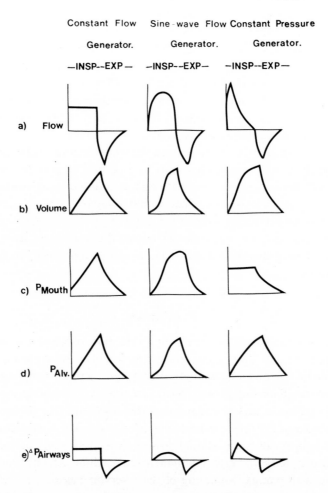

Fig. 146.—Characteristics of three types of lung ventilators. (a) Flow pattern; (b) Volume change in the lung; (c) Pressure change at the mouth; (d) Pressure changes in the alveoli; and (e) Pressure gradient across the airway.

istics. The most commonly used pressure generator probably consists of a weight or spring arranged to act on a bellows.

Changeover from inspiration to expiration may be (a) time cycled, (b) pressure cycled, (c) volume cycled or (d) mixed—e.g. a volume stop on a pressure or time cycled machine.

(a) *Time cycled*: The changeover from inspiration to expiration takes place after a pre-set time interval during which the inspiratory gas flow occurs. The most vital function, the delivery of the tidal volume, is brought about by the application of flow or pressure during the inspiratory period. In other words, the tidal volume is indirectly achieved.

(b) *Pressure cycled*: The changeover occurs when a preset pressure is attained, irrespective of the tidal exchange and the time of inspiratory flow. Again the tidal volume is achieved indirectly. In animals with a high airway resistance the cycling pressure may be reached well before an adequate volume has been delivered into the lungs.

(c) *Volume cycled*: The changeover only occurs when a preset volume has been delivered, irrespective of the pressure or time necessary for its delivery. In these machines the tidal volume is directly achieved.

(d) *Mixed cycling*: Many machines have hybrid or alternative cycling mechanisms.

Each type of apparatus has its own advantages and disadvantages and discussion of their relative merits is outside the scope of this book.

In the expiratory phase of the respiratory cycle the machine may act as a flow generator (e.g. an injector) or a pressure generator—the commonest arrangement is a constant (i.e. atmospheric) pressure of zero. The changeover from expiratory phase to inspiratory phase may be time cycled or patient cycled.

Provided a machine conforms favourably with the following requirements it may be termed 'an adequate ventilator' no matter what its mode of operation or cycling mechanism may be.

Essential Characteristics of an Adequate Ventilator

For use in cats, dogs, sheep, goats, small calves and small pigs, a ventilator needs to have a range of tidal volumes up to 1000 ml. Whenever possible the expired volume should be monitored since the 'stroke volume' of the ventilator may not represent the tidal volume delivered to the animal. A very good machine will have an infinitely variable cycling rate from, say, 8 to 60 cycles/ minute, but a stepwise adjustment such as 10, 14, 18, 22, 24, 28 cycles may often be adequate. The inspiratory phase should be variable, independent of the expiratory time, and range from 0·5 to about 3 seconds' duration. While a relatively long inspiratory time (e.g. at least 1·5 seconds) permits better gas distribution in the lungs, prolonging the inspiratory phase beyond the minimum necessary to introduce the tidal volume may cause circulatory embarrassment which may be especially noticeable and dangerous in animals in which the systemic and pulmonary circulations are impaired. Expiration should begin immediately after the required tidal volume has entered the lungs. The expiratory phase is the time interval from the beginning of expiration to the onset of the inspiratory phase. It should be variable and independent of the duration of inspiration. The ventilator must permit inspiratory:expiratory ratios of at least 1:3. The machine should be capable of producing pressures up to 50 cm H_2O in the upper airway in order to deliver adequate tidal volumes in diseased lungs. The resistance to expired gas flow through the expiratory side of the ventilator circuit and the ventilator itself should be low. It is probable that it should not exceed 2 cm H_2O at a flow rate of 0·5 litre/second. A ventilator should be capable of producing a high instantaneous, or peak, inspiratory flow rate in order to achieve inflation of the lungs during a short inspiratory phase. A ventilator with a high peak flow rate can easily be adapted for low flow rate use, whereas the converse is never true. If a sub-atmospheric pressure phase is incorporated in the cycle, it should be controllable, independent of the respiratory rate and positive pressure of the inspiratory phase, while its inception along the expiratory phase should be under the control of the operator.

Provided the ventilator complies with the clinical criteria set out above, the method of its cycling can be regarded as largely irrelevant. However, one or two practical points should also be taken into account before a ventilator is purchased. It should be possible to change to manual ventilation if any mechanical fault develops during the course of an anaesthetic. If electrically operated, safety from explosion and electrocution must be guaranteed. The machine should not be noisy, and should be as small and light as possible. If free-standing it should occupy minimal floor space. Finally, it is worth noting that price is probably the least important guide to the utility of a ventilator, since machines may cost from £20 to £2000!

The basic clinical criteria for ventilators for adult horses, cattle and large pigs are similar to those set out above. A useful ventilator has a tidal volume of between 2 and 20 litres, with a cycling rate of between 8 and 18/minute, and an inspiratory phase of 2 to 4 seconds. It should be capable of sustaining pressures of up to 60 cm H_2O in the upper airway during inspiration. The inspiratory : expiratory ratio should be at least 1 : 2.

Ventilators designed for use in man have given very satisfactory results when used on small animals and there is no need to develop special machines for small animal patients. Among the very many which have performed consistently are the Bird, the Cyclator, the Fazakerly, the Manley and the Pulmomat. The three small, inexpensive ventilators (Minivent, Automatic Vent and Microvent) described by Hall and Massey (1969) are suitable for use anywhere supplies of compressed air or oxygen are available (Fig. 147).

Special machines have had to be developed for use with large animals and, at the moment, most workers use machines constructed to their own specifications. An attempt by Hansson and Johannisson (1958) to produce a ventilator for large animals was only partially successful for while it proved to be adequate for cattle it failed to ventilate horses in a satisfactory manner. The ventilator described by Fowler, Parker, McLaughlin and Tyler (1963) is quite widely used in the United States of America, but possesses a number of disadvantages. Weaver (1967) developed the use of a Monaghan machine designed for human use as a cuirass ventilator for the ventilation of horses, but commented that she was unable to obtain a large enough reserve of volume output for extensive use on large horses. At the Cambridge School, Carolyn

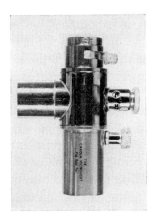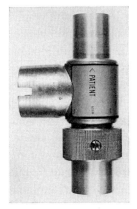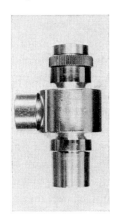

Fig. 147.—Three miniature lung ventilators—the Minivent, East's Automatic Vent and the Microvent.

Monahan designed a cam-operated leather bellows mechanism which compresses the reservoir bag of an anaesthetic apparatus to produce a very good pattern of lung inflation. This machine has proved adequate for ponies weighing up to 300 kg but again the volume output is not great enough for large horses, although it is possible that this limitation may be overcome by a minor modification. The best ventilator available for horses is, at present, undoubtedly that of Møgens-Smith (Royal Veterinary College, Copenhagen). His machine is driven by compressed air and may be used for assisted as well as for full controlled respiration, because it possesses a very sensitive patient trigger device.

Tidal and Minute Volumes of Controlled Respiration

In veterinary anaesthesia there are, as yet, no accepted standards for the tidal and minute volumes of controlled respiration. Ventilation through a breathing circuit which incorporates an absorber can easily lead to hypocapnia or hypercapnia and it is difficult to maintain a normal arterial carbon dioxide tension without actual direct monitoring of the blood gases or the continuous estimation of the percentage of carbon dioxide in the end-tidal expired air. Such monitoring is not generally possible and because hyperventilation is much less harmful than underventilation, it is always better to overventilate. This may be achieved by ventilating at tidal and minute volumes well in excess of those observed during spontaneous breathing. The rate is set at about twice the spontaneous breathing rate, and the chest wall is observed to gauge the tidal volume delivered at each inflation. Inflation should cause the chest wall to move much more than was observed when the animal was breathing quietly at rest before anaesthesia.

In spite of the apparent lack of harm resulting from hypocapnia, however, it would seem more desirable to maintain the arterial carbon dioxide tension at around the normal value of 40 mm Hg. In large animals, when the blood gases or end-tidal gas carbon dioxide concentration cannot be measured, this can only be achieved by chance because for reasons of economy in the use of gases, rebreathing circuits with carbon dioxide absorption must be employed. Small animal patients, however, can be ventilated economically on a non-rebreathing circuit and there are then two ways in which a normal carbon dioxide tension can be maintained throughout the period of controlled ventilation. The apparatus dead space can be increased to provide a calculated amount of rebreathing during hyperventilation; or, 4 to 5% carbon dioxide can be added to the inspired gases during hyperventilation using a non-rebreathing circuit with the minimum of apparatus dead space. The second method is more practicable, for in the first the dead space volume has to be adjusted for each individual animal and respiratory volume. The second method is, of course, liable to give rise to hypercapnia unless very deliberate hyperventilation is practised, but it has been shown to be capable of maintaining normal arterial carbon dioxide tensions over several hours of controlled respiration.

Termination of Controlled Respiration

No difficulty should be experienced in terminating controlled respiration provided that the problem is approached in the following manner:

1. When hyperventilation has been practised, allow some accumulation of carbon dioxide by (a) removal of the soda lime canister or (b) if a non-rebreathing technique is being used add carbon dioxide to the respired gases.
2. When the arterial blood carbon dioxide tension has been maintained at around normal levels, break the rhythm of lung inflation.
3. When volatile anaesthetics have been used, dilute the anaesthetic mixture with oxygen.
4. Where possible counteract any residual curarization by the intravenous administration of atropine and neostigmine. The administration of neo-

stigmine may, of course, be unwise when depolarizing relaxants have been used.

It is important to note that while in most animals apnoea is established with the aid of relaxant drugs, in all cases at the end of operation, apnoea should be mainly due to inhibition of the Hering–Bruer reflex by the rhythmical over-inflation of the lungs and, possibly, hyperventilation with carbon dioxide removal. Thus, the prompt resumption of spontaneous breathing should follow on the adoption of measures (1) and (2). Anoxia must be avoided and ventilation of the lungs must be assisted until spontaneous respiratory movements are quite adequate for the provision of satisfactory gaseous exchange.

When residual curarization is to be counteracted by the intravenous injection of atropine and neostigmine, this procedure is best carried out before any carbon dioxide accumulation is encouraged. The reason for this is that neostigmine appears to be less likely to produce cardiac irregularities when the carbon dioxide tension is low.

REFERENCES

FOWLER, M. E., PARKER, E. E., MCLAUGHLIN, R. F. and TYLER, W. S. (1963). *J. Am. vet. med. Ass.* **143**, 272
GILLESPIE, J. R., TYLER, W. S. and EBERLY, V. E. (1966). *J. appl. Physiol.* **21**, 416
HALL, L. W. and MASSEY, G. M. (1969). *Vet. Rec.* **85**, 432
HANSSON, C. H. and JOHANNISSON, D. (1958). *Nord. Vet. Med.* **10**, 469
WEAVER, B. M. Q. (1967). *Vet. Rec.* **80**, 249

21

Anaesthesia for Intrathoracic and Cardiac Surgery

For reasons which have been discussed in the previous chapter, intrathoracic surgery demands the use of controlled respiration while the pleural cavity is open, but apart from this consideration, the anaesthetic methods employed are largely governed by the personal preferences and experience of the anaesthetist. The main anaesthetic problems centre around the elimination of any pneumothorax remaining after closure of the thoracotomy incision. Co-operation between the surgeon and anaesthetist is essential if these problems are to be satisfactorily resolved.

Closure of the Chest

The anaesthetic technique used while the chest is being closed varies with the nature of the operation and in particular depends on whether or not the pleural cavity is drained.

After a limited operation that does not involve injury to the lung tissue the chest may be closed without drainage. This demands full re-expansion of any collapsed area of lung tissue and the maintenance of full control until the chest is airtight. If portions of the lung are allowed to remain collapsed they may stay in that condition post-operatively and become a focus of infection. They can be re-expanded by prolonging the period of positive inflation while the surgeon restrains the overexpansion of the rest of the lung. Sometimes an increase in the inflating pressure of up to about 30 cm of water is also required. Control is necessary until the chest becomes airtight because if air is trapped in the pleural cavity movements of the chest wall are transmitted to the lung by negative intrapleural pressure and pleural exudation is likely to occur as a result of this. The following methods are used to minimize the amount of air left in the pleural cavity after operations where the chest is not drained:

1. Inflation of the lungs during the final closure of the pleura. The chest wall is closed until only a small opening remains. The bag is squeezed and the inflated lung is held against the chest wall until the opening is completely closed. A variation of this method is to suture the chest wall around a small catheter. When the closure of the chest wall is complete, the lungs are inflated and at the peak of inflation the catheter is jerked out, the skin having been sutured tightly to prevent air from entering along the track of the catheter.

2. Suction during or after closure. A catheter is inserted into the pleural cavity and suction is applied through it until after the chest wall is closed. It is then pulled out with a sharp tug. Alternatively, when the thoracotomy wound has been closed a large-bore needle connected to a suction apparatus is

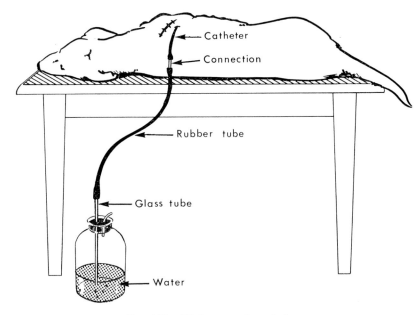

FIG. 148.—Underwater chest drain.

inserted into the pleural cavity and suction applied until there is a negative pressure present in the system. The needle or catheter may become blocked by the lung and the method is therefore not very satisfactory. Nevertheless this method is the only one of practical value for use in adult horses and cattle.

When there is injury to a lung which could cause an air leak the chest must be drained. The drain is connected to a water seal (Fig. 148); this acts as a non-return valve and allows air or fluid to be expelled from the pleural cavity but prevents the indrawing of air during inspiration. The drain tube dips about 2·5 cm below the surface of the water and should have an internal diameter of about 0·5 cm. The bottle must have an internal diameter of not less than 15 cm. When the closure of the chest is complete, inflation of the lung, or spontaneous respiratory movements of the animal, forces air out of the pleural cavity whenever the pressure within the pleural sac is greater than about 2·5 cm of water (i.e. the depth which the tube dips below the surface of the water). Provided that the bottle is kept at least 80 cm below the level of the animal's body, water cannot be aspirated into the chest for no effort of the animal can lift the water up this distance. The large diameter of the bottle ensures that no matter how high the level rises in the drainage tube the end of this tube will always be below the water surface.

When the animal breathes spontaneously the water level in the drainage tube rises on inspiration (as the cavity between the lung and chest wall increases) and falls on expiration. When the lung occupies the whole of the pleural space the pressure does not show marked fluctuations during the respiratory cycle. If, however, the lung is not completely expanded large variations in pressure occur. Observation of the behaviour of the water level in the glass tube thus provides useful information as to the state of expansion of the lung—the greater the amplitude of the swing of the water level, the poorer is the expansion of the lung. The drain should be allowed to remain in the pleural cavity until the lung is fully expanded. It is then pulled out, and a skin suture, which has been laid for the purpose, tied tightly to occlude the hole in the skin.

After any operation which has involved stripping of the visceral layer of pleura from the area of the lung there will be an air leak from the raw surface of the lung. In such circumstances suction may have to be applied to the far side of the underwater seal apparatus to control the pneumothorax. This suction must be maintained until there is no bubbling of air through the water indicating that the leak has been sealed off by inflammatory reaction. It may not be possible to remove the drain tube for up to 48 hours after operation and during this time the animal must be kept well sedated. Experience has shown that this sedation is best achieved by the use of combinations of phenthiazine ataractic drugs and pethidine in such a way that respiratory depression is avoided. After any thoracotomy the animal must be examined (radiologically whenever possible) for evidence of lung collapse. Collapse of a lung, or of a lobe of a lung, may necessitate immediately intrabronchial suction for the removal of any material which is occluding the bronchus to the lung or lobe.

It is often possible after the first few hours to clamp the drain tube, disconnect it from the bottle, and strap it to the chest wall to facilitate nursing care. Should a pleural effusion or a pneumothorax develop subsequently, the tube may then be reconnected to the bottle and the clamp removed. The drain tube should never be withdrawn from the chest until it is certain that it will be of no further use.

Thoracotomy for Non-pulmonary Lesions

Thoracotomies for non-pulmonary lesions present few special anaesthetic problems. Large neoplasms within the thorax can cause an animal considerable respiratory difficulty but removal of the space-occupying lesion eases the respiration at once. In removing some of the more extensive mediastinal tumours the surgeon may open both pleural cavities but with the maintenance of controlled respiration no trouble is encountered.

Oesophageal Surgery

The problems in oesophageal surgery arise from the danger of regurgitation of food and saliva which have been retained in the oesophagus. Thoracotomy for oesophageal surgery presents no special anaesthetic problems that have not already been discussed.

Repair of Ruptures of the Diaphragm

Although the majority of diaphragmatic ruptures are best repaired through an abdominal incision (Walker and Hall, 1965) the pleural cavity is, of course, opened to the atmosphere during the course of the operation. The anaesthetic management of these cases is not always easy.

Diaphragmatic rupture produces respiratory inefficiency which results both from reduced breathing capacity and from an unbalanced distribution of air and blood within the lungs. The presence of abdominal viscera and effusion within the chest reduces the vital capacity; the absence of effective diaphragmatic movement limits the enlargement of the thoracic cavity. Twisting or displacement of the lung lobes causes partial obstruction of the bronchi, leading to the uneven distribution of the inspired air. The blood passing through overventilated areas of lung will lose more carbon dioxide than it would under normal conditions, but it cannot become more fully oxygenated. In the underventilated areas of lung both oxygenation and carbon dioxide removal are impaired. Because of these effects the mixed blood returning from the lungs usually has a carbon dioxide tension near to normal, but its oxygen tension is low, i.e. the main threat to the life of animals suffering from rupture of the diaphragm is hypoxia. Anything which distresses the animal and thus increases its oxygen requirements may prove fatal. When most of the thoracic cavity is occupied by abdominal viscera and/or effusion, the animal can only survive by making maximal breathing efforts and the use of a respiratory depressant sedative or analgesic is most unwise. In dogs, phenothiazine ataractics such as acetylpromazine together with small doses of pethidine produce useful, safe sedation, and in cats small (10 mg) doses of pethidine are useful.

Anaesthesia for animals suffering from diaphragmatic rupture may be managed in a variety of ways. No hard and fast rules can be given and each individual case must be treated on its own merits. All cases must be handled very quietly and gently before anaesthesia is induced, and a smooth induction of anaesthesia with an intravenous agent is advisable. Some animals do not resent the application of a face-mask and such animals may be given oxygen to inhale for 2 to 3 minutes before the induction of anaesthesia. In dogs, whenever it can be done without undue disturbance of the animal, an intravenous drip should be set up before anaesthesia, otherwise it is set up as soon as possible during the course of the operation. This drip is often needed to remedy the fall in blood pressure seen when re-expansion of the lungs alters the haemodynamic state of the body (presumably due to re-opening of areas of the pulmonary vascular bed). Endotracheal intubation is, of course, essential in all cases.

Post-operative pain, which limits breathing to rapid, very shallow movements of the chest wall, is best controlled by the injection of pethidine hydrochloride, or in large dogs morphine, in the appropriate doses given as required.

Cardiac Surgery

In considering anaesthesia for cardiac surgery it is essential to look beyond the problems associated with thoracotomy. The action of the anaesthetic drugs may affect the heart and alter the vascular tone generally. Equally, disorders of the circulatory system may modify the absorption and action of anaesthetic drugs. The problems that arise are often particular to each lesion but certain general principles of anaesthetic management can be enunciated.

If thiopentone is used for the induction of anaesthesia two points must be noted. First, slowing of the circulation due to the disease process causes a considerable lag between the administration of the drug and the development of its effect. This makes it very easy to give too much, for it may give the impression that the animal is resistant to the drug. Secondly, thiopentone depresses the myocardium and produces peripheral vasodilatation. In animals where the cardiac output is fixed by valvular stenoses, the vasodilatation may produce a very marked fall in blood pressure. The drug should always be administered very slowly and in very dilute solutions.

If it does not excite the animal, oxygen should be administered through a face-mask before anaesthesia is induced, but in every case it should be administered as soon as consciousness is lost. A perfect airway is essential and a large-bore endotracheal tube must be introduced into the trachea as soon as possible.

Constrictive pericarditis and cardiac tamponade are very crippling conditions because they limit the cardiac output and depress the tissue respiration by the widespread action of the raised venous pressure. Associated ascites and pleural effusions reduce the vital capacity and venous back pressure may damage the liver. Careful pre-anaesthetic preparation of these cases is necessary. Pleural and peritoneal effusions must be tapped and fluid retention reduced by the use of mercurial diuretics. Cardiac tamponade must be relieved by paracentesis under local analgesia.

Operations on the heart and great blood vessels which necessitate a short period of circulatory arrest are already being undertaken in canine surgery and it is likely that as diagnostic methods improve many more will be attempted. Since it is most unlikely that pump-oxygenators will ever be freely available for veterinary surgery it is probable that the techniques of hypothermia will be employed to enable the circulatory arrest to be tolerated by the animal.

Hypothermia in Canine Surgery

Provided that it has no work to do, the heart muscle itself is not harmed by short periods of circulatory arrest but the brain cells are extremely sensitive to oxygen lack and cannot survive if the circulation stops for more than 3 to 4 minutes. Reducing the temperature of the brain cells depresses their metabolism and enables them to withstand the effects of longer periods of circulatory arrest. For example, at 30°C the brain will survive and function after a circulatory arrest of 10 minutes.

Body Temperature Measurement

During the rapidly changing conditions of body cooling and rewarming associated with hypothermia techniques, a temperature measurement made in the mouth or rectum fails to provide an adequate index of temperature in other regions of the body. There is ample evidence, however, that the oesophageal temperature at heart level is a most reliable measure of the heart and blood temperature. For this reason a suitable calibrated thermocouple or thermistor device, obtained commercially or made in the laboratory, introduced correctly into the oesophagus, should always be used for temperature measurement.

Reaction to Cold

In a conscious dog vasoconstriction in the skin is the first reaction of the body to a cold environment. Adrenaline is released from the adrenal glands and this, besides causing vasoconstriction, stimulates cellular metabolism, mobilizing glycogen and increasing heat production. Other responses include the release of thyrotrophic hormone and adrenal corticoids both of which result in greater heat production. If these reactions are insufficient to maintain the normal body temperature shivering occurs and a tremendous increase in heat production results. Shivering is by far the most effective means of maintaining the body temperature.

Physiology of Hypothermia

For an introduction to the now voluminous literature on hypothermia reference should be made to *The Physiology of Induced Hypothermia* (edited by R. D. Dripps) and to articles such as that of Cooper (1959). In the account which follows reference can only be made to a few of the physiological consequences of body cooling which are of practical interest in anaesthesia.

As the body cools, the heart rate falls and it is about halved when the body temperature reaches 25°C. This slowing is apparently due to cooling of the pacemaker and is accompanied by a prolongation of systole and isometric contraction. Changes in the electrocardiogram include prolongation of the P-R interval and a lengthening of the QRS complex. Elevation of the S-T segment or the appearance of a wave rising steeply from the S-wave is said to herald the onset of ventricular fibrillation. The onset of ventricular fibrillation, when it occurs in hypothermia, is influenced by a number of factors:

(a) The type of anaesthetic. Of the barbiturates, thiopentone sodium seems the least likely to cause fibrillation.

(b) Mechanical stimulation. Stimulation of the heart by catheters in the ventricles or by surgical procedures may induce fibrillation.

(c) Underventilation. Underventilation of the lungs, with a consequent rise in the carbon dioxide content of the blood and a fall in pH, predisposes to fibrillation.

(d) Changes in the ionic equilibrium. The ionic equilibrium in the blood plays a part in the initiation of cardiac arrhythmias and the relative concentrations of potassium and calcium are particularly important.

(e) Sympathetic discharge. There is some evidence which suggests that blocking the sympathetic nerves to the heart protects this organ against fibrillation under hypothermia.

(f) Blood pressure. Abrupt falls in blood pressure which give rise to a sharp drop in the coronary blood flow can, during hypothermia, precipitate ventricular fibrillation.

The blood flow in the brain, kidney and splanchnic region is reduced as the body temperature falls. In dogs the femoral vascular bed dilates down to oesophageal temperatures of about 34°C then vasoconstriction occurs and later at 20° to 25°C a second vasodilatation takes place. One of the common uses of hypothermia is in circumstances which require clamping of the aorta for a considerable time. The reactive hyperaemia which follows the release of the clamp is only reduced by hypothermia when the circulatory arrest is of short duration. After occlusions lasting more than about 30 minutes, the vaso-dilatation which follows the release of the clamp is large and lasts as long when the body is cold as when it is warm. This must be remembered as vasoconstrictor substances or blood transfusion may have to be used to counteract this effect during cardiac surgery.

A fall in the body and brain temperature results in a decrease in cerebral oxygen consumption. At 25°C the oxygen uptake of the dog's brain is about one-third of that at 37°C and over this range the oxygen consumption is a linear function of temperature. A matter of major importance is the degree of protection afforded to nervous tissue from the effects of circulatory arrest by hypothermia. At 25°C the circulation can be stopped for 15 minutes without damage to the brain cells and for various reasons this time of 15 minutes seems to be the maximum which can be achieved by surface cooling (between 28°C and 25°C the incidence of ventricular fibrillation rises steeply). The electro-encephalogram begins to change as the body temperature falls to 36° to 32°C. The potential recorded shows a decreased amplitude and large delta waves appear, particularly in the frontal area, at about 30°C. The electrical activity then declines until between 18° and 20°C no activity is recorded on an electro-encephalogram.

Technique for the Production of Hypothermia

Various methods including body surface cooling, body cavity cooling, intragastric cooling and bloodstream cooling have been used to induce hypothermia in anaesthetized dogs. Of these only the techniques of body surface cooling and intragastric cooling have been found to be really practic-able in *clinical* canine surgery.

Before hypothermia can be produced by surface cooling the animal's natural defence reaction to cold must be obtunded. Otherwise, attempts at reducing the body temperature are likely to increase, rather than decrease, the cellular metabolism. The efficacy of surface cooling therefore depends on maintaining a coincident vasodilatation of the superficial blood vessels and preventing shivering. Fortunately, the anaesthetic drugs which affect one reaction generally modify the other. Many systems of anaesthesia may be used quite satisfactorily but the one to be described below has proved to be quite adequate. It not only facilitates the induction of hypothermia but also ensures a rapid return of consciousness at the end of operation.

The dog is premedicated with 0·65 mg of atropine sulphate, 0·2 mg/kg of chlorpromazine hydrochloride and 4 mg/kg of pethidine about one hour before anaesthesia is to be induced. The chlorpromazine and pethidine both produce vasodilatation and help to prevent shivering. Larger doses of chlorpromazine should not be used for they may result in undesirable hypotension and tachycardia. Acetylpromazine may be used as an alternative to chlorpromazine.

Anaesthesia is induced with thiopentone sodium given by slow intravenous injection until the jaw muscles are relaxed and the tongue does not curl when the mouth is opened. After intubation with a large cuffed endotracheal tube, anaesthesia is maintained with nitrous oxide and oxygen. The nitrous oxide also helps to prevent shivering during the cooling process. An indwelling intravenous needle is inserted into a suitable vein or a very slow intravenous infusion of 5% dextrose is set up and 0·08 mg/kg of pancuronium is given intravenously. Controlled respiration is commenced as soon as spontaneous respiration ceases. (By paralysing the muscles shivering is made impossible.)

The temperature measuring device is introduced into the oesophagus and the dog's body is immersed in a bath of water at 15° to 20°C. The head is not immersed (Fig. 149) but no harm results if it is accidentally submerged at any time. It is important that the water should be circulated over the body and manual stirring of the water has not been found to be very effective. Agitation of the water is best performed by using a jet of water from a hose connected to a cold water tap. The jet of water is moved slowly over the submerged part of the animal's body. Cooling is rapid and there is no need to use ice to lower the temperature of the water. The body temperature falls to 30° to 25°C within about 30 minutes in most dogs. The dog is removed from the bath when the oesophageal temperature is about 30°C and dried with towels. One of the principal dangers of surface cooling is the 'after-drop' that occurs when the dog is removed from the bath. The 'after-drop' reduces the oesophageal temperature by up to 2°C and it is important to allow for this, for ventricular fibrillation is common at temperatures below 28°C. Between 28° and 25°C the incidence of ventricular fibrillation rises steeply. The reason why the after-drop occurs is that when the dog is removed from the bath the skin and neighbouring tissues are extremely cold. In fact they are much colder than the temperature of the circulating blood and as the blood reaches these parts it continues to cool long after the active cooling measures have been stopped.

In many cases the dog has rewarmed sufficiently by the end of the operation but if it has not done so it may be partially immersed in a bath of warm water. Anaesthesia is terminated when the dog's temperature reaches 35°C and recovery of consciousness should be almost immediate. It is only rarely that it is necessary to use atropine and neostigmine to reverse the paralysis produced by the relaxant, but these drugs should not be withheld if there is any evidence of residual curatization.

A simple refinement of this technique is the use of a collapsible plastic bath on the actual operating table, together with a circulating pump to circulate cold or warm water around the dog (Fig. 149). The sides of such a bath can be

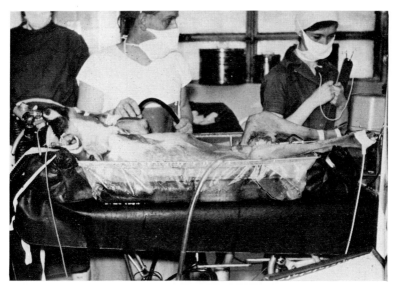

FIG. 149.—The use of a plastic bath with collapsible sides for the induction of moderate hypothermia.

lowered to enable the surgeon to work once the desired degree of hypothermia has been obtained. Partial raising of the sides of the bath and the circulation of water at 0°C or 40°C enables the anaesthetist to control the temperature of the dog during surgery and to ensure that rewarming is complete by the end of the operation.

The method which has been described above does not involve the use of any complicated apparatus and it can be applied by even inexperienced personnel with a fair degree of safety. Obviously, the best results will only be obtained by an experienced surgical team using devices such as electrocardiographs and electro-encephalographs to monitor the process. Absence of such monitoring apparatus will, of course, increase the risks involved but if the condition of the animal is such that it will die unless operation is performed and operation necessitates the use of hypothermia, then these increased risks may be accepted as being reasonable ones.

When a suitable instrument is available, the electrocardiogram is recorded using needle electrodes and it is observed closely throughout the cooling

15*

process. A surgeon should be standing by, scrubbed up and ready to operate, for if ventricular fibrillation occurs during the cooling process immediate thoracotomy and cardiac massage must be performed. One disadvantage of immersion cooling is that there is likely to be a little delay before cardiac massage can be carried out.

If the electro-encephalogram is to be recorded needle electrodes are inserted into the dog's scalp as soon as the dog is removed from the bath. The electrodes are not inserted while the dog is in the bath as the agitation of the water causes too much disturbance and the electrical activity of the brain cannot be recorded. During hypothermia it is most helpful to have the arterial blood pressure, the E.E.G. and the E.C.G. displayed on an oscilloscope.

Intragastric cooling is a slower but much more sophisticated process. A very good, relatively inexpensive apparatus for use in dogs has been described by Schneider and Pyenson (1965). Cold water is circulated through an intragastric balloon which is introduced into the stomach via the oesophagus after the induction of anaesthesia. The average length of time required to lower the rectal temperature of dogs weighing about 30 kg to 25°C is about 2 hours. This may seem to be rather a long time, but during the cooling process monitoring devices such as electrocardiographic leads and blood pressure transducers can easily be attached, vascular cannulations can be made and surgical procedures started. Rewarming can be started at any time during surgery. (without interrupting its progress) by circulating warm water through the balloon, and rewarming is more rapid than can be achieved by any other method.

REFERENCES

COOPER, K. E. (1959). *Br. J. Anaesth.* **31**, 96

DRIPPS, R. D. (1956). *The Physiology of Induced Hypothermia.* Symposium convened by the Division of Medical Sciences, National Research Council. Publication No. 451, Washington D.C.

HOWELLS, T. H. (1963). *Br. J. Anaesth.* **35**, 272

SCHNEIDER, H. P. and PYENSON, J. I. (1965). *J. Am. vet. med. Ass.* **147**, 828

SMITH, A. C. (1962). Lecture, May Scientific Meeting, Faculty of Anaesthetists, Royal College of Surgeons

WALKER, R. G. and HALL, L. W. (1965). *Vet. Rec.* **77**, 830

WATSON, W. E. (1962). *Br. J. Anaesth.* **34**, 502

Accidents and Emergencies associated with Anaesthesia

When the profound physiological changes initiated by the drugs used in anaesthesia are considered it is surprising that serious accidents and emergencies are not common. Familiarity with these drugs can lead to an attitude which may be described as nonchalant and it is easy to forget that the anaesthetic may be a greater hazard to an animal than the operation. During anaesthesia many accidents occur suddenly and the reason for the mishap must be recognized immediately so that the appropriate remedy can be applied at once. Other accidents are less dramatic and their results may only become apparent during the post-operative period. Moreover, one kind of emergency may lead to another. It is fortunate that today most disasters can be avoided, for the conditions which give rise to the occurrence of the more common accidents and emergencies are known. Nevertheless, prevention is not always possible and serious consequences may ensue if the anaesthetist is not always ready to apply the appropriate remedy in any difficult situation which may arise quite unexpectedly. Anaesthesia is still an art, and there is no substitute for experience, but even the inexperienced anaesthetist can deal successfully with most mishaps if aware of the nature of the more common accidents and emergencies.

Failure of the Circulation under General Anaesthesia

Failure of the circulation under general anaesthesia is usually due to the loss of blood. There may be either a sudden effusion of blood or, more commonly, an almost imperceptible loss which occurs during the course of a long operation. Unless blood loss is actually measured it is very difficult to estimate the amount of haemorrhage caused by trauma or operation. In an emergency due to the loss of blood, compatible whole blood, plasma or a plasma volume expander must be given rapidly and the quantity and speed of replacement are the factors which determine the fate of the patient. Dextran solutions which are often used in veterinary practice as plasma volume expanders should always be used with caution, because the infusion of large quantities of dextran results in a failure of the blood clotting mechanism.

Elderly animals and animals which have lost fluid due to their pre-operative condition do not tolerate haemorrhage well. In these animals an apparently moderate blood loss may result in circulatory failure. Fluid replacement should be carried out before operation and blood lost during operation replaced by transfusion of whole blood or these animals will not survive even moderately severe surgical interferences.

A sudden fall in blood pressure during operation sometimes occurs without warning in an animal whose cardiovascular system is apparently healthy and where there has been but little loss of blood. The pulse becomes imperceptible, respiration ceases and the veins (noticeably in the tongue) are dilated. The pupils remain normal in size and this may be the only indication that the heart has not stopped beating. This rather alarming reaction appears to be initiated by certain surgical manipulations. For example, it may be seen during Caesarean hysterotomies in cattle and sheep when traction is exerted on the mesovarium or on the broad ligament of the uterus. It may also be seen in dogs and cats when swabs or retractors are allowed to press upon the coeliac plexus, or when the stomach and liver are handled by the surgeon. When it arises the surgeon should stop and not recommence operating until recovery has occurred. The reaction may be avoided by gentle surgery and the anaesthetist should note that gentle surgery is only possible when the patient's muscles are adequately relaxed.

Shock

Shock is a term which is notoriously difficult to define, but all clinicians are familiar with its manifestations. The major factors in its initiation and maintenance are decreased cardiac output, increased vascular resistance and decreased effective circulating blood volume. Each of these feeds back, either directly or through the sympathetic nervous system, to perpetuate the condition of shock. Reduction in cardiac output leads to increased sympatho-adrenal activity which leads in turn to a selective reduction of blood flow in the splanchnic and cutaneous circulations, thereby producing the clinical signs of shock. Hypotension is not a primary manifestation or feature, and only occurs when the increased sympatho-adrenal activity fails to compensate for losses in effective circulating blood volume and decreased myocardial contractile force.

The most common and dramatic cause of shock is sudden external haemorrhage, but a similar state can arise if blood is lost internally or if large quantities of electrolytes and water are lost to the body through vomiting and diarrhoea or intestinal obstruction. Estimation of blood loss during surgery is difficult and most surgeons tend to grossly underestimate the blood loss they cause, but when the circulating blood volume is maintained during surgery by adequate transfusion, surgical shock is seldom encountered. Nearly all cases of surgical or traumatic shock respond to prompt transfusion and a fatal outcome is usually due to undiagnosed complications such as pneumothorax, fulminating cerebral fat embolism, cardiac tamponade, bilateral adrenal haemorrhage, air embolism or pre-existing cardiac, pulmonary or other diseases, such as diabetes mellitus.

Sometimes, however, shock is unresponsive to treatment and the condition is said to be 'irreversible'. This state is not uncommon in animals suffering from systemic bacterial infection or peritonitis. It can also arise from undertransfusion or too long a delay before replacing fluid losses. Dogs bled until they have become severely hypotensive recover if the blood is replaced within a certain time but after a delay of 2 to 4 hours transfusion has little or no effect. The animals die and their intestinal mucosa is found to be haemorrhagic and necrotic, especially in the ileum, and haemorrhages are found under the endocardium and elsewhere.

The processes which lead to irreversibility are complex and difficult to unravel, but if peripheral circulatory failure is the mechanism, then the final common pathway should be found in the microcirculation. It has been suggested that irreversibility begins when ischaemic anoxia changes to stagnant anoxia in certain tissues, and prolonged vasoconstriction is thought to be the key factor. After severe haemorrhage sympathetic activity and catecholamine secretion produce vasoconstriction and ischaemic anoxia in the splanchnic bed, liver and kidneys. This regional vasoconstriction enables the circulation to be maintained through the unconstricted cerebral and coronary vessels in spite of any reduction in cardiac output. Transfusion at this stage improves the cardiac output, relieves any hypotension and much of the vasoconstriction, allowing tissue perfusion to be restored. If transfusion is delayed, the constricted arterioles become less and less responsive to adrenaline, apparently due to accumulation of metabolites in the tissues. Eventually the capillaries become engorged and flow stagnates because, it is suggested (Lillehei, Longerbeam, Bloch and Manox, 1964), the venules remain constricted. The reason for the persistence of venular spasm when the arterioles become paralysed is not at all clear, however. Capillary engorgement then raises the hydrostatic pressure so that fluid exudes from the capillary beds and oligaemia becomes more severe. Anoxia changes become serious, local haemorrhages appear and the cycle to death begins. Transfusion is now of no avail, because it merely engorges further the stagnant capillary bed. The venous return and the cardiac output continue to fall and the heart stops or fibrillates as the coronary flow is reduced.

This hypothesis brings together two much older ideas about shock—one which postulated prolonged sympathetic vasoconstriction as causing or increasing the circulatory failure (Malcolm, 1905; Freeman, 1933; Tomb, 1937) and the other which regarded extensive capillary congestion of viscera and leakage of fluid from the bloodstream as essential mechanisms (Moon, 1936, 1942). Fine and his colleagues (1959) agree that changes in abdominal viscera and sympathetic activity are of importance in irreversibility; they also blame an endotoxin of Gram-negative bacilli. This toxin is absorbed from the damaged (anoxic) bowel, acts on the nervous system, produces a relentless abdominal sympathetic induced vasoconstriction, and then cannot be detoxicated because of failure of a reticuloendothelial enzyme in the hypoxic spleen and liver. Endotoxin action certainly has an important adrenergic component; its lethal effect is counteracted by adrenolytic compounds and it potentiates the pressor responses to catecholamines (Gourzis, Hollenberg and Nickerson, 1961).

Long continued vasoconstriction is undoubtedly harmful to the liver, bowel and kidney. Indeed, infusion of adrenaline to intact animals can itself produce lethal shock, even though there is a rise in blood pressure (Erlanger and Gasser, 1919; Smiddy and Fine, 1957). Preoccupation with hypotension in the presence of vasoconstriction has sometimes led clinicians to use adrenaline, noradrenaline, synthetic adrenergic substances or other vaso-pressors to raise the arterial pressure of shocked animals. Temporary benefit from an increase in cerebral and coronary blood flow is not sustained and harm can result from increased vasoconstriction which aggravates tissue anoxia and throws a further load on the heart. These vasopressors are much more likely to be harmful than beneficial in shocked animals and are no substitute for transfusion of the appropriate fluid in traumatic and other forms of shock associated with loss of blood volume.

The only measures which consistently reduce mortality are those which increase blood volume or reduce vasoconstriction (Nickerson, 1955) and this leads to the inference that vasodilators may have a place in the treatment of shock. Although they must not be used when the blood volume is already reduced and they are not substitutes for correct fluid therapy, there are some encouraging reports that anti-adrenergic drugs and other methods of in-hibiting sympathetic activity improve survival after haemorrhage or trauma (Wiggers, Ingraham, Roemheld and Goldberg, 1948), provided further transfusion is also given to cover the increased capacity of the vascular system. It is extremely doubtful if the adrenal cortex plays any part in shock but hydrocortisone (itself a vasodilator) given in massive doses of 50 mg/kg has been successfully used in this way (Lillehei et al., 1964).

Much work has been done to establish the best methods of estimating the severity of shock. Undoubtedly the most useful single determination is that of the central venous pressure (page 18). It provides a beat-to-beat assessment of the ability of the heart to propel the volume of blood constituting the venous return. Thus, it reflects both cardiac function and the adequacy of the blood volume in relation to the volume of the vascular bed. Capillary refilling time in the lips and the state of distension of the peripheral veins may also assist in the diagnosis and management of shock. The urinary output is also a sensitive indicator of the circulatory state because glomerular filtration depends on the renal blood flow which in turn depends on the circulating blood volume and cardiac output.

Obviously, the best treatment for shock is to prevent it from occurring. Early transfusion to restore the blood volume and expeditious operation to arrest bleeding, remove damaged tissue and, if necessary, fix broken bones, will prevent shock from becoming irreversible.

Disturbances of Cardiac Rhythm

Tachycardia is usual in young animals, but in adults the pulse rate increases in shock or after the administration of drugs such as atropine. It must be emphasized too, that in cases where relaxant drugs are being used tachycardia may indicate an insufficient depth of anaesthesia.

Cardiac arrhythmias are common in all kinds of animal under all forms of anaesthesia but they are frequently unrecognized since unless persistent gross irregularities of the peripheral pulse occur the anaesthetist is not likely to become aware of the disturbance. Electrocardiograms of animals under general anaesthesia often show arrhythmias while on clinical examination the animal appears normal.

The origin of these disturbances of cardiac rhythm is still uncertain. If the anaesthetic agent is known to depress the functional capacity of the heart muscle it is natural to assume that the direct action of the drug on the myocardium is the cause, but serious arrhythmias can be caused by the action of the autonomic nerves to the heart. The nervous system is often hyperactive immediately before operation, especially if the animal is frightened, and stimulation of the sympathetic nerves to the heart may cause ventricular ectopic beats or even ventricular fibrillation if the heart muscle is sensitized by hydrocarbon anaesthetic agents. The combination of adrenaline with chloroform, cyclopropane, trichloroethylene or ethyl chloride is known to cause serious cardiac arrhythmias, and the amount of adrenaline which may be released into the circulation when an animal is frightened is near to that necessary to produce ventricular fibrillation in the presence of these anaesthetic agents. Carbon dioxide accumulation in the body, and mild degrees of hypoxia may cause stimulation of the sympathetic nervous system, so arrhythmias are common when respiration is depressed or obstructed.

Treatment of cardiac arrhythmias will depend on the cause and an accurate diagnosis can only be made when an electrocardiograph is available. The use of drugs for the treatment of cardiac irregularities is not justified in the absence of an exact diagnosis. *However, most cardiac arrhythmias disappear once adequate respiratory exchange has been established.* An unobstructed airway must be ensured and pulmonary ventilation assisted by intermittent pressure on the chest wall or reservoir bag whenever respiratory depression is encountered.

Heart Failure

There are two distinct types of heart failure: the first is ventricular fibrillation which is comparatively uncommon. The second and more common type is ventricular asystole, frequently termed 'arrest of the heart'.

It has been known since 1911 that chloroform sensitizes the heart so that a mechanical, chemical or endocrine stimulus not normally sufficient to cause harm produces ventricular fibrillation, and more recently it has been shown that cyclopropane, trichloroethylene and ethyl chloride have a similar action. Fibrillation is more common under conditions of oxygen lack—e.g. in shocked or anaemic animals.

Cardiac arrest or asystole is the type of heart failure associated with overdosage of anaesthetic agents. Gross overdosage is probably rare, but relative overdosage is more frequent—e.g. the use of normal doses or concentrations of anaesthetic agents in old, shocked or debilitated animals.

If counter measures are to be effective, diagnosis of heart failure must be rapid. The brain cells are very sensitive to hypoxia and circulatory arrest of more than 3 to 4 minutes' duration causes irreversible brain damage. Respiration does not fail as soon as the circulation stops; it continues until the respiratory centre becomes anoxic. This must be remembered and cardiac arrest should be diagnosed, even when respiratory movements are present, when the peripheral pulse is absent, the mucous membranes an ashen colour and the pupils widely dilated. Conservative treatment is not only useless, it wastes valuable time. The only way of restoring the circulation is to institute effective cardiac massage immediately.

If not already in place an endotracheal tube should be introduced to ensure patency of the airway, any inhalation anaesthetics discontinued, and positive pressure respiration, preferably with pure oxygen, commenced at once.

Compression of the Heart through the Intact Chest Wall

Effective compression of the heart through the intact chest wall is possible in all animals. In cats and small dogs the chest walls over the region of the heart are compressed between the fingers and thumb of one hand. Compression must be forcible and fairly rapid (more than 60 times/minute). Larger animals are quickly placed on their side on a hard, unyielding surface. The upper chest wall over the region of the heart is then forced inward and allowed

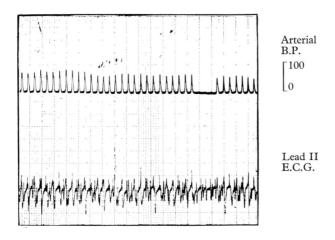

Fig. 150.—Tracing of the arterial blood pressure produced by cardiac compression through the intact chest wall in a dog suffering from ventricular fibrillation.

to recoil outwards, movement of the lower chest wall being restricted by the hard surface on which the animal is lying. In dogs and other small animals pressure on the uppermost chest wall with the hand is adequate, but in adult horses and cattle the knee or foot is used. Ribs may be fractured, but such fractures must be ignored, and the rate of compression should be above 60 compressions/minute in dogs, or 30 or 40/minute in adult horses and cattle. The rate of compression must, of course, allow for filling of the heart between compressions. An effective circulation can be maintained in this way (Fig. 150). Regular spontaneous respiratory movements may return, and the size of the pupils should remain small.

If, for some reason, an effective circulation cannot be produced by massage through the chest wall then the heart must be exposed by a thoracotomy incision.

Direct Cardiac Massage

No time should be lost in 'scrubbing up' or in preparing the site before making an intercostal incision and when the heart is exposed the ventricles must be squeezed rhythmically. The squeezing should be carried out with a gliding or milking motion from the apex towards the base of the heart. The rate of compression should not be too rapid for the chambers must have time to fill with blood between compressions and a slight head-down inclination of the body aids the filling of the heart. In small animals the ventricles can be compressed by the grasp of one hand but in larger animals both hands must be used. In every case care must be taken to avoid rupture of the heart—particularly of the atria—by the finger-tips. The effectiveness of the artificial circulation produced by the massage may be gauged by the maintenance of a small pupil size which indicates that the cerebral circulation is adequate. Once an artificial circulation has been established there is no longer any necessity for haste and there is time for a considered approach. Further treatment depends on whether the heart is at a standstill or is in ventricular fibrillation.

When the chest is open and the heart is visible, differentiation between standstill (asystole) and fibrillation is obvious, but when the heart is being compressed through the intact chest wall an electrocardiogram may be necessary for this differentiation.

In the case of cardiac standstill adrenaline or calcium chloride may be injected into the heart and massaged into the circulation. There is no general agreement about the best place for injection but when drugs are injected into the left ventricle they will quickly be massaged into the coronary vessels and myocardium. A large dog may be given 5 ml of 1:10,000 adrenaline hydrochloride or 2 to 3 ml of 10% calcium chloride solution and both drugs may be repeated in these doses.

Fibrillation may be present when cardiac arrest occurs or may be precipitated in a heart by the effects of drugs or even of massage. The best and most specific treatment is to pass an electric shock through the myocardium so that when the contraction which this causes passes off the whole muscle remains in a relaxed state of asystole. Then, it is hoped, normal contractions will start either spontaneously or after a brief period of further massage. Electrical defibrillation should only be attempted with properly constructed apparatus such as that in Fig. 151—*improvised apparatus connected to the mains supply of electricity is most dangerous*. Attempts at electrical defibrillation are much more likely to be successful if the myocardium is well oxygenated from effective massage before the shock is applied.

Procaine depresses cardiac contraction, decreases excitability and prolongs the refractory period of heart muscle so that it may be used to overcome fibrillation. In large dogs the dose is of the order of 5 to 10 ml of a 1% solution of procaine hydrochloride injected into a cavity of the heart and massaged into the circulation.

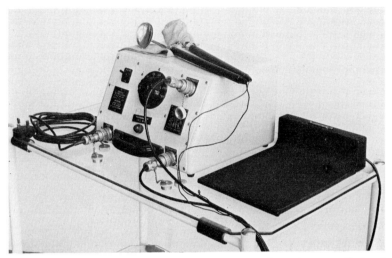

FIG. 151.—A type of 'internal' defibrillator in which the electrodes are applied to the heart itself.

The foot-switch is shown on the right of the picture and the spoon-shaped electrodes are covered with saline-soaked gauze before being applied. ('External' defibrillators are also available in which the electrodes are applied to the outside of the intact chest wall.)

Once normal cardiac action has been restored the ventilation of the lungs with oxygen must continue until all evidence of circulatory failure has vanished. The chest should not be closed until spontaneous heart beats have been present for 20 minutes.

It is fairly obvious that cardiac failure is likely to be treated with any consistent measure of success only in the smaller animals. Prophylaxis is therefore of major importance. A stormy induction of surgical anaesthesia should always be avoided and the one common factor in many anaesthetic fatalities—hypoxia—must never be allowed to occur.

Respiratory Acidosis

Serious consequences are seen when the minute volume of respiration is decreased since this causes a diminished excretion of carbon dioxide from the lungs and therefore results in the development of respiratory acidosis. This state is commonly seen when the total gas flow rate in a semi-closed circuit is too low, or when the soda lime in an absorber is exhausted. It also occurs when the airway is obstructed or when the respiratory movements are hampered by the position of the animal's body on the bed or operating table. Usually the disturbance of the acid–base balance of the blood results in very little harm when the duration of anaesthesia is short, but it may have serious effects if the anaesthetic period is prolonged. Death occurs when the pH of the blood falls below about 6·7.

The signs of respiratory acidosis are not always obvious, for the animal's mucous membranes remain pink and its pulse slow and of good volume. It is important to note that, although in the normal animal an increase in the alveolar carbon dioxide content causes a frank increase in the tidal volume, in the anaesthetized animal this may not be seen. The blood pressure first rises, then returns to normal and finally falls. Circulatory failure, when it occurs, is rapid and is due to heart failure. When respiratory acidosis has developed, the animal may collapse after the end of the operation, for the excess carbon dioxide is rapidly excreted as respiratory depression decreases and the circulatory pressure reflexes are not active enough to compensate for the sudden change in acid–base balance in the blood. The condition may be diagnosed as shock, but unlike shock, is characterized by a slow pulse and, in fit animals, by rapid spontaneous recovery.

Hypoxia

During anaesthesia, hypoxia is most commonly encountered when the oxygen content of the inspired gases is low, when the airway is obstructed, or when relaxant drugs weaken the respiratory muscles. It is also met during intra-thoracic surgery when portions of a lung are collapsed.

Mild degrees of hypoxia may be very hard to recognize. Cyanosis is usually regarded as the commonest sign of hypoxia, but not only is it an unreliable sign, it is not always easy to detect. It will be masked by pigmentation of the skin and mucous membranes, and may not be seen at all in anaemic or in shocked animals.

The brain cells are easily damaged by hypoxia and prolonged coma after anaesthesia should arouse suspicion of hypoxic brain damage. To prevent the progression of cellular damage from the early stage of oedema to an irreversible condition, treatment must be commenced as soon as possible after the hypoxic episode. It consists of the intravenous injection of a hypertonic solution of sucrose (50% sucrose) to promote absorption of oedema fluid. A dog may be given up to 50 ml/hour of the sucrose solution.

Hypoxia also has the effect of increasing the extent of liver and kidney damage caused by anaesthetic drugs while its effects on the heart have already been discussed.

Laryngeal and Bronchial Spasm

Laryngeal spasm appears to be seen more commonly than bronchial spasm, but both conditions can occur together during general anaesthesia. Laryngeal spasm can occur in all kinds of animal but is perhaps most frequently encountered in cats under ether anaesthesia when attempts are made to force the animal to breathe high concentrations of the ether vapour before the protective laryngeal reflexes have been subdued. Another common complication of ether anaesthesia in cats is laryngeal 'crowing'—the crowing noise being caused by a partial spasm of the vocal cords due to irritation by a blob of mucus, saliva, blood or vomit.

When laryngeal spasm is troublesome the best treatment is to administer a relaxant drug, in order to relax the spasm, and then to intubate with an endotracheal tube. Attempts at intubation without the aid of relaxant drugs will usually be unsuccessful and will prolong the spasm. Forcible intubation through a closed glottis may result in oedema of the mucous membrane of the larynx and necessitate subsequent tracheotomy.

Constriction of the bronchioles or 'bronchial spasm' is occasionally seen in all kinds of animal but ruminants appear to be particularly liable to develop this complication of general anaesthesia. This may well be due to unsuspected regurgitation and inhalation of fluid from the rumen. Bronchial spasm may be initiated during light anaesthesia reflexly by stimuli from the site of operation and there is some evidence which suggests that the passage through the brain of blood deficient in oyxgen and rich in carbon dioxide causes bronchoconstriction.

The first warning sign that bronchial spasm is imminent is a bout of coughing and if an endotracheal tube is not in use the larynx closes. Complete respiratory arrest follows. The chest is rigid and the lungs cannot be inflated by pressure on a rebreathing bag, nor can they be deflated by pressure applied to the chest wall. Cyanosis sets in and is soon replaced by a grey pallor. If ill, the animal may die, but usually the severe hypoxia releases the spasm and the animal gasps. The gasp is followed by normal spontaneous respiration and the animal recovers. Unfortunately bronchial spasm may recur if the stimulus responsible for the first attack is still present. In all cases where bronchial spasm occurs the anaesthetist must ensure that the upper airway is clear and that the first gasp of the animal will be of an oxygen enriched atmosphere whenever this is possible. The intravenous injection of pethidine hydrochloride or of aminophylline will often relieve and prevent the recurrence of bronchial spasm.

Obstruction to Respiration

Respiratory obstruction is usually due to the base of the tongue or the epiglottis coming into contact with the posterior wall of the pharynx. This type of obstruction may be overcome by extending the head and drawing the tongue forwards out of the mouth. In pigs overextension of the head will also cause respiratory obstruction and in these animals care should be taken to keep the head in a normal position in relation to the neck.

Brachycephalic dogs may develop respiratory obstruction due to the ventral border of the soft palate coming into contact with the base of the tongue for many of these animals are almost unable to breathe through their nostrils. This type of obstruction can only be overcome by endotracheal intubation.

Large blood clots may accumulate in the pharynx after tonsillectomy, tooth extraction or endotracheal intubation when the tube has been passed through the nostril. These blood clots must be found and removed at the end of operation. Animals unconscious after mouth, nose or throat operations should be placed in a position of lateral recumbency during the recovery period.

The fact that an endotracheal tube is in position in the trachea does not necessarily mean that the airway is clear. Endotracheal tubes may kink (particularly if the head is flexed), they may become blocked with mucous and in the case of cuffed tubes a faulty cuff may actually occlude the end of the tube. Obstruction may also be caused by the animal biting on the tube.

An uncommon but serious cause of respiratory obstruction is impaction of the epiglottis in the glottic opening. This may occur during 'blind' endotracheal intubation in horses and sheep, when a soft, flexible epiglottis is forced backwards into the laryngeal opening by the forcible passage of a endotracheal tube. Unless the epiglottis is dislodged by the withdrawal of the tube at the end of anaesthesia, it can give rise to serious respiratory obstruction in the recovery period until either coughing occurs, or the cause of the obstruction is diagnosed and overcome by the anaesthetist hooking the epiglottis out of the airway.

Respiratory Arrest

Apnoea during general anaesthesia is very common, and if means of carrying on artificial respiration are available, need give rise to little concern.

Respiratory failure due to an overdose of chloroform is especially dangerous because of the concurrent circulatory depression which exists and it is likely that cessation of breathing will be quickly followed by cardiac failure. With ether and other inhalation anaesthetics and with the barbiturates, it is probable that resuscitative measures will be successful. Respiratory failure is much more likely to occur in aged, debilitated and toxaemic animals than in healthy ones and thus in these the induction and maintenance of anaesthesia must be conducted with the greatest of care if respiratory arrest is to be avoided.

The immediate requirement in the treatment of respiratory failure is that oxygenation of the tissues shall be maintained and thus artificial respiration must be applied. The airway must be cleared and if necessary an endotracheal tube should be introduced to maintain a free airway. Artificial respiration is carried out by the application of intermittent pressure to the chest, abdomen or reservoir bag of the anaesthetic circuit. The rationale of using carbon dioxide in the treatment of respiratory failure due to an overdose of anaesthetic agent is doubtful, owing to the degree of central depression already present. Indeed, it has been shown experimentally that in deep narcosis with thiopentone sodium the administration of carbon dioxide may cause further depression instead of stimulating respiration.

The place of respiratory stimulant drugs in the treatment of respiratory failure during anaesthesia is debatable. In any case there are few effective respiratory stimulant drugs. It is perhaps fortunate that this is so, for there is nothing more conducive to the use of skill and care in the administration of potent anaesthetic drugs than the knowledge that they have no very satisfactory antagonists. It is often said that to need an antidote such as a respiratory stimulant at all in anaesthesia is to confess to lack of skill, and it is undoubtedly true that an experienced anaesthetist finds it necessary to use such drugs only on rare occasions. However, no anaesthetic drug is perfect and the use of analeptics to counteract the effects of an unintentional overdose, or certain undesirable properties of the anaesthetic drugs, may be regarded as being reasonable.

Picrotoxin has long been recognized as a powerful stimulant to the respiratory centre and was one of the first agents to be used in cases of severe respiratory depression or respiratory failure in barbiturate anaesthesia. It is administered by intravenous injection, generally in a dosage of about 1 mg/kg. It is, however, a toxic agent in that a large single dose or repeated smaller doses will produce convulsions. Regurgitation and inhalation of stomach contents may occur during these convulsions and cause the death of the animal. Leptazol (Cardiozol, Metrazol) is also used as a respiratory stimulant. It too is a convulsant when given in large doses. Leptazol is generally used in dogs and cats in a dose of 2 to 4 mg/kg by intravenous injection, while horses and cattle may be given up to 1 g by the same route of administration. Nikethamide

(Coramine) is another drug which increases the frequency and depth of respiration but it is less effective than picrotoxin or leptazol for counteracting the depressant effects of anaesthetics. Horses and cattle may be given 10 to 25 ml of nikethamide, dogs 1 to 3 ml and cats 1 to 2 ml by intravenous injection.

When overdosage is small, treatment with an analeptic will restore respiratory function and a single dose may overcome all danger. When, however, overdosage has been large, the duration of action of the analeptic may be too transient to restore completely the respiratory activity and respiratory failure may recur. Thus it becomes necessary to maintain a careful watch on the animal until signs of recovering consciousness are evident and should breathing again become alarmingly shallow or cease, repeated doses should be given.

Harthoorn (1956) studied restorative therapy in dogs grossly overdosed with pentobarbitone sodium. He found that using artificial respiration, infusion therapy and where necessary analeptics, breathing would recommence even after large overdoses of the barbiturate. In so far as resuscitation was concerned, the composition of the fluid infused made no significant difference provided, of course, that it was a compatible liquid isotonic with the body fluids. Thus similar results were obtained when using 20 ml/kg of physiological saline, Ringer's solution, or artificial plasma volume expanders. From this finding it would seem that the resuscitation of the animal was due to dilution of the drug rather than to the excretion of the solution containing the drug from the blood.

Since the report of Turner and Hodgetts in Australia in 1956 there have been many reports of the usefulness of Megimide ($\beta\beta$-methylethylglutarimide) in combating the depressant effects of pentobarbitone. It appears to be an innocuous drug which has no side effects and it is claimed that it is a specific antagonist to the barbiturate drugs. Megimide itself is only sparingly soluble in water and today the sodium salt is used. This sodium salt is known in Great Britain as Bemegride Sodium. It is a powerful stimulant of the central nervous system and overdosages will produce tremors, twitching and epileptiform convulsions. Given intravenously in doses of about 20 mg/kg to all species of animal it reverses depression due to all barbiturate drugs. In dogs, sheep and rabbits it usually reverses barbiturate depression to such an extent that the animals awaken. In cats, although narcosis is lightened and respiration and circulation are improved, consciousness is not restored even with convulsive doses. The duration of full action is only about 30 minutes and treated animals must be kept under observation since a relapse may occur, even after narcosis has been lightened to an apparently safe level.

Since 1951 the compound nalorphine hydrobromide (Lethidrone) has been given extensive trials as an antagonist to the opiate drugs. It is thought to compete with these drugs for the cell membrane receptor sites. When given to the normal animal it has a weak morphine-like action. When given to an animal under the influence of morphine, the narcotic effect of the morphine is lessened and may be abolished. The efficiency of the antagonism depends on the dose of nalorphine relative to the dose of morphine; large doses of morphine require large doses of nalorphine. Nalorphine also antagonizes the actions of all morphine-like analgesics, including pethidine, diethylthiambutene and codeine. It is not effective against the emetic action of apomorphine and does not reverse the central depression produced by barbiturates. In excessive dosage it will produce respiratory depression. The dose for the dog is of the order of 0·5 to 1·5 mg. The antagonistic action is not very sustained and there are many reports from veterinarians of dogs which have been aroused from diethylthiambutene narcosis by the injection of nalorphine relapsing into a state of deep unconsciousness as soon as the initial action of the antagonist has subsided. In anaesthesia nalorphine may be given when respiratory failure occurs in an animal which has been premedicated with morphine or a morphine-like drug, and to puppies born from a bitch which has been given one of these drugs during labour.

Aspiration of Material from the Oesophagus and Stomach

This accident probably occurs more frequently than is commonly realized for material from the oesophagus and stomach may reach the pharynx as a result of vomiting or passive regurgitation.

Vomiting

This is an active process and occurs in light anaesthesia. It is often preceded by swallowing or 'gagging' movements.

When vomiting occurs the protective mechanisms of laryngeal closure, coughing and breath-holding are present and the accident should not have serious consequences. All that is necessary is for the anaesthetist to clear the pharynx of the vomited material by swabbing or suction and to allow the animal to cough vigorously before proceeding with the further administration of the anaesthetic.

It is obvious that if anaesthetics are not given to animals whose stomachs *might* contain food then aspiration is unlikely to occur, but this is counsel of perfection which cannot always be realized in veterinary practice. The stomach may contain material many hours after the eating of a meal, particularly if an accident has occurred in the meanwhile or if the animal has gone into labour.

16

Passive Regurgitation

This is most commonly seen in ruminant animals but it also occurs in horses, pigs, dogs and cats. It usually happens when the animal is in a head down position, or lying horizontally on its side, and relaxation is induced by deep anaesthesia or the use of relaxant drugs. In these circumstances the protective reflexes are not active and aspiration occurs all too readily.

In cases of oesophageal dilatation or obstruction there may be an accumulation of fluid in the oesophagus, while the stomach may contain fluid material if there is an obstruction of the pylorus or small intestine. In deeply anaesthetized ruminants any increase in intra-abdominal pressure will force fluid ingesta up the oesophagus into the pharynx, and this regurgitation is frequently seen in adult cattle when anaesthesia is induced with a small, rapidly injected dose of thiopentone sodium.

Often, the first sign that aspiration has occurred is the unexpected appearance of cyanosis, dyspnoea and tachycardia. Obviously the severity of the condition depends on the quantity of fluid aspirated and the extent of the lung area involved.

Immediate treatment consists of thorough aspiration of the tracheobronchial tree—although this is often more easily advised than performed. Oxygen should be administered and attention directed towards the relief of bronchiolar spasm. If, after operation, the animal develops bronchopneumonia the appropriate treatment must be instituted.

The most certain practical way of preventing the aspiration of material from the oesophagus and stomach is to perform endotracheal intubation with a cuffed tube immediately anaesthesia has been induced.

Anaesthetic Explosions and Fires

The *Report of a Working Party on Anaesthetic Explosions including a Safety Code for Equipment and Installations* (H.M.S.O., London) emphasizes that one of the chief difficulties to be overcome if explosions and fires are to be avoided is the lack of any general consciousness of danger.

Probably the main cause of explosions in operating rooms is to be found in static electricity, and it is very difficult to ensure that conditions are always such that a dangerous discharge of static electricity is absolutely impossible. However, other more obvious causes, such as smoking and the use of gas and electric fires in locations where inflammable anaesthetics are used, can easily be eliminated.

Accidents associated with Posture

In horses, partial paralysis of the fore-limb is not uncommon after anaesthesia. It occurs in the limb which was lowermost during a period of lateral recumbency under deep anaesthesia and is most commonly seen in the heavier type of horse (Fig. 152). Recovery of function usually takes 24 to 48 hours. There is a clinical impression that this complication is seen more frequently when halothane is the anaesthetic agent, and its incidence appears to be decreased when thick soft padding is placed under the shoulder region of the recumbent

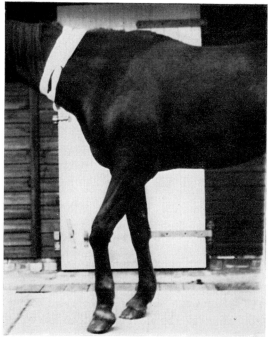

FIG. 152—Post-anaesthetic fore-limb lameness in the horse. This complication is associated with prolonged recumbency in the lateral position. Characteristic posture and hard swelling of the shoulder muscles and triceps.

animal, but this precaution does not entirely prevent its occurrence. While there is no doubt that it occurs much more commonly in horses it has been observed in small, light-weight ponies. Various hypotheses have been put forward to explain this unfortunate complication of general anaesthesia but it seems most likely that it is due to ischaemic muscle damage, for myoglobinuria may be observed in the post-operative period. At the moment, there appears to be no way of predicting when this complication will be encountered and the value of measures such as alteration of posture during anaesthesia and padding around the shoulder region remains speculative.

Intravenous Injections

The commonest mishap associated with the performance of an intravenous injection is the accidental injection of an irritant solution such as chloral hydrate or thiopentone sodium into the perivascular tissues. When this happens the injected irritant solution should be diluted by the immediate injection of a large volume of saline into the site. Hyaluronidase may be dissolved in the saline and this enzyme will hasten the absorption of the irritant drug. No other treatment is required.

Venous thrombosis is common after the injection of 5% solutions of thiopentone sodium but, as it does not appear for 5 to 10 days, it may be missed unless the anaesthetist has occasion to give another injection after that time. Whenever possible thiopentone should be used as a 2·5% solution and care should be taken to see that the venous return is not obstructed when the injection is made. Venous obstruction caused by acute flexion of the elbow or unnatural positions of the limbs will result in thiopentone being retained in the limb veins and this may give rise to thrombosis.

Permanent obliteration of vessels results from repeated, clumsy attempts at venepuncture, the use of unnecessarily large needles, and from allowing large haematomata to form at the site of venepuncture. In animals superficial veins are not too plentiful and their preservation is important.

Local Analgesia

Toxic reactions to local analgesic drugs arise when the drugs are absorbed into the general circulation at a rate greater than that at which they can be broken down by the body. Rapid absorption occurs from any hyperaemic or inflamed tissue and the rate of absorption is increased by the use of solutions which contain spreading agents such as hyaluronidase. Accidental intravascular injection may occur even though no blood can be aspirated into the syringe. The rate of absorption is decreased by the addition of vasoconstrictor drugs to the solution.

Local analgesic drugs both stimulate and depress the activity of the central nervous system. Often the toxic effects are manifested by stimulation of one part of the brain while another part is depressed. Obviously the effects will vary according to the area of the brain which is affected. Cortical stimulation produces generalized clonic convulsions, while stimulatory effects on the medulla cause an increase in the rate and depth of respiration, tachycardia and vomiting. Typical general anaesthesia with respiratory and vasomotor depression usually follows. It is uncertain whether death is due to cardiac or to respiratory failure, but it seems probable that intravascular injection causes sudden primary cardiac failure, while rapid absorption from the tissues results in depression of the central nervous system and respiratory failure.

The minimum lethal doses of the various agents for the different species of animal encountered in veterinary practice are apparently unknown and it is probable that insufficient attention is given to the quantities of local analgesics used in clinical anaethesia.

In every case where collapse has occurred after the use of a local analgesic drug artificial respiration must be commenced at once. Analeptic drugs increase the oxygen requirement of the brain and should be withheld. Convulsions should be controlled by the injection of *hypnotic* doses of short or ultra-short-acting barbiturates. Any fall in blood pressure due to peripheral or central vasomotor failure may be treated by the intravenous injection of vasopressor drugs such as methoxamine. Primary cardiac failure must be treated by cardiac massage.

Complications associated with Spinal and Epidural Analgesia

Drugs used to produce spinal analgesia may cause a reaction which affects the meninges and nerves. Clinical signs resulting from damage to nerves appear rather rapidly after the effects of the nerve block should have passed off and the nerves and region of the spinal cord subjected to the greatest concentration of the drug show the most marked pathological changes. When the main damage is to the meninges clinical signs appear later and the reaction to the drug takes the form of an aseptic meningitis which may be mild or severe. These complications do not appear to be due to faults in technique. Injection of solutions of local analgesic drugs into the substance of the spinal cord produces a severe myelitis and neuritis.

In man, post-lumbar puncture headache is a well-known complication and it has been observed that sheep which have been subjected to spinal analgesia behave in a manner which suggests that they too suffer from headache. The headache is believed to be due to a low cerebrospinal fluid pressure caused by leakage of the fluid through the needle puncture in the dura mater. It does not occur after epidural analgesia.

Infection of the epidural space is fortunately rare, but has been reported after caudal epidural block in cattle. The prognosis appears to be better than in those cases in which the infection is within the dura for it usually remains localized. Strict aseptic precautions should be employed whenever a spinal or epidural block is attempted.

The rapid injection of a large volume of fluid into the epidural space may cause arching of the back and opisthotonus. This reaction is presumably due to a rapid increase in the pressure in the epidural space and is usually of short duration. No treatment is required.

REFERENCES

ERLANGER, J. and GASSER, H. (1919). *Am. J. Physiol.* **49**, 345
FINE, J. (1960). *Surgery Gynec. Obstet.* **110**, 628

FINE, J. (1964). *J. Am. med. Ass.* **188**, 127

————— FRANK, E. D., RAVIN, H. A., RUTENBURG, S. H. and SCHWEINBURG, F. B. (1959). *New Engl. J. Med.* **260**, 214

FREEMAN, N. E. (1933). *Am. J. Physiol.* **103**, 185

GOURZIS, J. T., NOLLENBERG, M. W. and NICKERSON, M. (1961). *J. exp. Med.* **114**, 593

HARTHOORN, A. M. (1956). 'A Therapy for Anaesthetic Overdosage in the Dog', Fellowship Thesis, Royal College of Veterinary Surgeons

LILLEHEI, R. C., LONGERBEAM, J. K., BLOCH, J. H. and MANOX, W. G. (1964). *Ann. Surg.* **160**, 682

MALCOLM, J. D. (1905). *Lancet*, **ii**, 573

MOON, V. H. (1936). *Archs Path.* **22**, 325

————— (1942). *Am. J. med. Sci.* **203**, 1

NICKERSON, M. (1955). *J. Mich. St. med. Soc.* **34**, 45

SMIDDY, F. G. and FINE, J. (1957). *Proc. Soc. exp. Biol. N.Y.* **96**, 558

TOMB, J. W. (1937). *Lancet*, **ii**, 1416.

TURNER, A. W. and HODGETTS, V. E. (1956). *Aust. vet. J.* **32**, 49

WIGGERS, H. C., INGRAHAM, R. C., ROEMHILD, F. and GOLDBERG, H. (1948). *Am. J. Physiol.* **153**, 571

Needle Sizes in Relation to British Wire Gauge

| | External diameter |
Metric gauge (mm)	British wire gauge
0·35	28
0·40	27
0·45	26
0·50	25
0·55	24
0·65	23
0·70	22
0·80	21
0·90	20
1·10	19
1·25	18
1·45	17
1·65	16
1·80	15
2·10	14
2·40	13
2·80	12
3·00	11
3·25	10
3·65	9
4·06	8

Metric–British Weights and Measures

Conversion data

1	milligram—mg	equals	$\frac{1}{65}$ grain	
65	,,	,,	1 ,,	
1	gramme (1000 mg)—g	,,	$15\frac{1}{2}$,,	
28·3	,,	,,	1 oz	
453·6	,,	,,	1 lb	
1	kilogram (1000 g)—kg	,,	2·2 lb	
50	,,	,,	110·2 ,, (approx. 1 cwt)	

1	millilitre—ml or cc	,,	16	minim
28·4	,,	,,	1	fluid oz
568·2	,,	,,	1	pint
1	litre (1000 ml)—l	,,	32·8	fluid oz
				(approx. $1\frac{3}{4}$ pt)
4·5	,,	,,	1	gallon

Approximate equivalents

Milligrams per kilogram	Grains per lb
1	$\frac{1}{160}$
2	$\frac{1}{80}$
3	$\frac{1}{55}$
4	$\frac{1}{40}$
5	$\frac{1}{32}$
6	$\frac{1}{27}$
7	$\frac{1}{23}$
8	$\frac{1}{20}$
9	$\frac{1}{18}$
10	$\frac{1}{15}$

Approximate equivalents—(contd.)

Milligrams per kilogram	Grains per lb
12	$\frac{1}{12}$
15	$\frac{1}{9}$
20	$\frac{1}{7}$
24	$\frac{1}{6}$
29	$\frac{1}{5}$
35	$\frac{1}{4}$
45	$\frac{1}{3}$
70	$\frac{1}{2}$
142	1

Grammes per 50 kilograms	Grains per cwt	Ounces per 10 cwt
3	46	1·05
3·5	54	1·23
4	62	1·4
4·5	70	1·6
5	77	1·8
5·5	85	1·9
6	93	2
6·5	101	2·3
7	108	2·5

Standardization of Cone and Socket Unions

The following note has been prepared by Mr. A. J. Juby, and is included by the kind permission of the British Oxygen Company Limited.

'For many years the incompatibility of breathing attachment components of mixed manufacture has been a source of inconvenience to the anaesthetist and a potential danger to the patient. The first practical steps to remedy this undesirable state of affairs were taken when the British Standards Institution, at the request of the Ministry of Health and with the support of the professional and medical defence organizations, set up a technical committee with the object of evolving a national standard for the cone and socket couplings of anaesthetic apparatus outlets and breathing attachment components. This was followed by the establishment of a similar committee within the American Standards Association. Work proceeded in close collaboration and Anglo-American agreement was reached on a cone and socket specification as well as on a gender sequence which would ensure full interchangeability.

'Details will be found in British Standard 3849: 1965. Specification for breathing attachments for anaesthetic apparatus is obtainable from British Standards Institution, 2 Park Street, London W.1.

'The scope of British Standard 3849: 1965 extends from the outlet of the anaesthetic apparatus (the term "anaesthetic apparatus" includes circle type carbon dioxide absorption units) through to the face mask or endotracheal connector. All components of the Waters' type "to-and-fro" carbon dioxide absorption assemblies are also included. The Standard specifies gender sequence and recommends that outlets of anaesthetic apparatus have a cone, i.e. male fitting. This is the reverse of past practice where a socket, i.e. female, fitting has been employed. In the case of breathing attachments the Standard recommends that each component has a socket fitting at the gas entry and a cone fitting at the other end. This sequence is carried through to the face mask which has a socket fitting. Dimensions specified for cone and socket unions are

22 mm nominal diameter for adult equipment and 15 mm nominal diameter for paediatric equipment.

'Although it is the product of an Anglo-American agreement, B.S. 3849 contains minor points of difference from the American counterpart. However, these do not detract from full interchangeability of equipment made to the British and American Standards. B.S. 3849 has the support of the Commonwealth, Scandinavia and other countries in Europe and is expected to become an international standard through the offices of the International Standards Organization in Geneva.

'It is strongly recommended that all existing anaesthetic apparatus should be modified to accept breathing attachments made to the new British Standard. This can be achieved quite simply by fitting an adaptor to the outlet of the apparatus.'

Index

Index